ORTHOPEDIC CLINICS OF NORTH AMERICA

www.orthopedic.theclinics.com

Fracture Care

October 2021 • Volume 52 • Number 4

Editor-in-Chief

FREDERICK M. AZAR

Editorial Board

MICHAEL J. BEEBE
CLAYTON C. BETTIN
TYLER J. BROLIN
JAMES H. CALANDRUCCIO
CHRISTOPHER T. COSGROVE
BENJAMIN J. GREAR

BENJAMIN M. MAUCK
WILLIAM M. MIHALKO
BENJAMIN SHEFFER
DAVID D. SPENCE
KIRK M. THOMPSON
PATRICK C. TOY

ELSEVIER

1600 John F. Kennedy Boulevard • Suite 1800 • Philadelphia, Pennsylvania, 19103-2899.

http://www.orthopedic.theclinics.com

ORTHOPEDIC CLINICS OF NORTH AMERICA Volume 52, Number 4
October 2021 ISSN 0030-5898, ISBN-13: 978-0-323-98681-6

Editor: Lauren Boyle
Developmental Editor: Ann Gielou Posedio

Orthopedic Clinics of North America (ISSN 0030-5898) is published quarterly by Elsevier Inc., 360 Park Avenue South, New York, NY 10010-1710. Months of issue are January, April, July, and October. Business and Editorial Offices: 1600 John F. Kennedy Blvd., Suite 1800, Philadelphia, PA 19103-2899. Customer Service Office: 3251 Riverport Lane, Maryland Heights, MO 63043. Periodicals postage paid at New York, NY and additional mailing offices. Subscription prices are $347.00 per year for (US individuals), $1,003.00 per year for (US institutions), $411.00 per year (Canadian individuals), $1,028.00 per year (Canadian institutions), $476.00 per year (international individuals), $1,028.00 per year (international institutions), $100.00 per year (US students), $100.00 per year for (Canadian students), $220.00 per year for (international students). Foreign air speed delivery is included in all *Clinics* subscription prices. All prices are subject to change without notice. **POSTMASTER:** Send change of address to *Orthopedic Clinics of North America*, **Elsevier Health Sciences Division, Subscription Customer Service, 3251 Riverport Lane, Maryland Heights, MO 63043. Customer Service (orders, claims, online, change of address): Elsevier Health Sciences Division, Subscription Customer Service, 3251 Riverport Lane, Maryland Heights, MO 63043. Tel: 1-800-654-2452 (U.S. and Canada); 314-447-8871 (outside U.S. and Canada). Fax: 314-447-8029. E-mail:** journalscustomerservice-usa@elsevier.com **(for print support);** journalsonlinesupport-usa@elsevier.com **(for online support).**

Reprints. For copies of 100 or more, of articles in this publication, please contact the Commercial Reprints Department, Elsevier Inc., 360 Park Avenue South, New York, NY 10010-1710. Tel.: 212-633-3874; Fax: 212-633-3820; E-mail: reprints@elsevier.com.

Orthopedic Clinics of North America is covered in *MEDLINE/PubMed (Index Medicus)*, *Cinahl, Excerpta Medica,* and *Cumulative Index to Nursing and Allied Health Literature.*

EDITORIAL BOARD

CONTRIBUTORS

EDITOR

FREDERICK M. AZAR, MD
Professor, Department of Orthpaedics,
Department of Orthopaedic Surgery and
Biomedical Engineering, Chief-of-Staff,
Campbell Clinic, University of Tennessee–
Campbell Clinic, Memphis, Tennessee, USA

AUTHORS

AMIT ATREY, MBBS, MRCS, MSc, FRCS
Assistant Professor, Division of Orthopedic
Surgery, St. Michael's Hospital, University of
Toronto, Toronto, Ontario, Canada

ZACHARY C. BAILEY, MD
Department of Orthopaedic Surgery,
University of Nebraska Medical Center,
Omaha, Nebraska, USA

CHARLES LOWRY BARNES, MD
Department Chairperson, Department of
Orthopaedic Surgery, University of Arkansas
for Medical Sciences, Little Rock, Arkansas,
USA

LORENA BEJARANO-PINEDA, MD
Fellow, Foot and Ankle Research and
Innovation Laboratory - Harvard Medical
School, Division of Foot and Ankle Surgery,
Department of Orthopaedic Surgery,
Massachusetts General Hospital - Newton-
Wellesley Hospital, Boston, Massachusetts,
USA; Foot and Ankle Service, Department of
Orthopaedic Surgery, Massachusetts General
Hospital, Waltham, Massachusetts, USA

KEITH R. BEREND, MD
Vice President, Orthopedic Surgeon, JIS
Orthopedics, New Albany, Ohio, USA

RICHARD BRANSFORD, MD
Professor, Department of Orthopaedics and
Sports Medicine, Adjunct Professor,
Department of Neurological Surgery,
Director, University of Washington, Spine
Fellowship Program, Seattle, Washington,
USA

DANIEL A. COHEN, MBBS, FRACS, MSc
Clinical Fellow, Division of Orthopedic
Surgery, St. Michael's Hospital, University of
Toronto, Toronto, Ontario, Canada

DAVID A. CRAWFORD, MD
Orthopedic Surgeon, JIS Orthopedics, New
Albany, Ohio, USA

JUSTIN DEANS, DO
Adult Reconstruction Fellow, Department of
Orthopaedic Surgery, Lenox Hill Hospital,
New York, New York, USA

**CHRISTOPHER W. DIGIOVANNI, MD,
FAOA**
Professor, Foot & Ankle Research and
Innovation Laboratory - Harvard Medical
School, Division of Foot and Ankle Surgery,
Department of Orthopaedic Surgery,
Massachusetts General Hospital - Newton-
Wellesley Hospital, Boston, Massachusetts,
USA; Foot and Ankle Service, Department of
Orthopaedic Surgery, Massachusetts General
Hospital, Waltham, Massachusetts, USA

MATHEW H. FREEMAN, MD
Department of Orthopaedic Surgery,
University of Nebraska Medical Center,
Omaha, Nebraska, USA

KEVIN L. GARVIN, MD
Department of Orthopaedic Surgery,
University of Nebraska Medical Center,
Omaha, Nebraska, USA

RISHABH GUPTA, BA
Research Analyst, Department of
Orthopedics, Vanderbilt University Medical
Center, Nashville, Tennessee, USA

DANIEL GUSS, MD, MBA
Assistant Professor, Foot and Ankle Research and Innovation Laboratory - Harvard Medical School, Division of Foot and Ankle Surgery, Department of Orthopaedic Surgery, Massachusetts General Hospital - Newton-Wellesley Hospital, Boston, Massachusetts, USA; Foot & Ankle Service, Department of Orthopaedic Surgery, Massachusetts General Hospital, Waltham, Massachusetts, USA

WILLIAM HOZACK, MD
Walter Annenberg Professor of Joint Replacement Surgery, The Rothman Institute, Thomas Jefferson University, Philadelphia, Pennsylvania, USA

PHILIP B. KAISER, MD
Department of Orthopaedic Surgery, Foot and Ankle Service, Foot and Ankle Research and Innovation Laboratory - Harvard Medical School, Division of Foot and Ankle Surgery, Department of Orthopaedic Surgery, Massachusetts General Hospital - Newton-Wellesley Hospital, Boston, Massachusetts, USA

AMIR KHOSHBIN, MD
Assistant Professor, Division of Orthopedic Surgery, St. Michael's Hospital, University of Toronto, Toronto, Ontario, Canada

BEAU J. KILDOW, MD
Department of Orthopaedic Surgery, University of Nebraska Medical Center, Omaha, Nebraska, USA

JOHN Y. KWON, MD
Associate Professor, Foot and Ankle Research and Innovation Laboratory - Harvard Medical School, Division of Foot and Ankle Surgery, Department of Orthopaedic Surgery, Massachusetts General Hospital - Newton-Wellesley Hospital, Boston, Massachusetts, USA; Foot and Ankle Service, Department of Orthopaedic Surgery, Massachusetts General Hospital, Waltham, Massachusetts, USA

TYLER J. LARSON, MD
Department of Orthopaedic Surgery, University of Nebraska Medical Center, Omaha, Nebraska, USA

ELIZABETH R. LYDEN, MS
Department of Orthopaedic Surgery, University of Nebraska Medical Center, Omaha, Nebraska, USA

BASSAM A. MASRI, MD, FRCSC
Department of Orthopaedics, University of British Columbia, Vancouver, British Columbia, Canada

SIMON C. MEARS, MD, PhD
Professor, Department of Orthopaedic Surgery, University of Arkansas for Medical Sciences, Little Rock, Arkansas, USA

SAMANTHA A. MOHLER, MS
Medical Student, Department of Orthopaedic Surgery, University of Arkansas for Medical Sciences, Little Rock, Arkansas, USA

SPENCER J. MONTGOMERY, MD, FRCSC
Clinical Fellow, Division of Orthopedic Surgery, St. Michael's Hospital, University of Toronto, Toronto, Ontario, Canada

CHAD MYEROFF, MD
TRIA Orthopedic Center, Woodbury, Minnesota, USA

CATHERINE OLINGER, MD
Acting Instructor, Harborview Medical Center, University of Washington Department of Orthopaedics and Sports Medicine, Seattle, Washington, USA

NAOKO ONIZUKA, MD, PhD, MPH
Department of Orthopaedic Surgery, University of Minnesota, Minneapolis, Minnesota, USA; Department of Orthopaedic Surgery, Methodist Hospital, Saint Louis Park, Minnesota, USA

EDWARD SCOTT PAXTON, MD
Brown University, East Providence, Rhode Island, USA

STEFAN RAMMELT, MD, PhD
Professor, Head, Foot and Ankle Center, University Center of Orthopaedics, Trauma and Plastic Surgery, University Hospital Carl Gustav Carus at TU Dresden, Dresden, Germany

GILES R. SCUDERI, MD
Professor, Orthopaedic Surgery, Donald and
Barbara Zucker School of Medicine at Hofstra/
Northwell, Vice President, Orthopaedic
Service Line at Northwell Health, Northwell
Orthopaedic Institute, New York, New York,
USA

ARESH SEPEHRI, MD, MSc
Department of Orthopaedics, University of
British Columbia, Vancouver, British
Columbia, Canada

GERARD A. SHERIDAN, MD, FRCSI
Department of Orthopaedics, University of
British Columbia, Vancouver, British
Columbia, Canada

JEFFERY B. STAMBOUGH, MD
Assistant Professor, Department of
Orthopaedic Surgery, University of Arkansas
for Medical Sciences, Little Rock, Arkansas,
USA

ALEXANDRA STAVRAKIS, MD
Assistant Professor, Division of Orthopedic
Surgery, University of California Los Angeles,
Santa Monica, California, USA

BYRON FITZGERALD STEPHENS II, MD
Chief of Spine Surgery, Department of
Orthopedics, Vanderbilt University Medical
Center, Nashville, Tennessee, USA

KARL STOFFEL, MD, PhD, FRACS
Department of Orthopaedics and
Traumatology, University Hospital Basel,
Basel, Switzerland

BENJAMIN M. STRONACH, MD, MS
Associate Professor, Department of
Orthopaedic Surgery, University of Arkansas
for Medical Sciences, Little Rock, Arkansas,
USA

JULIE SWITZER, MD
Department of Orthopaedic Surgery,
University of Minnesota, Minneapolis,
Minnesota, USA; Department of Orthopaedic
Surgery, Methodist Hospital, Saint Louis Park,
Minnesota, USA

MICHAEL P. SWORDS, DO
Michigan Orthopedic Center, Chair,
Department of Orthopedic Surgery, Director
of Orthopedic Trauma, Sparrow Hospital,
Lansing, Michigan, USA

DAVID CLAYTON TAPSCOTT, MD
Brown University, East Providence, Rhode
Island, USA

WILLIAM HUNTER WADDELL, MD
Resident Physician, Department of
Orthopedics, Vanderbilt University Medical
Center, Nashville, Tennessee, USA

GREGORY WARYASZ, MD
Instructor, Foot and Ankle Research and
Innovation Laboratory - Harvard Medical
School, Division of Foot and Ankle Surgery,
Department of Orthopaedic Surgery,
Massachusetts General Hospital - Newton-
Wellesley Hospital, Boston, Massachusetts,
USA; Foot and Ankle Service, Department of
Orthopaedic Surgery, Massachusetts General
Hospital, Waltham, Massachusetts, USA

STEVEN YACOVELLI, MD
Clinical Research Fellow, The Rothman
Institute, Thomas Jefferson University,
Philadelphia, Pennsylvania, USA

CONTENTS

Knee and Hip Reconstruction

The direct anterior approach (DAA) is gaining popularity in primary total hip arthroplasty (THA). Although DAA has demonstrated many advantages over other surgical approaches, periprosthetic femur fractures (PPFF) rates continue to be higher. Femoral stem designs that allow for easier insertion via a DAA may contribute to the higher rates of fracture seen in this approach. Certain stem designs and fixation methods may reduce the risk of PPFF via a DAA in primary THA.

Periprosthetic fracture around a femoral component is a potentially devastating complication after total hip arthroplasty. Surgical treatment is often technically demanding and requires a thorough understanding of fracture care and revision joint reconstruction. Advancements in femoral component designs for revision total hip arthroplasty have improved management of this challenging complication. It is important for surgeons to understand which femoral component design might best suit their needs. We present an overview of revision total hip arthroplasty in the setting of periprosthetic fracture, focusing on comparing the 2 most popular femoral component revision models, the modular and monolithic tapered fluted conical prostheses.

This article is a retrospective review of a consecutive series of 401 primary total hip arthroplasties with the use of cementless, ream and broach Synergy stem (Smith & Nephew, Memphis, TN, USA) with minimal 10-year follow-up. We report an overall 10-year survivorship of 99.6% with a total of 15 fractures during the study period. Six of these fractures occurred intraoperatively. This is the largest series to our knowledge reporting greater than 10-year follow-up. This stem has excellent survivorship with overall low risk of periprosthetic fracture

> Optimal management of acetabular fractures (AF) in the elderly has not been clearly defined. The incidence of such fractures is rising in the aging population. Advancements in implant technology have improved the longevity of combined or staggered total hip arthroplasty procedures for this patient population, thus allowing earlier weight bearing and continued functional independence. Perioperative/postoperative complication rates remain significantly high in all treatment arms. Overall, the best outcomes with the lowest complication rates are achieved when AF are treated by a surgeon or a team of surgeons who specialize in both orthopedic traumatology and adult reconstruction.

> The burden of periprosthetic distal femoral fractures is projected to increase accordingly with the increase in total knee arthroplasties (TKAs) performed globally in the future. Less invasive plating and intramedullary (IM) nailing techniques still seem to provide similar outcomes based on current literature. Double-plating and combination techniques may prove to be beneficial in the future pending further large-scale studies but currently have not demonstrated superiority over single plating and IM nailing based on current evidence. Distal femoral replacement may provide a useful option for future treatment, provided it is performed by a trained knee arthroplasty surgeon.

> Complications related to the extensor mechanism and patellofemoral joint continue to be the most common cause of pain and indication for surgical revision following total knee arthroplasty. Numerous risk factors related to the patient, implant, and technical performance of the procedure have been identified. The Ortiguera and Berry classification system is widely used for the systematic classification and management of these fractures. Because of the difficult nature of revision surgery for fracture and the high risk of complication, a careful assessment of the fracture and implants is vital to determining the best course of treatment.

> Periprosthetic fracture occurring during or after total knee arthroplasty is a rare injury. Literature concerning periprosthetic tibial factures is sparse, and there is limited guidance for evidence-based management. This review aims to provide readers with an overview of the epidemiology, risk factors, and classification of these fractures. Management includes nonoperative treatment of nondisplaced fractures, fixation for those with stable implants, and revision for those with loose implants.

Shoulder and Elbow

Proximal humerus fracture nonunions are heterogenous group of posttraumatic sequelae in both the operatively and nonoperatively treated proximal humerus fracture. The management of these fractures is largely based on the residual morphology. Understanding the relationship of the nonunited and malunited fragments, anatomic location of the fracture, and viability of the residual bone stock will allow for better surgical planning. Patient optimization with nonoperative care, open reduction internal fixation, intramedullary nailing, and shoulder arthroplasty, all have a role in the treatment of proximal humerus fracture nonunions.

Approximately 4.1% of all fractures in the elderly involve the elbow. Most elbow injuries in geriatric patients occur as the result of low-energy mechanisms such as falls from standing height. Elbow injuries in elderly patients present complex challenges because of insufficient bone quality, comminution, articular fragmentation, and preexisting conditions, such as arthritis. Medical comorbidities and baseline level of function must be heavily considered in surgical decision making.

Foot and Ankle

Ankle fractures are common injuries to the lower extremity with approximately 20% sustaining a concomitant injury to the syndesmosis. Although the deltoid ligament is not formally included in the syndesmotic complex, it plays an important role in the mortise stability. Therefore, its integrity should be always evaluated when syndesmotic injury is suspected. Given the anatomic variability of the syndesmosis between individuals, bilateral ankle imaging is recommended, especially in cases of subtle instability. Diagnostic tests that allow dynamic assessment of the distal tibiofibular joint in the 3 planes are the most reliable in determining the presence of syndesmotic injury.

Syndesmotic injuries in the setting of ankle fracture are critically important to diagnosis and treat to restore an anatomic tibiotalar relationship. Physical examination and clinical suspicion remain critically important for diagnosis. Ultrasound examination and weight-bearing computed tomography scans are evolving to help diagnosis more subtle injuries. Although flexible syndesmotic fixation may decrease malreduction rates, the benefits over rigid fixation is the subject of ongoing study. Anatomic reduction remains critical regardless of fixation choice. Routine removal of rigid syndesmotic hardware does not seem to offer substantial clinical improvement in pain or range of motion; however, broken hardware may cause irritation.

Treatment of calcaneal fractures has to be tailored to the individual pathoanatomy. If operative treatment is chosen, anatomic reconstruction of the calcaneal shape and joint surfaces is mandatory. For most of the displaced, intraarticular fractures, this can be achieved by less invasive reduction and fixation via a sinus tarsi approach, which may be extended along the "lateral utility" line for calcaneocuboid joint involvement or calcaneal fracture-dislocations. Purely percutaneous fixation is the treatment of choice for displaced extraarticular fractures and simple intraarticular fractures with adequate control of joint reduction. Specific approaches are used for rare calcaneal fracture variants.

Spine Section

Craniocervical injuries (CCJs) account for 10% to 30% of all cervical spine trauma. An increasing number of patients are surviving these injuries due to advancements in automobile technology, resuscitation techniques, and diagnostic modalities. The leading injury mechanisms are motor vehicle crashes, falls from height, and sports-related events. Current treatment with urgent rigid posterior fixation of the occiput to the cervical spine has resulted in a substantial reduction in management delays expedites treatment of CCJ injuries. Within CCJ injuries, there is a spectrum of instability, ranging from isolated nondisplaced occipital condyle fractures treated nonoperatively to highly unstable injuries with severely distracted craniocervical dissociation. Despite the evolution of understanding and improvement in the management of cases regarding catastrophic failure to diagnose, subsequent neurologic deterioration still occurs even in experienced trauma centers. The purpose of this article is to review the injuries that occur at the CCJ with the accompanying anatomy, presentation, imaging, classification, management, and outcomes.

Thoracolumbar spine trauma can result in potentially life-threatening consequences and requires careful management to ensure good outcomes. The purpose of this chapter is to discuss the anatomy, diagnostic tools, non-operative, and operative treatments important when addressing thoracolumbar trauma.

FRACTURE CARE

PREFACE

This issue of *Orthopedic Clinics of North America* contains a comprehensive collection of information on periprosthetic fractures, including those of the proximal and distal femur, patella, and tibia. The first seven articles discuss periprosthetic fractures after total hip arthroplasty (THA) and total knee arthroplasty (TKA).

Drs Crawford and Berend point out the frequency of periprosthetic fractures after THA done through a direct anterior approach and suggest stem designs and fixation methods that may reduce the risk. Drs Yacovelli and Hozack present an overview of revision THA after use of cementless, ream and broach Synergy stem (Smith and Nephew, Memphis, TN, USA). Freeman and colleagues report an overall 10-year survivorship of 99.6% at 10 years.

Periprosthetic fracture occurring during or after TKA is a relatively rare injury. Mohler and colleagues provide an overview of the epidemiology, risk factors, classification, and management of these fractures. Sheridan and colleagues note that less invasive plating and Intramedullary nailing techniques still appear to provide similar outcomes and discuss the possibilities of double-plating and combination techniques and distal femoral replacement. In their review of infrapatellar fractures after TKA, Deans and Scuderi note risk factors related to the patient, implant, and technical performance of the procedure. Cohen and colleagues discuss acetabular fractures in geriatric patients and suggest that advancements in implant technology have improved the longevity of combined or staggered THA procedures in these patients by allowing earlier weight-bearing and continued functional independence.

Proximal humeral fracture nonunions are a heterogenous group of posttraumatic sequelae in both operative and nonoperatively treated proximal humeral fractures. Tapscott and Paxton emphasize that understanding the relationship of the nonunited and malunited fragments, anatomic location of the fracture, and viability of the residual bone stock will allow for better surgical planning. Elderly patients are at risk for elbow injuries following low-energy falls and, as noted by Onizuka and colleagues, can impact mobility, function, and ultimately, independence.

Ankle fractures are common injuries to the lower extremity with approximately 20% sustaining a concomitant injury to the syndesmosis. Bejarano-Pineda and colleagues describe the anatomy, injury mechanism, diagnosis, and classification of syndesmosis injuries, and Kaiser and colleagues discuss surgical treatment strategies. Together, these two articles provide an in-depth review of syndesmosis injuries. Rammelt and Swords note that, if operative treatment is chosen, anatomic reconstruction of the calcaneal shape and joint surfaces is mandatory, they and describe fixation options.

Olinger and Bransford review craniocervical injuries with the accompanying anatomy, presentation, imaging, classification, management, and outcomes, while Waddell and colleagues discuss the anatomy, diagnostic tools, and nonoperative and operative treatment of thoracolumbar trauma.

This issue provides a wealth of information, which we hope will be useful to readers in their treatment of these injuries.

Frederick M. Azar, MD
Department of Orthopaedic Surgery &
Biomedical Engineering
University of Tennessee–Campbell Clinic
1211 Union Avenue, Suite 510
Memphis, TN 38104, USA

E-mail address:
fazar@campbellclinic.com

https://doi.org/10.1016/j.ocl.2021.06.001
0030-5898/21/© 2021 Published by Elsevier Inc.

Knee and Hip Reconstruction

Reduction of Periprosthetic Proximal Femur Fracture in Direct Anterior Total Hip According to Stem Design

David A. Crawford, MD*, Keith R. Berend, MD

KEYWORDS

• Total hip arthroplasty • Direct anterior • Periprosthetic femur fracture • Stem design
• Cemented • Cementless

KEY POINTS

• The incidence of periprosthetic proximal femur fractures (PPFF) is higher in direct anterior approach because of challenges in femoral exposure and broaching trajectory.
• Cemented stems have a low risk of PPFF, however, are less commonly used worldwide.
• Single-wedge taper stem designs appear to have the highest rate of PPFF.
• Proximal fit and fill stems have a lower risk of PPFF than single-wedge taper.
• The addition of a collar in cementless femoral fixation may reduce the risk of PPFF.

INTRODUCTION

Total hip arthroplasty (THA) remains one of the most successful of all orthopedic surgeries,[1-3] and outcomes continue to improve with implant design modifications, enabling technologies and surgical approach. The direct anterior approach (DAA) has garnered much attention over the past decade for its muscle-sparing nature, rapid recovery, and ability to easily use intraoperative fluoroscopy to assess component positioning, limb length, and offset. The utilization of the DAA in primary THA is increasing rapidly. A recent survey of the members of the American Association of Hip and Knee Surgeons found that utilization of the DAA was up 333% from 8 years before.[4]

The DAA has demonstrated a more rapid recovery[5] and improved component positioning over other approaches[6,7]; however, studies have consistently shown a higher risk of femoral complications, such as periprosthetic proximal femur fracture (PPFF) and femoral aseptic loosening.[8-10] Intraoperative fracture rates with the anterior approach have been reported between 2.2% and 4.4%,[11-14] with early postoperative periprosthetic femur fractures between 0.83% and 2%.[12,15] Despite longstanding awareness of the consequences of PPFF, the prevalence of this complication appears to be increasing.[16] A recent analysis from multiple joint registries found that the rate of periprosthetic fractures is projected to increase by 4.6% every decade over the next 30 years.[17] These fractures can have devastating complications with 1-year mortalities reported from 13% to 18% in the year following revision for PPFF.[18-20]

Aside from surgical approach, other variables can contribute to femoral complications in THA. These variables include patient factors, such as elevated body mass index, diabetes, female gender, older age, and bony morphology.[15,21,22,23] However, one of the primary areas of focus to decrease periprosthetic femur fracture is changes in design of the femoral component. The focus of this review is on the impact of femoral stem design and fixation method on PPFF in primary direct anterior THA.

JIS Orthopedics, 7277 Smith's Mill Road, Suite 200, New Albany, OH 43054, USA
* Corresponding author.
E-mail address: Crawfordda@JISOrtho.com

Orthop Clin N Am 52 (2021) 297–304
https://doi.org/10.1016/j.ocl.2021.05.002
0030-5898/21/© 2021 Elsevier Inc. All rights reserved.

BRIEF EVOLUTION OF FEMORAL STEM DESIGN

There have been numerous changes in both femoral stem designs and fixation methods over the past 60 years of THA. Sir John Charnley[24] was the pioneer of THA and the first surgeon to use bone cement for femoral fixation in the 1960s. Cemented fixation remained the primary mode of femoral fixation into the 1980s. In 1983, the Food and Drug Administration approved the first uncemented porous-coated femoral implant, the anatomic medullary locking stem (AML; Depuy Synthes, Warsaw, IN, USA). This stem is a circumferentially porous coated, nontapered distal cylindrical design with a proximal porous coated triangular shape. Survivorship with the AML stem has been reported to be 98.3% at 22-year follow-up.[25] Similar stem designs, such as the Mallory-Head prosthesis, also gained popularity (Fig. 1). Despite the success of extensively porous coated cylindrical stems, they have been associated with thigh pain and osteolysis.[26] These concerns led to the evolution of other cementless designs.

Shorter and more "anatomic" stems were constructed to match the anatomic metadiaphyseal contour of the femur and provide metaphyseal rather than diaphyseal fixation. Early designs, however, had high complication rates of thigh pain and aseptic loosening.[27,28] These issues then led to manufacturing of tapered stem designs to allow 3-point fixation with endosteal contact posterior proximally, anterior midportion, and posterior distally.[29] Evolutions of the taper design included double- and triple-wedge designs with a more proximal filling nature along with shorter bone-conserving implants.

Aside from achieving biologic fixation and reducing the incidence of thigh pain, stem designs have also changed to allow insertion through more minimally invasive surgical approaches. The need for stems that can be inserted through minimally invasive approaches has held especially true with the popularization of the DAA and challenges with femoral exposure. To this end, femoral component design is increasingly more important in the minimization of femoral complication in the DAA.

CHALLENGES OF FEMORAL PREPARATION AND STEM INSERTION IN DIRECT ANTERIOR APPROACH TOTAL HIP ARTHROPLASTY

Although the DAA lends itself to relatively straightforward acetabular exposure, the femoral exposure and preparation can be more challenging. Regardless of whether a DAA surgery is performed on or off a specialized table, the femur needs to be delivered anteriorly, adducted, and externally rotated for optimal exposure and broaching (Fig. 2). With the abductors posteriorly in the surgical field and extension of the femur, the angle of broaching tends to err in a more varus position. Furthermore, broaching trajectory is not always linear, which may be secondary to patient body habitus, femoral exposure, or the patient's proximal femoral anatomy.

Fractures can occur during broaching, final impaction of the implant, or postoperatively because of either unrecognized intraoperative fracture, stem subsidence, or trauma. The risk of fracture can be further compounded with the DAA during the learning curve when the highest rate of femoral complications occurs.[30,31] Jewett and Collis[30] reported a 10% incidence of intraoperative fractures in the first 200 direct anterior cases. Furthermore, with the minimally invasive DAA technique, surgeons may elect to use offset broach handles and inserters. In a finite element analysis, large offset handles increased the moment-to-force ratios up to 163% to 235%.[32] Although the DAA offers many advantages, surgeons must be cognizant of the femoral complication profile, and choosing the appropriate stem design and fixation can mitigate these risks.

CEMENTED STEMS

Cementation was the principal mode of fixation for femoral components in primary THA for many decades. However, widespread use of cementing has declined and varies across the world. From the 2019 annual report of the American Joint Replacement Registry, cemented stems accounted for only 4.3% of primary THA stems in the United States.[33] This finding differs from European trends, of which data from the National Joint Registry reported that in 2019 about 25% of femoral components were cemented.[34] There are 2 general designs of cemented femoral components: taper loaded (Fig. 3A) and composite beam (see Fig. 3B).

Compared with cementless stems, cemented stems have shown a lower rate of PPFF in various surgical approaches.[35-37] In a systematic review, Carli and colleagues[35] found that cemented stems had the lowest rate of periprosthetic fracture compared with all designs of cementless stems. Furthermore, the investigators found the taper-loaded designs were associated with

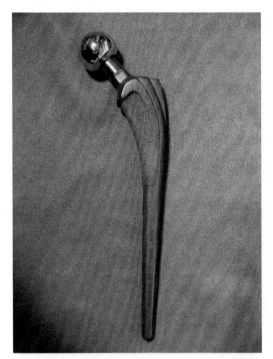

Fig. 1. Image of an extensively porous coated cylindrical stem.

significantly higher incidence of PPFF compared with the composite beam. Review of the Nordic Arthroplasty Register Association database found the incidence of PPFF in cemented stems as 0.07% compared with 0.47% with cementless stems (P<.005). Thien and colleagues[37] went on to note that again taper-loaded cemented designs had a 5-fold increased risk of fracture when compared with the composite beam stems. Herndon and colleagues[38] in a retrospective review of complications with various stem designs found an overall intraoperative and postoperative fracture rate of 8.3%; however,

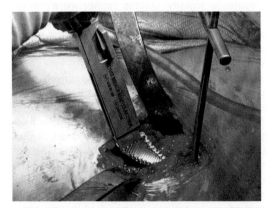

Fig. 2. Clinical picture of femoral exposure in off-table direct anterior approach total hip replacement.

there were no fractures when cemented stems were used.

Unlike cementless periprosthetic fractures that typically occur in the early perioperative period, fracture around cementless stems more often occurs 5 or more years after the index procedure.[39]

CEMENTLESS STEMS

Cementless femoral stems are used in many primary THAs in the United States and around the world.[33,34,40] Cementless stems can be inserted with less operative time than cemented,[41] and once biologic fixation is achieved, can produce durable long-term survivorship.[34] Khanuja and colleagues[29] classified cementless femoral stem designs into 6 distinct types: (1) Single wedge; (2) double wedge, metaphyseal filling; (3) smooth tapered; (4) cylindrical distally fixed; (5) modular; (6) curved, anatomic. These stem designs are classified based on the contact area of the bone as well as the fixation sites. Changes in cementless design have focused on bone preservation and allowing insertion through minimally invasive techniques, such as direct anterior. To that end, this article focuses on type 1 and type 2 stems, as they are the cementless stems that are most commonly used in a DAA for primary THA.

Single-Wedge Taper

Single-wedge taper designed stems are a very popular option and one that the authors' institution has been using for more than a decade. These type 1 tapered designs, however, rely solely on mediolateral cortical fixation. Especially in thin osteoporotic bone, there is a fine line in choosing a large enough stem that achieves fixation without too firm of impaction creating fracture. In cadaveric osteoporotic testing, single-wedge tapered designs create higher rates of fractures than more proximal filling design.[42]

The authors' institution has extensive experience with single-wedge cementless stems used during DAA THA. The authors have previously published 2 articles evaluating the rate of early PPFF with the DAA and a single-wedge tapered stem and have noted a 0.9% and 0.83% incidence of PPFF (Fig. 4).[15,43] Furthermore, older age and female gender had an increased incidence of fracture.[15] In a systematic review of 34 articles, single-wedge stems were associated with the highest incidence of PPFF at 1.48% compared with other cementless designs.[44] Similarly, Cidambi and colleagues[45] found a

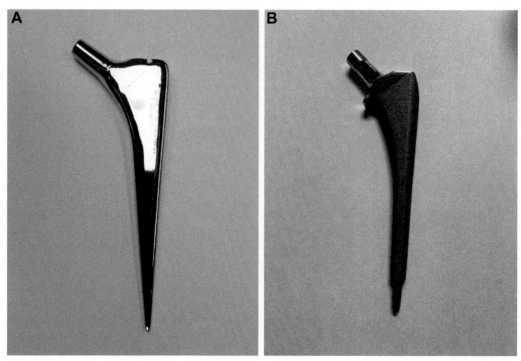

Fig. 3. (A) Image of the "taper-loaded" cemented stem. (B) Image of the "composite beam" cemented stem.

significantly higher revision rate for tapered wedge (1.3%) over hip arthroplasty–coated, compaction broached stems (0%) (P<.005) via DAA THA.

One hypothesis for the higher incidence of PPFF with a thin, collarless tapered stem design is that nonlinear broach insertion and extraction can create an anterior metaphyseal gap that compromises initial stability leading to subsidence, distal potting, and failure of proximal ingrowth.[45] Furthermore, the increased rate of loosening with the tapered wedge inserted via a DAA can be due to failure to obtain adequate initial stability and subsequent ingrowth.

Changes to single-wedge stem geometry have decreased the fracture rates in certain designs. For example, Fleischman and colleagues[46] found a 7.5-fold reduction in risk of intraoperative fractures going from a first-generation to the second-generation single-wedge stem. These second-generation designs with a reduced distal geometry and lateral relief can reduce fracture risk.[47,48]

Short Versus Long Single-Wedge Taper
The shift toward shorter stem lengths was greatly driven by the anterior approach. These shorter designs allowed for easier broaching and stem insertion. The reduced length and tapered stem diameter make it less likely that the implant will prematurely engage the diaphysis before fully achieving a metaphyseal press-fit.[29] However, specifically with the single-wedge design, these shorter stems have come at the cost of increased femoral fractures.[15,49] A possible explanation is that short stems have been shown to be more rigid in mediolateral bending than longer stems of the same material composition.[50] The difference in geometric rigidity creates higher intrafemoral stresses, which may lead to the cortical thickening and fracture.[51] Fig. 5 illustrates the differences in design between a short and long single-wedge taper implant.

Tamaki and colleagues[49] retrospectively evaluated 850 THAs performed via DAA with a single-stem design that had both a short- and full-length design. The occurrence of femur fracture was significantly higher in the short design versus full length (2.7% vs 0%, P = .02). The authors' institution published more than 5000 THA done via a DAA with a single-wedge taper design and found a 0.31% incidence of periprosthetic femur fracture with standard length stems and 1.27% with short stems (P = .054).[15]

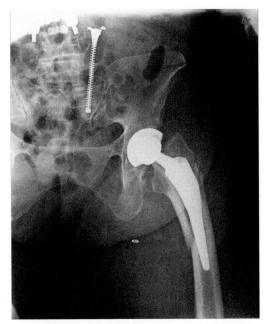

Fig. 4. A PPFF with a single-wedge taper stem.

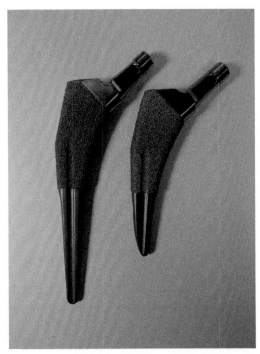

Fig. 5. Comparison image of the single taper wedge full length stem (*left*) and shorter stem (*right*).

Although this difference was not statistically different, it does highlight a trend seen in other studies.

Proximal Fit and Fill Stems

The type II double- and triple-wedge proximal metaphyseal filling implants are designed to contact the medial and lateral metaphyseal cortex as well as the anterior and posterior portion of the metaphyseal cortex. This category of stems is quite broad and includes stems with varying degrees of anterior/posterior size growth. In recent years, many companies have developed newer stems around this design, such as the Zimmer Biomet Avenir Complete (Zimmer Biomet, Warsaw, IN, USA) (Fig. 6A), the Total Joint Orthopedics Klassic Blade (Park City, UT, USA) (see Fig. 6B), and the Depuy Synthes Actis (see Fig. 6C).

Since 2015, the authors have experience using a triple-wedge broach only short-stem implant and have published their experience with this stem in a DAA. In a series 245 patients, no patients sustained an early postoperative periprosthetic femur fracture, and no femoral revisions were performed.[52] In a national registry review, a type II double-taper stem had the lowest hazard ratio of PPFF between the cementless stems.[37] Sershon and colleagues[53] performed a retrospective analysis on 6309 THA that were performed with either single-wedge taper design or a proximal fit and fill.

The authors found with Cox regression analysis that single-wedge taper designs had a 2.3 times risk of proximal femur fracture than the proximal fit and fill stems. A newer medial calcar triple wedge design implant was shown in a series of 144 patients to have no intraoperative or perioperative fractures.[54]

Collared Versus Noncollared

The use and popularity of collared cementless stems have waxed and waned over the years. As designs shifted toward more tapered wedge designs, there was concern that a collar would prevent the stem from fully seating and engaging the metaphysis. However, a collared stem offers numerous advantages, such as reduced subsidence, better rotational stability, and lower risks of calcar fracture propagation.[45] In a cadaveric study, Demey and colleagues[55] found that collared stems were able to withstand greater vertical and horizontal forces before the initiation of subsidence and subsequent fracture. As the femoral stem is at greatest risk of subsidence or early fracture before osseointegration, it is possible that the improved immediate stability conferred by collared stems allows more rapid bony ingrowth.

In a meta-analysis of femoral complications in primary THA, collared femoral stem had a lower

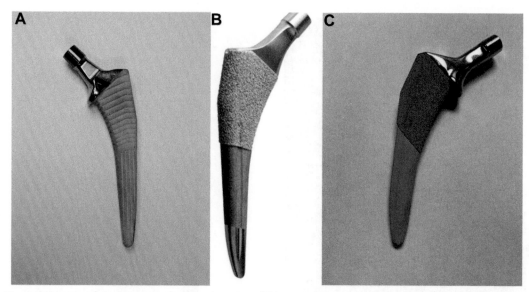

Fig. 6. (A) Image of double tapered cementless stem. (B) Image of the triple taper proximal fit and fill stem. (C) Image of the triple taper proximal fit and fill stem (© Depuy Synthes 2021. All rights reserved.).

relative risk of complications (0.02, 95% confidence interval, 0.001, 0.30) when compared with collarless femoral stem.[56] Similarly, in a meta-analysis of 337,647 primary THAs, Lamb and colleagues found that a collared stem had a significantly lower risk of PPFF compared with collarless stems.[57] A recent single-institution retrospective analysis found that collarless stems had a relative risk of 2.3 times for PPFF than collared stem.[53]

SUMMARY

The literature demonstrates that femoral stem design has in impact on the risk of PPFF in a DAA primary THA. Cemented stems and collared proximal fit and fill cementless stems appear to have the lowest risk of PPFF. Surgeons should carefully evaluate their stem choice, especially in osteoporotic bone.

CLINICS CARE POINTS

- The incidence of PPFF fracture in THA is reported between 2.2% and 4.4%.
- Taper-loaded cemented stems have a 5-fold increased risk of PPFF compared to composite-beam cemented stems.
- Single wedge taper stems with reduced distal geometry have a 7.5-fold lower risk of PPFF than non-reduced distal singe wedge designs.

- Compared to cementless proximal fit and fill designs, cementless single wedge stems have 2.3 fold increase in PPFF.
- Collard cementless stems have a 0.02 relative risk of PPFF compared to collarless cementless stems.

DISCLOSURE

1) For Dr Crawford D Consultant Depuy Synthes, Institutional research support from Zimmer Biomet, SPR Therapeutics.

2) For Dr Berend K Royalties Zimmer Biomet, Innomed. Stock/Stock options: SPR therapeutics, Joint Development Corporation, Elute Inc, VuMedi, Prescribe Fit, Parvizi Surgical Innovation. Institutional research support: Zimmer Biomet, SPR Therapeutics.

REFERENCES

1. Learmonth ID, Young C, Rorabeck C. The operation of the century: total hip replacement. Lancet 2007;370(9597):1508–19.
2. Kunkel ST, Sabatino MJ, Kang R, et al. The cost-effectiveness of total hip arthroplasty in patients 80 years of age and older. J Arthroplasty 2018; 33(5):1359–67.
3. Kamaruzaman H, Kinghorn P, Oppong R. Cost-effectiveness of surgical interventions for the management of osteoarthritis: a systematic review of

the literature. BMC Musculoskelet Disord 2017; 18(1):183.

4. Abdel MP, Berry DJ. Current practice trends in primary hip and knee arthroplasties among Members of the American Association of Hip and Knee Surgeons: a long-term update. J Arthroplasty 2019; 34(7S):S24–7.

5. Barrett WP, Turner SE, Murphy JA, et al. Prospective, randomized study of direct anterior approach vs posterolateral approach total hip arthroplasty: a concise 5-year follow-up evaluation. J Arthroplasty 2019;34(6):1139–42.

6. Rathod PA, Bhalla S, Deshmukh AJ, et al. Does fluoroscopy with anterior hip arthroplasty decrease acetabular cup variability compared with a non-guided posterior approach? Clin Orthop Relat Res 2014;472(6):1877–85.

7. Gromov K, Greene ME, Huddleston JI, et al. Acetabular dysplasia and surgical approaches other than direct anterior increases risk for malpositioning of the acetabular component in total hip arthroplasty. J Arthroplasty 2016;31(4):835–41.

8. Meneghini RM, Elston AS, Chen AF, et al. Direct anterior approach: risk factor for early femoral failure of cementless total hip arthroplasty: a multicenter study. J Bone Joint Surg Am 2017;99: 99–105.

9. Panichkul P, Parks NL, Ho H, et al. New approach and stem increased femoral revision rate in total hip arthroplasty. Orthopedics 2016;39(1):e86–92.

10. Angerame MR, Fehring TK, Masonis JL, et al. Early failure of primary total hip arthroplasty: is surgical approach a risk factor? J Arthroplasty 2018;33(6): 1780–5.

11. Lee GC, Marconi D. Complications following direct anterior hip procedures: costs to both patients and surgeons. J Arthroplasty 2019;30(9 Suppl):98–101.

12. Hartford JM, Knowles SB. Risk factors for perioperative femoral fractures: cementless femoral implants and the direct anterior approach using a fracture table. J Arthroplasty 2016;31(9):2013–8.

13. Cohen EM, Vaughn JJ, Ritterman SA, et al. Intraoperative femur fracture risk during primary direct anterior approach cementless total hip arthroplasty with and without a fracture table. J Arthroplasty 2017;32(9):2847–51.

14. Ponzio DY, Shahi A, Park AG, et al. Intraoperative proximal femoral fracture in primary cementless total hip arthroplasty. J Arthroplasty 2015;30(8):1418–22.

15. Greco NJ, Lombardi AV, Morris MJ, et al. Direct anterior approach and perioperative fracture with a single-taper wedge femoral component. J Arthroplasty 2019;34(1):145–50.

16. Yasen AT, Haddad FS. Periprosthetic fractures: bespoke solutions. Bone Joint J 2014;96-B:48–55.

17. Pivec R, Issa K, Kapadia BH, et al. Incidence and future projections of periprosthetic femoral fracture following primary total hip arthroplasty: an analysis of international registry data. J Long Term Eff Med Implants 2015;25:269–75.

18. Shields E, Behrend C, Bair J, et al. Mortality and financial burden of periprosthetic fractures of the femur. Geriatr Orthop Surgrehabil 2014;5: 147–53.

19. Drew JM, Griffin WL, Odum SM, et al. Survivorship after periprosthetic femur fracture: factors affecting outcome. J Arthroplasty 2016;31:1283–8.

20. Boylan MR, Riesgo AM, Paulino CB, et al. Mortality following periprosthetic proximal femoral fractures versus native hip fractures. J Bone Joint Surg Am 2018;100:578–85.

21. Cottino U, Dettoni F, Caputo G, et al. Incidence and pattern of periprosthetic hip fractures around the stem in different stem geometry. Int Orthop 2020;44(1):53–9.

22. Gromov K, Bersang A, Nielsen CS, et al. Risk factors for post-operative periprosthetic fractures following primary total hip arthroplasty with a proximally coated double-tapered cementless femoral component. Bone Joint J 2017;99-B(4):451–7.

23. Kim SM, Han SB, Rhyu KH, et al. Periprosthetic femoral fracture as cause of early revision after short stem hip arthroplasty-a multicentric analysis. Int Orthop 2018;42(9):2069–76.

24. Charnley J. Surgery of the hip-joint: present and future developments. Br Med J 1960;1(5176):821–6.

25. Belmont PJ Jr, Powers CC, Beykirch SE, et al. Results of the anatomic medullary locking total hip arthroplasty at a minimum of twenty years. A concise follow-up of previous reports. J Bone Joint Surg Am 2008;90(7):1524–30.

26. Eng CA Jr, Culpepper W, Eng CA. Long-term results of the anatomic medullary locking prosthesis in total hip arthroplasty. J Bone Joint Surg Am 1997;79(2):177–84.

27. Kawamura H, Dunbar MJ, Murray P, et al. The porous coated anatomic total hip replacement. A ten to fourteen-year follow-up study of a cementless total hip arthroplasty. J Bone Joint Surg Am 2001;83(9):1333–8.

28. Ferrell MS, Browne JA, Attarian DE, et al. Cementless porous-coated anatomic total hip arthroplasty at Duke: 18- to 24-year follow-up. J Surg Orthop Adv 2009;18(3):150–4.

29. Khanuja HS, Vakil JJ, Goddard MS, et al. Cementless femoral fixation in total hip arthroplasty. J Bone Joint Surg Am 2011;93(5):500–9.

30. Jewett BA, Collis DK. High complication rate with anterior total hip arthroplasties on a fracture table. Clin Orthop Relat Res 2011;469(2):503–7.

31. Masonis J, Thompson C, Odum S. Safe and accurate: learning the direct anterior total hip arthroplasty. Orthopedics 2008;31(12 Suppl 2). Available at: orthosupersite.com/view.asp?rID=37187.

32. Greenhill DA, Abbasi P, Darvish K, et al. Broach handle design changes force distribution in the femur during total hip arthroplasty. J Arthroplasty 2017;32(6):2017–22.

33. American Joint Replacement Registry 2019 report. Accessed January 2021. Available at: http://connect.ajrr.net/2019-ajrr-annual-report.

34. National Joint Replacement Registry England and Wales 2018 report. Available at: https://reports.njrcentre.org.uk/. Accessed January 2021.

35. Carli AV, Negus JJ, Haddad FS. Periprosthetic femoral fractures and trying to avoid them: what is the contribution of femoral component design to the increased risk of periprosthetic femoral fracture? Bone Joint J 2017;99-B(1 Supple A):50–9.

36. Jämsen E, Eskelinen A, Peltola M, et al. High early failure rate after cementless hip replacement in the octogenarian. Clin Orthop Relat Res 2014;472(9):2779–89.

37. Thien TM, Chatziagorou G, Garellick G, et al. Periprosthetic femoral fracture within two years after total hip replacement: analysis of 437,629 operations in the Nordic Arthroplasty Register Association database. J Bone Joint Surg Am 2014;96(19):e167.

38. Herndon CL, Nowell JA, Sarpong NO, et al. Risk factors for periprosthetic femur fracture and influence of femoral fixation using the mini-anterolateral approach in primary total hip arthroplasty. J Arthroplasty 2020;35(3):774–8.

39. Grammatopoulos G, Pandit H, Kambouroglou G, et al. A unique peri-prosthetic fracture pattern in well fixed femoral stems with polished, tapered, collarless design of total hip replacement. Injury 2011;42(11):1271–6.

40. Australian Orthopedic Association National Joint Replacement Registry 2020 Annual Report. Available at: https://aoanjrr.sahmri.com/annual-reports-2020. Accessed January 2021.

41. Bredow J, Boese CK, Flörkemeier T, et al. Factors affecting operative time in primary total hip arthroplasty: a retrospective single hospital cohort study of 7674 cases. Technol Health Care 2018;26(5):857–66.

42. Mears SC, Richards AM, Knight TA, et al. Subsidence of uncemented stems in osteoporotic and non-osteoporotic cadaveric femora. Proc Inst Mech Eng 2009;223(2):189–94.

43. Berend KR, Mirza AJ, Morris MJ, et al. Risk of periprosthetic fractures with direct anterior primary total hip arthroplasty. J Arthroplasty 2016;31:2295–8.

44. Carli AV, Negus JJ, Haddad FS. Periprosthetic femoral fractures and trying to avoid them: what is the contribution of femoral component design to the increased risk of periprosthetic femoral fracture? Bone Joint J 2017 Jan;99-B(1 Supple A):50–9.

45. Cidambi KR, Barnett SL, Mallette PR, et al. Impact of femoral stem design on failure after anterior approach total hip arthroplasty. J Arthroplasty 2018;33(3):800–4.

46. Fleischman AN, Schubert MM, Restrepo C, et al. Reduced incidence of intraoperative femur fracture with a second-generation tapered wedge stem. J Arthroplasty 2017;32(11):3457–61.

47. Sueyoshi T, Berend M, Meding J, et al. Changes in femoral stem geometry reduce intraoperative femoral fracture rates in total hip replacement. Open J Orthop 2015;5:115–9.

48. Molli RG, Lombardi AV Jr, Berend KR, et al. A short tapered stem reduces intraoperative complications in in primary total hip arthroplasty. Clin Orthop Relat Res 2012;470:450–61.

49. Tamaki T, Jonishi K, Miura Y, et al. Cementless tapered-wedge stem length affects the risk of periprosthetic femoral fractures in direct anterior total hip arthroplasty. J Arthroplasty 2018;33(3):805–9.

50. Sumner DR, Galante JO. Determinants of stress shielding: design versus materials versus interface. Clin Orthop Relat Res 1992;274:202–12.

51. Katsimihas M, Katsimihas G, Lee MB, et al. Distal femoral cortical hypertrophy: predisposing factors and their effect on clinical outcome. Hip Int 2006;16:18–22.

52. Crawford DA, Rutledge-Jukes H, Berend KR, et al. Does a triple-wedge, broach-only stem design reduce early postoperative fracture in anterior total hip arthroplasty? Surg Technol Int 2019;35:386–90.

53. Sershon RA, Mcdonald JF, Ho H, et al. Periprosthetic femur fracture risk: influenced by stem choice, not surgical approach. J Arthroplasty 2021;36(7S):S363–6.

54. Kaszuba SV, Cipparrone N, Gordon AC. The actis and corail femoral stems provide for similar clinical and radiographic outcomes in total hip arthroplasty. HSS J 2020;16(Suppl 2):412–9.

55. Demey G, Fary C, Lustig S, et al. Does a collar improve the immediate stability of uncemented femoral hip stems in total hip arthroplasty? A bilateral comparative cadaver study. J Arthroplasty 2011;26(8):1549–55.

56. Panichkul P, Bavonratanavech S, Arirachakaran A, et al. Comparative outcomes between collared versus collarless and short versus long stem of direct anterior approach total hip arthroplasty: a systematic review and indirect meta-analysis. Eur J Orthop Surg Traumatol 2019;29(8):1693–704.

57. Lamb JN, Baetz J, Messer-Hannemann P, et al. A calcar collar is protective against early periprosthetic femoral fracture around cementless femoral components in primary total hip arthroplasty: a registry study with biomechanical validation. Bone Joint J 2019;101-B(7):779–86.

Modular or Monolithic Tapered Fluted Prostheses for Periprosthetic Fractures
Which One Could Work for You?

Steven Yacovelli, MD*, William Hozack, MD

KEYWORDS

- Periprosthetic fracture • Modular • Monolithic • Tapered • Fluted

---

KEY POINTS

- PPFx in the setting of THA is a technically challenging complication that requires an understanding of both fracture care and adult reconstruction.
- With a number of viable options to choose from, it is important for surgeons to understand which femoral component design might best suit their needs..
- While modular TFT prostheses have been and continue to be the work horse for the treatment of PPFxs, monolithic TFC prosthesis can be used for almost all PPFxs, but work best in the hands of an experienced revision arthroplasty surgeon.

INTRODUCTION

Periprosthetic fracture (PPFx) around a femoral component is a potentially devastating complication after total hip arthroplasty (THA), leading to significant morbidity and mortality. Surgical treatment is often technically demanding and requires a thorough understanding of fracture care and revision joint reconstruction. Fortunately, advancements in femoral component designs for the purpose of revision THA have improved management of this challenging complication. With a number of viable options to choose from, it is important for surgeons to understand which femoral component design might best suit their needs. We present an overview of revision THA in the setting of PPFx, with a focus on comparison between the 2 most popular femoral component revision models, the modular and monolithic tapered fluted conical (TFC) prostheses.

EPIDEMIOLOGY AND RISK FACTORS

- As the number of THAs performed in the United States increases, the incidence of femoral PPFx is expected to increase significantly as well. Studies report PPFx rates after primary and revision THA of 1.0% to 2.3% and 1.5% to 7.8%, respectively, making PPFx the third most common cause of reoperation after THA.[1,2]
- According to the Swedish National Hip Arthroplasty Registry, the breakdown of PPFx based on the Vancouver classification system was found to be as follows: 4% were type A fractures, 86% type B fractures, and 10% type C fractures. They found that the majority (70%) of type B fractures following primary THA occurred around a loose stem (type B2), whereas fractures after revision surgery are more commonly (51%) around a well-fixed prosthesis (type B1).[3]
- In their study, they found the most common mechanism of injury was found to be a fall from sitting or standing (85%), with spontaneous fractures and

---

The Rothman Institute, Thomas Jefferson University, Suite 1000, 125 South 9th Street, Philadelphia, PA 19107, USA
* Corresponding author.
E-mail address: stevenyaco@gmail.com

Orthop Clin N Am 52 (2021) 305–315
https://doi.org/10.1016/j.ocl.2021.05.004

Type	Location	Treatment
Table 1 Vancouver classification for periprosthetic femur fractures		
A	Fracture around the trochanter	
A_G	Greater trochanter	Non-operative or ORIF
A_L	Lesser trochanter	Non-operative or ORIF
B	Fracture around the prosthesis	
B1	With well-fixed stem	ORIF vs revision THA
B2	With loose stem	Revision THA
B3	With loose stem, poor proximal bone stock	Revision THA
C	Fracture distal to the tip of stem	ORIF

high-energy trauma accounting for the remaining 10% and 5%, respectively.[3]

- Risk factors for the development of PPFx after THA include osteolysis and loosening, trauma, age, gender, osteoporosis, index diagnosis, revision surgery, technique, and the type of implant used.[3,4]

VANCOUVER CLASSIFICATION

Although many classification systems have been proposed to describe femoral PPFx, the Vancouver classification system is used most commonly because it describes the fracture pattern and helps to guide treatment (**Table 1**).[5] This classification is based on 3 major features: (1) fracture location, (2) implant stability, and (3) integrity of the residual bone stock.

- Type A fractures are located around the trochanters and are further subdivided into type A_G (around the greater trochanter) and type A_L (around the lesser trochanter). Without evidence of stem loosening pre/intraoperatively, these fractures can be adequately managed without revision of the femoral component.
- Type B fractures are located around the femoral prosthesis itself and are further subdivided by stem stability and bone

stock. Type B1 fractures are fractures with a stable stem, type B2 fractures are fractures with a loose stem and supportive femoral bone stock, and type B3 fractures are fractures with a loose stem and poor integrity of the residual bone stock, wherein the metaphyseal and diaphyseal bone stock is deficient and unsupportive.

- Type C fractures are located distal to the tip of the stem, are typically not associated with a loose stem, and therefore do not require revision THA.

A careful evaluation of preoperative radiographs, clinical presentation, and intraoperative stability of the prosthesis are required to make an informed decision as to whether or not the femoral component is loose needs to be revised.[6,7] For the sake of simplicity, we focus primarily on Vancouver B2 and B3 fractures because they are associated with a loose stem and therefore uniformly require revision of the femoral component.[8]

PAPROSKY CLASSIFICATION FOR FEMORAL BONE DEFECTS

Regardless of whether a PPFx is present or not, it is important to assess both preoperative and intraoperative (after removal of the stem) femoral bone loss when planning and executing a revision THA. The Paprosky classification system is the most widely used system to describe femoral bone loss and serves as a useful reference for the remainder of this article because bone loss, likelihood of remodeling, and intact diaphyseal bone that can be used for bicortical scratch fit fixation, are all important factors to consider when choosing an ideal implant.[9,10] In the context of PPFx, the residual diaphyseal bone stock that is most clinically relevant is that which is distal to the fracture line, because distal fixation is necessary for fracture and implant stability. However, proximal metaphyseal bone loss is also relevant, for example, when one is considering using a TFC stem, which requires some degree of medial bone support at the level of the stem–body junction. In these situations, a proximal femoral replacement type stem might be the best choice.[11] The Paprosky system is based on 3 factors: (1) the location of femoral bone loss, (2) the degree of residual proximal femoral bone stock, and (3) the amount of residual isthmus available for diaphyseal fixation. Bone loss is categorized into 4 different types as shown in **Table 2**.

Table 2
Paprosky classification system for femoral bone loss defects

Paprosky Grade	Femoral Bone Loss
Type I	Minimal metaphyseal bone loss
Type II	Extensive metaphyseal bone loss, minimal diaphyseal bone loss
Type IIIa	Extensive metaphyseal bone loss and diaphyseal bone loss, >4 cm intact diaphyseal bone
Type IIIb	Extensive metaphyseal bone loss and diaphyseal bone loss, <4 cm intact diaphyseal bone
Type IV	Extensive metaphyseal bone loss and diaphyseal bone loss, nonsupportive isthmus

PRIOR FEMORAL REVISION COMPONENT MODELS

To better understand the modern femoral revision components it is helpful to have a better understanding of the historical progression of revision component designs. Over the past 40 years, improvements in implant technology, coupled with better understanding of reconstructive principles, have led to the rapid improvement in femoral component revision design regardless of revision indication. This point is especially true for the treatment of highly complex revision cases, such as those involving severe bone loss and PPFxs. Although most investigators agree that modular and monolithic Tapered, fluted, Titanium (TFT) components are the new standard of care, both long cemented femoral and the fully porous coated cylindrical (FPCC) femoral components represent advancement milestones that ultimately led to where we are today.

Long Cemented Femoral Component

- The first component design described for use in revision THA for PPFx provided diaphyseal fixation by bypassing the fracture site by means of a long, cemented stem.[12] Unfortunately, a number of studies began to report high rates of fracture nonunion and loosening with use of these components, and they eventually fell out of favor as we better understood the drawbacks of a cemented technique.[13]

Fully Porous Coated Cylindrical Femoral Component

- FPCC femoral component designs, initially made of cobalt–chrome, were developed as a means to provide adequate diaphyseal fixation beyond the fracture site without the use of cementation. For the most part, FPCC components provided satisfactory outcomes, with survivorship, functional scores, and radiographic stability all adequate at the long-term follow-up. However, the drawbacks of the FPCC prosthesis, including high rates of iatrogenic PPFx, subsidence, proximal stress shielding, and thigh pain present opportunities for improvement.[9,14] Most prostheses of this type still in use are now made from a titanium alloy, rather than cobalt chromium alloy, in an attempt to decrease the stiffness mismatch between the stem and the bone. However, the biggest issue with FPCC prostheses is that they may fail with less than 4 to 6 cm of scratch fit to provide stable fixation, making them less useful in cases with Paprosky IIIB or IV defects and many PPFx fractures (Fig. 1).[15]

Tapered Fluted Conical Components

- TFC component designs were first popularized by Wagner in 1987.[16] The original design was a monolithic-type prosthesis. The biggest problem with the original design was subsidence. Initial short-term results with a first-generation monolithic TFC stem showed a rate of radiographic subsidence of 21% at 1 year, with more than 5 mm occurring in between 21% and 34% of procedures and more than 10 mm in 15% to 20%.[17] Subsidence and subsequent instability also led to significant rates of dislocation, reported as high as 14% in the earlier literature.

- TFC prostheses all are based on a similar design principle for fixation, which is to create axial stability through proper distal bone preparation of a taper, thus limiting subsidence. Rotational stability then is achieved through longitudinal flutes, which typically increase in height and width from proximal to distal along the stem. The flutes also provide an advantage by engaging the diaphyseal

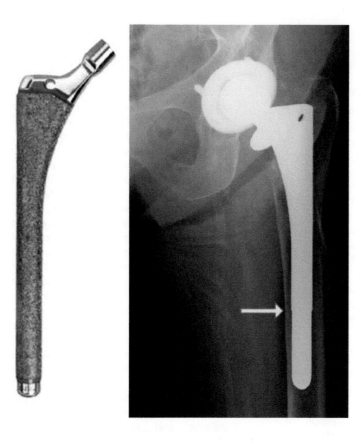

Fig. 1. Example of a fully porous coated cylindrical prosthetic design. Radiograph of a well-fixed fully porous coated cylindrical femoral stem. This stiff cobalt–chromium stem transfers weight bearing stresses distally resulting in proximal bone atrophy. Notice the proximal bone atrophy especially in the medial calcar area. The bone atrophy extends into the diaphyseal area until the point at which the porous coating ends (*arrow*).

cortex circumferentially to promote preferential biologic ingrowth at the sharp bone-implant interface (Fig. 2).[18] Proximal biologic fixation can vary between stem types based on the geometry and surface characteristics of the proximal segment. There is variation in taper angle and spline geometry between manufacturers, with no specific design showing superior clinical results despite some differences in laboratory testing.[19,20]

- The TFC prostheses have some specific advantages over other stem choices.
  - The most important advantage is that the axial stability provided by the TFC design allows for stable fixation over a relatively short segment of diaphyseal bone, as little as 4 cm or even less.[21] Of course, this factor requires careful and precise preparation of the bony

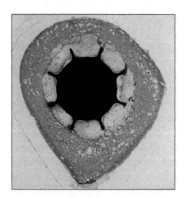

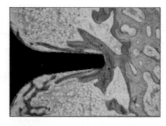

Fig. 2. Histologic view of conical stem with splines integrated into the bone.

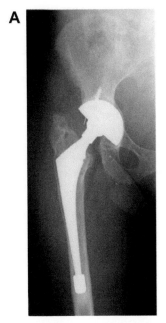
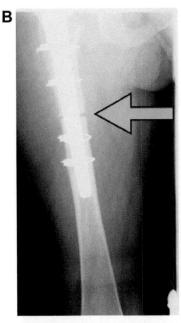
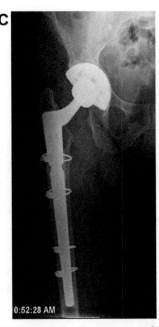

Fig. 3. Preoperative (*A*), initial postoperative (*B*), and 2-year postoperative (*C*) radiographs showing successful initial fixation with minimal diaphyseal support. *Arrow* shows the level of extended osteotomy, with fixation of conical stem achieved distal to the osteotomy site.

bed to maximize the effect of the taper stem design. As a result, TFC prosthesis can be used in patients with significant femoral bone loss or distal PPFx patterns in which there is only a short segment of available bone distally (Fig. 3). As one might expect, the risk of subsidence is higher as the bone stock diminishes.

○ Because a TFC prosthesis provides surgeons with the ability to address all PPFx cases (and all femoral revisions as well) with the 1 component design. This versatility allows the surgeon quickly to gain familiarity with the techniques and instruments for preparation and implantation and subsequently master its use for a variety of situations. This versatility also allows the operating room staff quickly to become comfortable with the instrumentation and components. The simplification that this provides the surgeon and the operative room staff cannot be understated (Fig. 4).

○ The ability to use a TFC prosthesis in a variety of bone loss situations also eliminates intraoperative shuffles or changes in the surgical plan, resulting in more instruments and different components being opened. This easily

can happen with PPFx because bone loss can be significantly underestimated preoperatively or may change intraoperatively.

MODERN FEMORAL REVISION COMPONENT DESIGNS: MONOLITHIC AND MODULAR TAPERED FLUTED CONICAL PROSTHESES

Key Issue 1: Achieve Solid Initial Fixation

The most important surgical goal with a TFC prosthesis is to achieve solid initial axial and rotational fixation for the distal conical stem (Fig. 5). Subsidence can be minimized by placing a cerclage cable around the femur distal to the fracture site so as to allow more aggressive bone preparation and firm impaction of the tapered conical trial or stem (depending on the specifics of the surgical technique for the specific prosthesis being used). It is the authors' experience that reaming with power works best at achieving this goal. Direct visualization of the bone distal to the PPFx improves the chance of achieving solid initial fixation for the stem. Fortunately, for the most part, this is already the case with a PPFx.

Key Issue 2: Reproduce the Mechanics of the Hip Joint

Another key goal of the surgery is to restore the mechanics and stability of the hip joint through

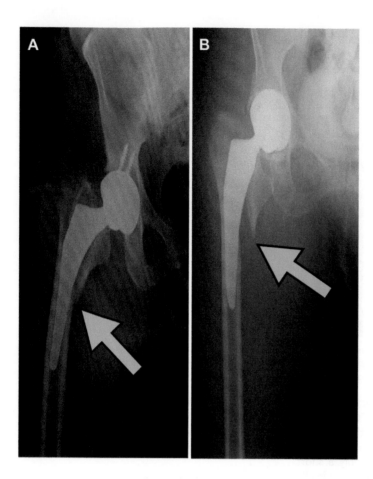

Fig. 4. Examples of PPFx treated at our institution in a 71-year-old woman (A) and a 66-year-old woman (B) Arrows depicts fracture site location.

restoration of leg lengths and hip offset. Likely the greatest advantage of the TFC prosthesis is the ability to separate completely the task of fixation from other tasks such as restoring offset, leg length, and obtaining stability. The ability to do this potentially allows the surgeon to minimize patient restrictions postoperatively. Whether done through a distal stem trial (when using the monolithic stems) or through insertion of the actually final distal fluted conical stem (when using the modular stems), the important sequence is to obtain distal fixation first. The modular proximal trials then enable the surgeon to easily increase the length of the proximal body, change the neck–shaft angle, and change the femoral version. These maneuvers allow for optimization of the component fit for each patient situation to maximize anatomic reconstruction of hip mechanics.

Key Issue 3: Maximize the Potential for Fracture Healing
Minimizing damage to the blood supply of the fracture fragments during exposure and close

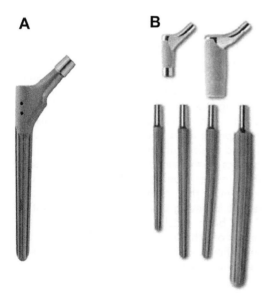

Fig. 5. Examples of the tapered conical prosthetic design for both monolithic (A) and modular (B) prostheses (Zimmer Biomet, Warsaw, IN, and Stryker, Mahwah NJ).

attention to fracture reduction not only improves the chance of fracture healing but also, with fracture healing, can decrease stresses at the modular junction.

SURGICAL TECHNIQUE: MONOLITHIC VERSUS MODULAR

The monolithic prosthesis has 2 segments—a proximal body and distal stem. The sequence in surgery is to ream aggressively the diaphysis distal to the fracture site to create secure initial stem fixation (key issue 1). A trial conical stem then is inserted after reaming. The subsequent reconstruction of the hip stability and mechanics (key issue 2) is then done using proximal body trials with the trial stem in place. Once the trialing is complete, all the trials are removed and the final monolithic prosthesis is inserted. The only modular choice left, after removal of the trials, is at the head–neck interface.

The modular stem is made of 2 independent and separate components—a proximal body and a distal conical stem. As with the monolithic procedure, the sequence in surgery is to ream aggressively the diaphysis distal to the fracture site to create secure initial stem fixation (key issue 1). Unlike the monolithic technique, the final stem is then inserted immediately after reaming. The subsequently reconstruction of hip stability and mechanics (key issue 2) is then done using proximal body trials with the final stem already in place. Once the trialing is complete, the final proximal body is assembled in vivo.

Monolithic Tapered Fluted Conical Components and Periprosthetic Fracture

With extensive experience, a monolithic TFC component can be used for most femoral revisions. Long-term clinical outcomes have been favorable for monoblock TFC stems for use in revision THA overall. Regis and colleagues[22] reported on a consecutive series of 66 patients who underwent femoral revision using a cementless Wagner tapered stem at a mean follow-up of 13.9 years and found survivorship of the femoral stem to be 96.6%. The mean Harris hip scores improved from 33 points preoperatively to 75 points postoperatively.[22]

Unfortunately, the use of monolithic TFC stems in the setting of PPFxs has minimal support in the literature at this time. To our knowledge, no study has published outcomes specifically in a cohort of patients with PPFxs using monolithic TFC stems. The 1 reported series, reported by Menken and Rodriguez,[12] has only 11 cases and less than 1 year of follow-up.

The main potential benefit of the monolithic TFC stem arises from the simplicity of the design itself. There is no modular junction and therefore there is no risk of implant failure or corrosion at the stem–body junction, something that has been seen in some modular TFC components (Fig. 6).[23–25] Of course, if the monolithic stem fixates distally, and through lack of fracture healing, remains unsupported proximally, there is a theoretic risk of fracture as well.[26]

Another possible benefit of the monolithic design is that it can accommodate smaller bone sizes and smaller stem lengths, whereas the modular stems cannot, owing to the mechanical integrity of the modular junction.[17] Small stems like this are used most often in situations where a TFC prosthesis is being contemplated for a nonrevision situation. In the scenario of PPFx; however, this advantage over modular TFC prostheses is only theoretical.

Finally a cost analysis should be considered when choosing a stem. In reality, all revision stems are costly, but the monolithic prosthesis generally is less so. If a similar clinical outcome can be achieved, it would be reasonable to choose the least expensive prosthesis.

Sandiford and colleagues[21] evaluated a cohort of 104 patients who underwent revision THA and insertion of the Wagner SL femoral stem between 2011 and 2012, and confirmed this notion. They found only 6% of patients (6/104) to have exhibited radiographic subsidence of 10 mm to 15 mm. The remaining patients (98/104) who did not subsidence more than 10 mm were found to subside a mean of 2 mm (range, 0–9 mm). None of the patients required revision for a diagnosis of subsidence. They concluded that, although many patients experience subsidence, the majority subside a distance of less than 10 mm, are not associated with poor outcome scores, and stabilize by 1 year postoperatively.[21]

Currently, with the advancements in implant design, improved trials, access to a range of stem lengths and diameters, and high offset options, concerns of early subsidence and dislocation with monolithic TFC stems are decreased.

Modular Tapered Fluted Conical Components and Periprosthetic Fracture

At this time, modular TFC prostheses are the most common choice for PPFx. In the setting of a PPFx, these prostheses offer substantial advantages, especially in the operating room, over other prosthetic choices.

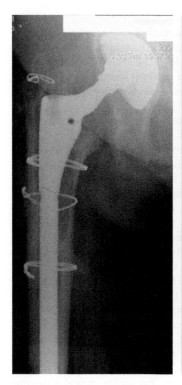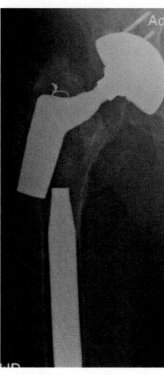

Fig. 6. Modular stem fracture. Note lack of bone support proximal to the modular junction. (*From* Lakstein et al JBJS 2011; 93:57-65.)

Overall clinical outcomes for modular TFC stems have shown it to be a successful implant option for revision THA, with improvements in postoperative outcome scores, low complication rates, and consistent restoration of proximal bone stock. The 5-year survivorship of modular TFC stems is reported as between 86% and 99%, with a low risk of clinically significant stem subsidence, aseptic loosening, instability, and dislocation.[27] Studies have shown modular stems to be particularly effective for Paprosky type III femoral defects, in which they have reported 75% to 94% survivorship rates at 4.5 to 10.0 years.[9,28–32]

A few studies have focused specifically on the use of modular TFC stems during revision THA for an indication of PPFx specifically. Abdel and colleagues[33] reported on a cohort of 44 patients (25 Vancouver type B2 and 19 Vancouver type B3), and found 98% (43/44) to have reached radiographic union at 4.5 years of follow-up, with an average Harris hip score of 83.5%; 2 of the 44 stems were revised during the period, both of which were for infection.[33] In a separate study by Munro and colleagues,[34] 55 patients (38 Vancouver type B2 and 17 Vancouver type B3) reported similarly positive outcomes at 4.5 years of follow-up; 98% (54/55) reached

radiographic union, with an average Western Ontario and McMaster Universities Osteoarthritis Index score of 76 for B2 fractures and 77 for B3 fractures. 4% (2/55) stems were revised overall (one for subsidence and one for infection).[34]

The greatest advantage of the modular TFC prosthesis (over the monolithic prosthesis) is that the proximal body size, length, and version is chosen after placement of the distal conical stem.[35] Even with the best of technique, there are times when the distal conical stem stabilizes in a deeper position than the reamer. This complication can be addressed immediately with a different length of proximal body trial. This condition is much more difficult to address in a monolithic prosthesis, because all the decisions are made off of a trial conical stem and it is possible that the final stem might become axially stable at a deeper depth. Making up this difference through head and neck trials (now the only choice other than choosing a bigger monolithic stem) is more difficult and results in changes in hip offset and hip mechanics. This situation is more common when the surgeon is in the learning curve or when the surgeon is an infrequent user of a TFC stem. It is also a common issue in PPFxs because of the poor bone quality that exists in these cases.

A modular prosthesis is useful in the setting of severe proximal bone loss because the custom fit of the body can be tailored directly to the patient's bone defects.[35] Any proximal or distal bone size mismatches can be accommodated, which is not possible with a monolithic prosthesis. Proper sizing of the proximal segment, such that it comes into contact with host bone, leads to biologic fixation of the proximal segment; this procedure also substantially decreases, if not completely removes, stresses at the modular junction.[35]

Although implant modularity is very helpful for the challenge of PPFxs, the surgeon needs to be mindful of the potential for fracture at the modular junction. Some modular prostheses have been withdrawn from the market because of a high incidence of implant fracture.[17] In contrast, there are other modular TFC prostheses with an impeccable clinical experience over many years with no issues related to implant fracture.[24]

OUR CLINICAL EXPERIENCE

Recently, our institution reported results from a retrospective study on clinical and functional outcomes for modular TFC (n = 225) and monolithic TFC (n = 63) prostheses.[36] Patients were included regardless of indication, with 25% of the cohort (80/325) being treated for PPFx. Of those who received a modular TFC stem, 46.7% had type IIIa 20.0% type IIIb, and 4.89% type IV femoral bone loss. Similarly, in those who received a monolithic TFC stem, 38.1% had type IIIa, 15.9% type IIIb, and 4.76% type IV bone loss. Radiographic subsidence of more than 5 mm occurred in 23.6% of patients with modular TFC, 16.1% with monolithic TFC, and 8.1% with FPCC stems. Of these patients with subsidence, 3 patients in the modular group and 1 patient in the monolithic group required re-revision. After controlling for potential confounding factors for subsidence including femoral bone loss and preoperative diagnosis, prosthesis type (modular vs monolithic) had no significant impact on the rate of subsidence. Aseptic revision rates and functional outcome scores were comparable between all 3 groups as well. In total, 10 patients with modular TFT stems (4.44%), and 2 patients with monolithic stems (3.17%) required re-revision for an aseptic cause.

These results are similar to those previously published our institution in 2010, in which we evaluated 118 patients who underwent revision using a modular TFC prosthesis for a diagnosis of PPFx. This study included patients across all Paprosky classifications 69 type I, 35 type II, 17 type III, and 1 type IV, and evaluated functional outcome scores as well as stem fixation, leg length discrepancy, and hip stability. At a minimum of 2 years of follow-up, we found that patients reported improvements in functional outcome, with 10% of patients showing distal bone ingrowth fixation of the prothesis. Furthermore, leg length discrepancy was corrected to within 5 mm in 78% of patients (95/118), and stability was achieved in 97% (114/118). None of the prostheses were noted to have failed and there were no implant fractures noted at the stem–body junction.[37]

SUMMARY

Modular TFC prostheses have been and continue to be the work horse for the treatment of PPFxs. Monolithic TFC prostheses also can be used for almost all PPFxs, but work best in the hands of an experienced revision arthroplasty surgeon. The infrequent revision arthroplasty surgeon (perhaps <10–15 cases per year) may find a modular TFC prosthesis to be a better option because the final proximal construct works off of an already well-fixed distal stem. We recommend considering modular TFC components if the surgeon is in the learning curve, or if proximal/distal bone size mismatch is present.

CLINICS CARE POINTS

- PPFx in the setting of THA is a technically challenging complication that requires an understanding of both fracture care and adult reconstruction.

- TFC prosthetic designs, in comparison with FPCC, designs have the advantage of obtaining adequate distal fixation over a shorter segment of bicortical fit. This makes TFC prostheses making them ideal revision THA in the setting of PPFx where bone loss can be substantial.

- Monolithic and modular TFC components share the same principles for obtaining fixation, minimizing subsidence, and restoring the mechanical integrity of the hip joint. Subsidence can be minimized by placing a cerclage cable around the femur distal to the fracture site so as to allow more aggressive bone preparation and firm impaction of the tapered conical stem.

- Modular TFC components have been, after in vivo distal fixation of the distal conical stem, able offer the ability to easily fine tune anteversion, leg length, and offset with trials. This process is not possible with a monolithic stem, where all choices, including distal conical stem size, are made before implantation. Therefore, the monolithic stem could be implanted immediately at a lower level than the trials, creating difficulty managing leg length and stability in the operative room.

- Monolithic TFC stems are less expensive and do not come with the risk of stem–body junction failure.

ACKNOWLEDGMENTS

This research was funded internally by Rothman Orthopaedics and Thomas Jefferson University.

DISCLOSURE

The authors have nothing to disclose.

REFERENCES

1. Fleischman AN, Chen AF. Periprosthetic fractures around the femoral stem: overcoming challenges and avoiding pitfalls. Ann Transl Med 2015;3(16): 234.

2. Berry DJ. Epidemiology: hip and knee. Orthop Clin North Am 1999;30(2):183–90.

3. Lindahl H, Malchau H, Herberts P, et al. Periprosthetic femoral fractures classification and demographics of 1049 periprosthetic femoral fractures from the Swedish National Hip Arthroplasty Register. J Arthroplasty 2005;20(7):857–65.

4. Shah RP, Sheth NP, Gray C, et al. Periprosthetic fractures around loose femoral components. J Am Acad Orthop Surg 2014;22(8):482–90.

5. Masri BA, Meek RM, Duncan CP. Periprosthetic fractures evaluation and treatment. Clin Orthop Relat Res 2004;(420):80–95.

6. Brady OH, Garbuz DS, Masri BA, et al. The reliability and validity of the Vancouver classification of femoral fractures after hip replacement. J Arthroplasty 2000;15(1):59–62.

7. Naqvi GA, Baig SA, Awan N. Interobserver and intraobserver reliability and validity of the Vancouver classification system of periprosthetic femoral fractures after hip arthroplasty. J Arthroplasty 2012;27:1047–50.

8. Parvizi J, Rapuri VR, Purtill JJ, et al. Treatment protocol for proximal femoral periprosthetic fractures. J Bone Joint Surg Am 2004;86-A(Suppl 2):8–16.

9. Chen AF, Hozack WJ. Component selection in revision total hip arthroplasty. Orthop Clin North Am 2014;45(3):275–86.

10. Valle CJ, Paprosky WG. Classification and an algorithmic approach to the reconstruction of femoral deficiency in revision total hip arthroplasty. J Bone Joint Surg Am 2003;85-A(Suppl 4): 1–6.

11. Fink B. What can the surgeon do to reduce the risk of junction breakage in modular revision stems? Arthroplast Today 2018;4(3):306–9.

12. Menken LG, Rodriguez JA. Femoral revision for periprosthetic fracture in total hip arthroplasty. J Clin Orthop Trauma 2020;11(1):16–21.

13. da Assunção RE, Pollard TC, Hrycaiczuk A, et al. Revision arthroplasty for periprosthetic femoral fracture using an uncemented modular tapered conical stem. Bone Joint J 2015;97-B(8):1031–7.

14. Richards CJ, Duncan CP, Masri BA, et al. Femoral revision hip arthroplasty: a comparison of two stem designs. Clin Orthop Relat Res 2010;468(2): 491–6.

15. Paprosky WG, Burnett RS. Extensively porous-coated femoral stems in revision hip arthroplasty: rationale and results. Am J Orthop (Belle Mead NJ) 2002;31(8):471–4.

16. Wagner H. Revisionsprothese für das Hüftgelenk bei schwerem Knochenverlust [Revision prosthesis for the hip joint in severe bone loss]. Orthopade 1987;16(4):295–300 [in German].

17. Van Houwelingen AP, Duncan CP, Masri BA, et al. High survival of modular tapered stems for proximal femoral bone defects at 5 to 10 years followup. Clin Orthop Relat Res 2013;471(2):454–62.

18. Bühler DW, Berlemann U, Lippuner K, et al. Three-dimensional primary stability of cementless femoral stems. Clin Biomech (Bristol, Avon) 1997;12(2): 75–86.

19. Gabor JA, Padilla JA, Feng JE, et al. Short-term outcomes with the REDAPT monolithic, tapered, fluted, grit-blasted, forged titanium revision femoral stem. Bone Joint J 2020;102-B(2):191–7.

20. Pierson JL, Small SR, Rodriguez JA, et al. The effect of taper angle and spline geometry on the initial stability of tapered, splined modular titanium stems. J Arthroplasty 2015;30(7):1254–9.

21. Sandiford NA, Garbuz DS, Masri BA, et al. Nonmodular Tapered 1 THAs. Clin Orthop Relat Res 2017;475(1):186–92.

22. Regis D, Sandri A, Bonetti I, et al. Femoral revision with the Wagner tapered stem: a ten- to 15-year

follow-up study. J Bone Joint Surg Br 2011;93(10): 1320–6.

23. Konan S, Garbuz DS, Masri BA, et al. Non-modular tapered fluted titanium stems in hip revision surgery: gaining attention. Bone Joint J 2014;96-B(11 Supple A):56–9.

24. Rodriguez JA, Deshmukh AJ, Robinson J, et al. Reproducible fixation with a tapered, fluted, modular, titanium stem in revision hip arthroplasty at 8-15 years follow-up. J Arthroplasty 2014;29(9 Suppl):214–8.

25. Abdel MP, Cottino U, Larson DR, et al. Modular fluted tapered stems in aseptic revision total hip arthroplasty. J Bone Joint Surg Am 2017;99(10): 873–81.

26. Lakstein D, Eliaz N, Levi O, et al. Fracture of cementless femoral stems at the mid-stem junction in modular revision hip arthroplasty systems. J Bone Joint Surg Am 2011;93(1):57–65.

27. Garbuz DS, Toms A, Masri BA, et al. Improved outcome in femoral revision arthroplasty with tapered fluted modular titanium stems. Clin Orthop Relat Res 2006;453:199–202.

28. Palumbo BT, Morrison KL, Baumgarten AS, et al. Results of revision total hip arthroplasty with modular, titanium-tapered femoral stems in severe proximal metaphyseal and diaphyseal bone loss. J Arthroplasty 2013;28(4):690–4.

29. Wang L, Dai Z, Wen T, et al. Three to seven year follow-up of a tapered modular femoral prosthesis in revision total hip arthroplasty. Arch Orthop Trauma Surg 2013;133(2):275–81.

30. Jibodh SR, Schwarzkopf R, Anthony SG, et al. Revision hip arthroplasty with a modular cementless stem: mid-term follow up. J Arthroplasty 2013; 28(7):1167–72.

31. Klauser W, Bangert Y, Lubinus P, et al. Medium-term follow-up of a modular tapered noncemented titanium stem in revision total hip arthroplasty: a single-surgeon experience. J Arthroplasty 2013;28(1):84–9.

32. Skyttä ET, Eskelinen A, Remes V. Successful femoral reconstruction with a fluted and tapered modular distal fixation stem in revision total hip arthroplasty. Scand J Surg 2012;101(3):222–6.

33. Abdel MP, Lewallen DG, Berry DJ. Periprosthetic femur fractures treated with modular fluted, tapered stems. Clin Orthop Relat Res 2014;472(2): 599–603.

34. Munro JT, Garbuz DS, Masri BA, et al. Tapered fluted titanium stems in the management of Vancouver B2 and B3 periprosthetic femoral fractures. Clin Orthop Relat Res 2014;472(2):590–8.

35. Shilling JW, Sharkey PF, Hozack WJ, et al. Femoral revision hip arthroplasty: modular versus nonmodular femoral component for severe femoral deficiency. Oper Tech Orthopaedic Surg 2000; 10(2):133–7.

36. Yacovelli S, Ottaway J, Banerjee S, et al. Modern revision femoral stem designs have no difference in rates of subsidence. J Arthroplasty 2021;36(1): 268–73.

37. Restrepo C, Mashadi M, Parvizi J, et al. Modular femoral stems for revision total hip arthroplasty. Clin Orthop Relat Res 2011;469(2):476–82.

Ten-Year Survivorship and Risk of Periprosthetic Fracture of a Cementless Tapered Stem

Mathew H. Freeman, MD, Beau J. Kildow, MD*,
Tyler J. Larson, MD, Zachary C. Bailey, MD,
Elizabeth R. Lyden, MS, Kevin L. Garvin, MD

KEYWORDS

- Periprosthetic fracture • SYNERGY • Survivorship • Total hip arthroplasty • Cementless
- Uncemented

KEY POINTS

- Overall 10-year survivorship of SYNERGY stem is 99.6%.
- There were a total of 6 (1.2%) intraoperative fractures and 9 (1.8%) during the study period.
- Ream and broach femoral stem reveals excellent long-term survivorship with low risk of periprosthetic fracture.

INTRODUCTION

Periprosthetic femur fractures have been reported more frequently with uncemented compared with cemented femoral stems in total hip arthroplasty (THA).[1] Despite the risk of this uncommon complication, uncemented fixation is performed much more commonly than cemented fixation.[2] Studies have shown the risk of intraoperative fractures occurring 14 times more often during uncemented stem placement compared with cemented stem placement (3.0% vs 0.2%). Postoperative fractures have also been shown to be increased at 10-year follow-up in uncemented hips (2.6% vs 0.9%).[1] In addition, uncemented stems have been reported to fail and require revision more frequently because of periprosthetic fracture during the first 2 postoperative years.[3]

Several factors have contributed to periprosthetic fractures, including the age of patients undergoing surgery, bone quality, and stem geometry.[1,4] Watts and colleagues[5] recently studied 736 cementless tapered stems with an exaggerated proximal taper compared with 3228 hips in which cementless, tapered stems were used. Stems with an exaggerated proximal taper had an increased cumulative probability of both early and late fractures. The cumulative probability of early and late fracture was higher with the exaggerated proximal taper (7.4% at 10-year follow-up) compared with standard, proximally fixed tapered stems (1.6%; $P<.001$). This increased fracture rate in exaggerated proximally tapered stems led to poor survival of 92.6% at 10-year follow-up compared with 98.4% survival in the nonexaggerated proximally tapered stems ($P<.001$). Additional studies have

---

The authors have not received grant support or research funding and do not have any proprietary interests in the materials described in this article. The authors have nothing to disclose.
This study was approved by the institutional review board at our institution.
Conflict of Interest: The authors declare that there is no conflict of interest.
Department of Orthopaedic Surgery, University of Nebraska Medical Center, 985640 Nebraska Medical Center, Omaha, NE 68198, USA
* Corresponding author.
E-mail address: kildow06@gmail.com

evaluated other problematic stem designs associated with factors such as poor fixation, pain, and increased osteolysis.[6–10]

The overall results of cementless fixation with short-, mid-, and long-term follow-up have been excellent with several studies in support. Belmont and colleagues[11] demonstrated a 97.8% survivorship of an anatomic medullary locking hip stem with minimum 20-year follow-up. In a study of 2000 tapered titanium porous plasma-sprayed femoral components, Lombardi and colleagues[12] demonstrated a 98.6% survival of the femoral component at 5 years and 95.5% survival at 20 years. McLaughlin and Lee[13] report the survivorship of a similarly designed Taperloc uncemented stem (Taperloc, Zimmer-Biomet, Warsaw, IN, USA) to be 98% at a mean follow-up of 24.5 years. Additional studies have reported high success ranging from 86% survival at 22 years to 99% at 20 years.[14–16]

The reported frequency of periprosthetic fractures associated with uncemented stems compared with cemented stems encouraged us to evaluate our results on this topic and identify if fractures were associated with failure. Therefore, the purpose of this study was to investigate the minimum 10-year risk of fracture and stem failure of an uncemented ream-and-broach tapered stem. In addition, we sought to determine if early or late perioperative fractures led to failure.

PATIENTS AND METHODS

A consecutive series of 475 hip arthroplasties performed using the ream-and-broach SYNERGY uncemented tapered stem (Smith and Nephew, Memphis, TN, USA) between January 1999 and March 2007 was identified. The SYNERGY stem is a ream-broach design with circulotrapezoidal taper proximally and cylindrical distally. The proximal portion has porous coating, whereas the distal cylindrical portion is grit-blast with 3 fins on the anterior and posterior aspects. The distal tip is polished. All arthroplasties were performed by a single surgeon at a single institution using the posterior approach. During this period, the indications for the uncemented stem included osteoarthritis (75%), osteonecrosis (9.3%), dysplasia (8.0%), posttraumatic arthritis (5.7%), and inflammatory arthritis (2.0%). Patients with Dorr C femoral morphology older than 80 years were considered candidates for cemented fixation and thus excluded from this cohort. The average age at time of primary surgery was 54.7 years (range = 20–93 years). A total of 401 patients had 10-year follow-up, and of those without 10-year follow-up, 27%

were deceased. No patients were lost to follow-up. If there was not a clinical visit follow-up, patients were able to be contacted for a phone survey. Average time to follow-up was 11.1 years. For the study stem, males accounted for 55.1% of cases.

All cases were templated. Posterior approach was used for all cases. Surgical technique involved preparing the acetabulum followed by the femur. Reamers were sequentially used up to the size that was templated and/or obtaining adequate endosteal fit for an appropriate sized stem; this was followed by sequential broaching to match proximal femur anatomy and version. The hip was reduced and checked for stability. The real stem was placed and seated to the exact position of the broach. In every case 28- to 32-mm cobalt-chrome heads were used. Postoperatively patients were allowed to weight bear as tolerated with posterior hip precautions. At the 6-week postoperative visit, hip precautions were discontinued.

We retrospectively reviewed operative notes and radiographs to identify intraoperative and postoperative fractures and classified these according to the Vancouver classification system.[17] Operative notes were used to discern the primary surgeon's technique for fixing intraoperative and postoperative fractures. We also identified revisions, defined as removal of the femoral component, and further quantified revision data with variables such as time to revision and cause for revision. Follow-up was conducted with use of questionnaires, clinic visit notes with physical examination, and postoperative radiographs. Institutional review board approval was obtained before initiation of this study.

STATISTICAL ANALYSIS

Descriptive statistics (means, standard deviations, medians, counts, and percentages) was used to summarize demographic and clinical characteristics. Hip survival with 95% confidence interval (CI) was estimated using the method of Kaplan and Meier for the end point of revision for any reason. All analyses were done using SAS, Version 9.4 (Cary, NC, USA). $P<.05$ was considered statistically significant.

RESULTS

There were 6 (1.2%) intraoperative fractures and 9 (1.8%) postoperative fractures. Intraoperative fractures occurred during impaction of the final component in 4 patients and broaching in 2 patients. Primary fixation for fractures included

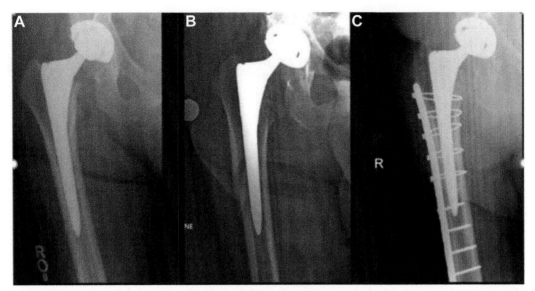

Fig. 1. Radiographs of a 76-year-old man who underwent cementless arthroplasty in the setting of osteoarthritis. (A) The postoperative radiograph of the right hip reveals a well-fixed primary, cementless tapered hip arthroplasty. (B) The radiograph demonstrates a postoperative B1 fracture occurring approximately 10 years following primary surgery. At the time of surgery the femoral component was well fixed to the proximal fragments. (C) The radiograph demonstrates open reduction internal fixation with use of cerclage wires and plate in the fixation of the postoperative fracture. The patient is asymptomatic 4-year status post open reduction internal fixation.

open reduction internal fixation in 10 patients (2.2%), nonoperative management in 3 patients (0.06%), and revision in 1 patient. Intraoperative fractures comprised 5 A2 and 1 A3, whereas postoperative fractures in this group consisted of 4 B1 (Fig 1), 4 AG, and 1C (Table 1). There were 3 total revisions, 2 (0.4%) for infection (same patient with acute myeloid leukemia with immunosuppression) and 1 (0.2%) for recurrent dislocation secondary to greater trochanteric fracture. Average time to revision was 6.61 years (minimum = 4.6 years, maximum = 10.3 years).

Kaplan-Meier analysis of the femoral component survival-free revision of all causes in uncemented (n = 401) was performed.[18] The overall 10-year survivorship for the uncemented

component was 99.6% (95% CI: 97%, 100%) (Fig. 2). Because the failure and fracture rate were so low, regression analysis was unable to identify any contributing factors, including age and comorbidities.

DISCUSSION

Uncemented tapered femoral components are widely used and have been reported to perform well in primary THA.[12,19–23] Numerous studies provide long-term outcomes of various stems including metrics such as revision-free survival, radiographic analyses, and patient-reported hip scores, such as Harris Hip Score, but few studies have evaluated the incidence and consequence of a periprosthetic fracture.[12,19,24] Periprosthetic fracture remains one of the most common complications associated with primary THA because intraoperative fractures have been reported to occur 14 times more frequently during uncemented hip arthroplasty compared with cemented.[1] The overall frequency of periprosthetic fractures associated with uncemented stems encouraged us to evaluate our results on this topic. Therefore, we investigated the minimum 10-year risk of fracture and stem failure of the SYNERGY uncemented tapered stem and determined if early periprosthetic fractures predicted failure.

Table 1 Classification of periprosthetic fractures				
Hip Characteristics	**Operation**	**N**	**Vancouver Class**	
Uncemented	6 Intraoperation	5	A2	
		1	A3	
	9 Postoperation	4	B1	
		4	AG	
		1	C	

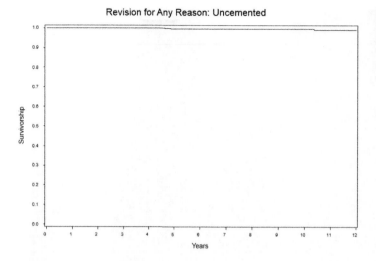

Fig. 2. Graph shows the Kaplan-Meier survivorship curve with femoral revision of uncemented tapered stems for any reason as the end point. Ten-year survival was estimated at 99.6% (95.5 CI).

The cementless tapered design we used demonstrated a low intraoperative fracture risk of 1.2% and postoperative fracture risk of 1.6%. Abdel and colleagues[1] demonstrated a 10-year intraoperative fracture risk of 2.6% and postoperative fracture risk of 0.9% with use of cementless tapered designs, whereas Schwarzkopf and colleagues[25] demonstrated 0.4% postoperative fracture rate in 2078 uncemented arthroplasties. Early studies of uncemented implants found intraoperative fracture rates to range between 3.7% and 5.4%.[26,27] These studies demonstrate variable results, which corroborates the need for additional literature as in the current study.

There were 15 periprosthetic fractures with follow-up of at least 10 years. No intraoperative (n = 6) and 1 postoperative fracture (n = 9) required revision of the femoral component. The survivorship at minimum 10-year follow-up was 99.6%. This cohort had a higher proportion of males (55.1%), and they were younger (mean = 54.7 years). Although there was no definitive criteria for which patient obtained a cementless implant, these results can be generally applied to younger patients with surgeon-determined adequate bone stock.

Limitations of our study include most importantly selection bias as it pertains to patient selection for the use of a cementless implant. Because this is a retrospective series, there were no defined parameters on which patients received cementless components other than the aforementioned exclusion criteria. In addition, not all hips are accounted for (<10-year follow-up), which is anticipated with 10-year longitudinal studies.[12,23] Finally, with our limited number of periprosthetic fractures (n = 25), the clinical significance of failure associated with fracture is difficult to ascertain. However, the number of patients in our study group was substantial and largest when compared with similar studies.[13,22,23,28–30]

In conclusion, we observed intraoperative fractures in 1.2% and postoperative fractures in 1.6% with the use of the cementless tapered ream-and-broach stem. Young age and the improved tapered design are 2 factors likely contributing to our results. Periprosthetic fracture necessitated revision of the stem in the ingrowth-tapered design in only 1 patient. Although we report excellent survivorship of a ream-broach cementless stem, caution should be taken with consideration of using cemented stems in older patients with less-than-optimal bone quality. Additional studies evaluating factors associated with periprosthetic fractures, including stem design and patient selection, may help lessen the complication and improve the outcome of patients undergoing THA.

FUNDING

This research received no specific grant from any funding agency in the public, commercial, or not-for-profit sectors.

CLINICS CARE POINTS

- Cementless tapered ream and broach stems have excellent long-term survivorship with minimal risk of fracture.
- This stem should however be used with caution in patients with poor bone quality.

REFERENCES

1. Abdel MP, Watts CD, Houdek MT, et al. Epidemiology of periprosthetic fracture of the femur in 32 644 primary total hip arthroplasties: a 40-year experience. Bone Joint J 2016;98-B:461–7.

2. Troelsen A, Malchau E, Sillesen N, et al. A review of current fixation use and registry outcomes in total hip arthroplasty: the uncemented paradox. Clin Orthop Relat Res 2013;471:2052–9.

3. Hailer NP, Garellick G, Karrholm J. Uncemented and cemented primary total hip arthroplasty in the swedish hip arthroplasty register. Acta Orthop 2010;81:34–41.

4. Lindahl H, Garellick G, Regner H, et al. Three hundred and twenty-one periprosthetic femoral fractures. J Bone Joint Surg Am 2006;88:1215–22.

5. Watts CD, Abdel MP, Lewallen DG, et al. Increased risk of periprosthetic femur fractures associated with a unique cementless stem design. Clin Orthop Relat Res 2015;473:2045–53.

6. Callaghan JJ, Dysart SH, Savory CG. The uncemented porous-coated anatomic total hip prosthesis. two-year results of a prospective consecutive series. J Bone Joint Surg Am 1988;70: 337–46.

7. Campbell D, Mercer G, Nilsson KG, et al. Early migration characteristics of a hydroxyapatite-coated femoral stem: an RSA study. Int Orthop 2011;35:483–8.

8. Capone A, Congia S, Civinini R, et al. Periprosthetic fractures: epidemiology and current treatment. Clin Cases Miner Bone Metab 2017;14:189–96.

9. Cook RE, Jenkins PJ, Walmsley PJ, et al. Risk factors for periprosthetic fractures of the hip: a survivorship analysis. Clin Orthop Relat Res 2008;466:1652–6.

10. Dodge BM, Fitzrandolph R, Collins DN. Noncemented porous-coated anatomic total hip arthroplasty. Clin Orthop Relat Res 1991;16–24.

11. Belmont PJ Jr, Powers CC, Beykirch SE, et al. Results of the anatomic medullary locking total hip arthroplasty at a minimum of twenty years. A concise follow-up of previous reports. J Bone Joint Surg Am 2008;90:1524–30.

12. Lombardi AV Jr, Berend KR, Mallory TH, et al. Survivorship of 2000 tapered titanium porous plasma-sprayed femoral components. Clin Orthop Relat Res 2009;467:146–54.

13. McLaughlin JR, Lee KR. Uncemented total hip arthroplasty with a tapered femoral component: a 22- to 26-year follow-up study. Orthopedics 2010;33:639.

14. Corten K, Bourne RB, Charron KD, et al. What works best, a cemented or cementless primary total hip arthroplasty?: minimum 17-year followup of a randomized controlled trial. Clin Orthop Relat Res 2011;469:209–17.

15. Streit MR, Innmann MM, Merle C, et al. Long-term (20- to 25-year) results of an uncemented tapered titanium femoral component and factors affecting survivorship. Clin Orthop Relat Res 2013;471: 3262–9.

16. Vidalain JP. Twenty-year results of the cementless corail stem. Int Orthop 2011;35:189–94.

17. Masri BA, Meek RM, Duncan CP. Periprosthetic fractures evaluation and treatment. Clin Orthop Relat Res 2004;420:80–95.

18. Kaplan E, Meier P. Nonparametric estimation from incomplete observations. Biometrics 1958;53:457.

19. Aldinger PR, Breusch SJ, Lukoschek M, et al. A ten- to 15-year follow-up of the cementless spotorno stem. J Bone Joint Surg Br 2003;85:209–14.

20. Berend KR, Lombardi AV, Mallory TH, et al. Cementless double-tapered total hip arthroplasty in patients 75 years of age and older. J Arthroplasty 2004;19:288–95.

21. Herrera A, Mateo J, Gil-Albarova J, et al. Cementless hydroxyapatite coated hip prostheses. Biomed Res Int 2015;2015:386461.

22. Hozack WJ, Rothman RH, Eng K, et al. Primary cementless hip arthroplasty with a titanium plasma sprayed prosthesis. Clin Orthop Relat Res 1996; 333:217–25.

23. Meding JB, Galley MR, Ritter MA. High survival of uncemented proximally porous-coated titanium alloy femoral stems in osteoporotic bone. Clin Orthop Relat Res 2010;468:441–7.

24. Song JH, Kim DH, Kim J. Total hip replacement arthroplasty with mallory-head system–minimum ten-year follow-up results. Int Orthop 2012;36: 2055–9.

25. Schwarzkopf R, Oni JK, Marwin SE. Total hip arthroplasty periprosthetic femoral fractures: a review of classification and current treatment. Bull Hosp Jt Dis (2013) 2013;71:68–78.

26. Berry DJ. Epidemiology: hip and knee. Orthop Clin North Am 1999;30:183–90.

27. Schwartz JT J, Mayer JG, Engh CA. Femoral fracture during non-cemented total hip arthroplasty. J Bone Joint Surg Am 1989;71:1135–42.

28. Burt CF, Garvin KL, Otterberg ET, et al. A femoral component inserted without cement in total hip arthroplasty. A study of the tri-lock component with an average ten-year duration of follow-up. J Bone Joint Surg Am 1998;80:952–60.

29. Parvizi J, Keisu KS, Hozack WJ, et al. Primary total hip arthroplasty with an uncemented femoral component: a long-term study of the taperloc stem. J Arthroplasty 2004;19:151–6.

30. Xu J, Xie Z, Zhao J, et al. Results of a hydroxyapatite-coated femoral stem (corail) in chinese: a minimum 10-year follow-up. Springerplus 2016;5:1983. eCollection 2016;1–5.

Treatment of Geriatric Acetabular Fractures—A Concise Review of the Literature

Daniel A. Cohen, MBBS, FRACS, MSc[a],
Spencer J. Montgomery, MD, FRCSC[a],
Alexandra Stavrakis, MD[b], Simon C. Mears, MD, PhD[c],
Amit Atrey, MBBS, MRCS, MSc, FRCS[a],
Amir Khoshbin, MD[a],*

KEYWORDS

- Acetabular fractures • Posttraumatic arthritis • Open reduction and internal fixation
- Total hip arthroplasty

KEY POINTS

- With the elderly population remaining active, the incidence of geriatric acetabular fractures is on the rise.
- There is no consensus on the acute management of geriatric acetabular fractures with most treated surgically by ORIF or combined ORIF and acute THA.
- ORIF is an appropriate treatment option in medically well patients with adequate bone stock in the absence of osteochondral impaction injury, instability and pre-existing osteoarthritis.
- Acute THA +/- ORIF is a technically demanding operation best performed by specialist surgeons and should allow for early mobility and unrestricted weight bearing.
- Acute and delayed THA after geriatric acetabular fractures result in acceptable PROM scores and functional outcomes but higher complication rates relative to THA for osteoarthritis.

INTRODUCTION

Posttraumatic arthritis (PTA) is a considerable cause of disability and accounts for approximately 20% to 40% of all total hip arthroplasty (THA) cases performed.[1] The incidence of PTA following acetabular fracture (AF) ranges from 12% to 67%.[2–4] As the population ages, low-energy fragility AFs in the elderly (defined as ≥60 years old) are becoming more common. Between 1980 and 2007, there was an estimated 2.4-times increase in the incidence of AFs in patients over the age of 60.[5] Elderly patients comprised 53.9% of AFs presenting to trauma centers in the United States between 1990 and 2007.[6] Most elderly AFs are low energy and are caused by a fall from standing height. Fracture patterns most commonly involve most commonly the anterior column with associated chondral injuries of the acetabulum and femoral head, in the possible setting of preexisting osteoarthritis (OA).[5,7–9]

Treatment of AFs in the geriatric population is associated with high rates of perioperative and postoperative complications.[10–12] Open reduction and internal fixation (ORIF) is the mainstay of treatment of displaced AFs in young patients; however, older patients remain a management dilemma due to concurrent osteoporosis,

---

[a] Division of Orthopedic Surgery, St. Michael's Hospital, University of Toronto, 55 Queen Street East - Suite 800, Toronto, Ontario M5C 1R6, Canada; [b] Department of Orthopaedic Surgery, University of California Los Angeles, UCLA Department of Orthopaedic Surgery, 1250 16th St, Santa Monica, CA 90404 USA; [c] Department of Orthopedic Surgery, University of Arkansas for Medical Sciences, 4301 W Markham Street, Little Rock, AR 72205, USA
* Corresponding author.
E-mail address: Amir.Khoshbin@unityhealth.to

Orthop Clin N Am 52 (2021) 323–333
https://doi.org/10.1016/j.ocl.2021.05.007
0030-5898/21/© 2021 Elsevier Inc. All rights reserved.

fracture comminution, articular impaction, significant rates of loss of reduction, preexisting OA, and the possible need for revision surgery, including a conversion to salvage THA.[13–17] Additionally, medical comorbidities and the sequelae of prolonged weight-bearing limitations can further complicate management and increase the morbidity and mortality in this vulnerable patient population.[10,14,18,19] The 1-year mortality in elderly patients who sustain an AF ranges between 8.1% and 33% and is highly dependent on concomitant injuries.[18,20,21]

Current treatment options include nonoperative treatment, ORIF, and THA (delayed or acute, with or without combined ORIF). The Major Extremity Trauma Research Consortium (METRC) surveyed 15 level-I trauma centers and reported significant variation in the management of geriatric AFs between sites, with no overriding clinical practice guidelines.[9] This likely relates to limited high-quality prospective studies examining surgical treatment of AFs in this patient population. The purpose of this article is to provide an overview of the available modern literature on the 3 main treatment modalities for geriatric AFs: nonoperative management, ORIF, and THA.

NONOPERATIVE MANAGEMENT

Nonoperative management of AFs is sparsely reported and historically required prolonged recumbency or traction and a period of weight-bearing limitations.[22] This is problematic particularly because it is difficult for elderly patients to adhere to a non–weight-bearing status, in addition to the morbidity associated with such restrictions.[22–24] As such, nonoperative management typically is reserved for undisplaced stable fracture patterns, frail or medically unfit patients, and patients who are nonmobile at baseline.[10,14,25,26]

Letournel[4] described the concept of "secondary congruency" in associated both column AFs where the comminuted acetabular dome remains reduced in an anatomic position around the femoral head, thus maintaining a congruent and stable joint.[4] Nonoperative management in this scenario showed very good to excellent results in 85% of patients at 4 years of follow-up.[25]

A retrospective review by Spencer[27] reported on the outcomes of 25 nonoperatively managed AFs and showed 30% of patients had "unacceptable" functional results. Similarly, studies report that only 60% of patients are able to ambulate independently at 1 year with nonoperative management, and as few as 35% return to their

baseline functional status.[28,29] The mortality rate, however, repeatedly has been reported to be independent of treatment strategy but more correlated with a patient's overall preexisting health and baseline functional status.[10,18,30,31] When choosing nonoperative management, strict bed rest is not indicated and thromboprophylaxis should be prescribed.

Indications for delayed THA after index nonoperative management include OA, avascular necrosis (AVN), ongoing pain or immobility, and patients who were medically unfit to undergo surgery due to intercurrent illness or injury[11] (Fig. 1). Prolonged periods of restricted weight bearing, associated deconditioning, and altered biomechanics (medialization of the hip center of rotation) have led to suboptimal outcomes with delayed arthroplasty in this group of patients.[14,24] The optimal timing for delayed THA is after consolidation of bone stock on imaging.

OPEN REDUCTION AND INTERNAL FIXATION

Operative treatment (encompassing of ORIF and/or closed reduction and percutaneous pinning [CRPP] of osteoporotic AFs) is challenging, with a high degree of variability in treatment approaches[9] (Fig. 2).The fracture pattern in elderly AFs has been reported to largely involve the anterior column (50%–60%) and often is associated with significant marginal impaction of the weight-bearing dome, in addition to medialization of the hip joint, because the quadrilateral plate usually is fractured.[10] In a meta-analysis by Capone and colleagues[32], an "anatomic reduction," as per the Matta criteria, was achieved in only 50% of patients with 35% of patients receiving a "satisfactory" reduction and 15% a "poor" reduction.[2] Despite these challenges, reasonable long-term results have been demonstrated, with up to 68% of patients not needing a conversion to salvage THA at approximately 10.3 years post-ORIF.[33]

CRPP of AFs also has been proposed as a means of providing fracture stability and earlier weight bearing without the morbidity associated with conventional open surgical approaches.[34] Percutaneous fixation is indicated primarily for fractures of the anterior or posterior columns and relies on the technical ability of the surgeon and operating room staff (x-ray technologists) as well as patient anatomy being amenable to screw fixation. It is not intended to achieve anatomic articular reduction but rather re-

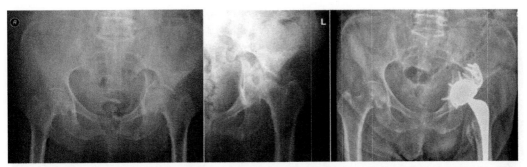

Fig. 1. An 83-year-old woman sustained an anterior column/posterior hemitransverse fracture of the left acetabulum after a fall from standing height. (Left) She was treated nonoperatively due to concurrent urosepsis requiring critical care admission after the index injury. At 6 months' postinjury (middle), she went on to have a delayed THA with acetabular reconstruction using an antiprotrusio cage with a cemented dual mobility cup. (Right) Femoral head autograft was used to help restore the native center of rotation.

establish column integrity and allow a stable hip joint for weight bearing.[34] In a retrospective review of 80 fractures treated with percutaneous fixation, Gary and colleagues[35] found a complication rate of 41%, a 25% conversion rate to THA, and an overall survival rate of 65% at 4.7 years.

In a retrospective analysis of 82 elderly AFs treated nonoperatively or with ORIF, at 2 years' follow-up, Harris Hip Score (HHS) and Postel–Merle d'Aubigné functional outcome scores were shown to be significantly higher in patients treated with ORIF irrespective of fracture pattern compared with patients treated nonoperatively.[36] Navarre and colleagues[37] reported on 72 elderly AFs treated with ORIF and showed that the Physical Component Summary score and 12-Item Short Form Health Survey score were comparable to age and sex-matched general population scores at 2 years' follow-up. O'Toole and colleagues[20] reported that elderly patients receiving ORIF for displaced AF at a high-volume level I trauma center had a mean Western Ontario and McMaster Universities Osteoarthritis Index score of 17 and 8-Item Short Form Health Survey score of 46.1, similar to outcomes in THA for OA and geriatric patient norms.

Perioperative complication rates have been reported as high as 40% after ORIF in elderly patients.[10] The 1-year mortality rate has also been shown to differ, depending on the presence of concomitant traumatic injuries and/or preexisting medical conditions, with isolated AFs having a 1-year mortality rate of 8%. When an elderly patient presents with multiple associated injuries, the mortality rate is reported between 22% and 24%.[18,32] In a matched cohort registry study comparing elderly patients with AFs versus hip fractures, patients with AFs were found to have longer wait times to surgery, longer in hospital admissions, higher rates of pulmonary embolism, and higher adjusted mortality rates.[19]

A recent population-based cohort-registry study reported rates of conversion to salvage THA following an acetabular ORIF were 8.6%,

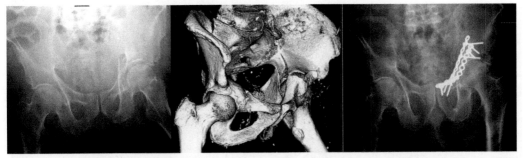

Fig. 2. An 82-year-old man sustained an anterior column/posterior hemitransverse acetabular fracture as a result of a low energy fall. (Left/Middle) He was treated with ORIF of his fracture through a Stoppa approach plus a lateral ilioinguinal window.[64] Fixation utilized infrapectineal and suprapectineal plates. At 3 months (Right), the patient was mobilizing fully and had a pain-free range of motion of the left hip.

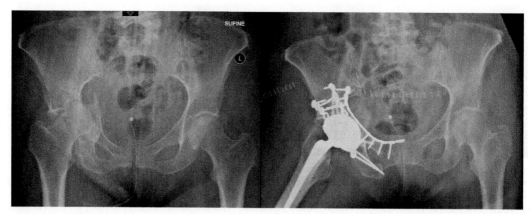

Fig. 3. A74-year-old healthy woman with comminuted bicolumnar AF and associated femoral head impaction injury. (Left) She was treated acutely with ORIF and a hybrid THA with multihole revision acetabular component. (Right) This operation was performed via dual anterior (Stoppa) and posterior approaches.[64]

12.4%, and 16.7% at 2 years, 5 years, and 10 years, respectively.[15] Patients who underwent ORIF were 25 times more likely to require THA compared with matched controls in the general population.[15] Similarly, a meta-analysis comparing ORIF and simultaneous ORIF and acute THA showed a conversion rate of 22.4% to salvage THA in the ORIF-only group at approximately 24.6 months.[10] Predictors of ORIF failure have included superomedial dome impaction (Gull sign), intra-articular comminution, femoral head impaction, preexisting OA, initial fracture displacement/dislocation, and ipsilateral femoral head and neck fractures.[38–41]

TOTAL HIP ARTHROPLASTY

There are 2 distinct groups of patients treated with THA after AFs: those treated with acute arthroplasty and/or fixation to restore column/ wall stability and those treated with delayed arthroplasty following a trial of nonoperative management or failed ORIF. Each group carries with it distinct advantages and disadvantages.

Acute THA with or without ORIF has gained popularity for treatment of geriatric AFs.[3,11,12,26,42–44] Indications for THA as the primary treatment of geriatric AFs include preexisting OA, osteoporosis, fracture comminution/ non-reconstructible fracture patterns, increased age, chondral injuries to the acetabulum and femoral head, and ipsilateral femoral head and neck fractures[16,42,45] (**Figs. 3 and 4**). Determination of the fracture pattern is critical to distinguish when additional fixation is indicated.

Posterior wall fractures may be amenable to more straightforward THA, with or without augmentation. Small fractures may be ignored, whereas larger posterior wall fractures may require either femoral head autograft or metallic

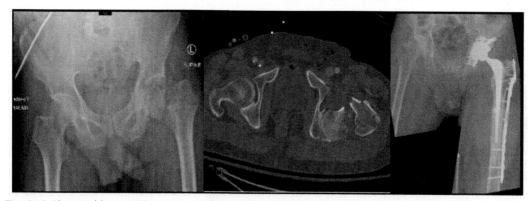

Fig. 4. A 63-year-old man with posterior wall/posterior column AF, femoral neck and greater trochanter fracture (Left/Middle). Patient was treated with ORIF of posterior AFs and an acute hybrid THA with multihole revision acetabular component and ORIF of the greater trochanter (Right).

augmentation to gain cup stability. Posterior patterns typically involve the posterior capsule; as such, care must be taken to prevent dislocation. Anterior or central fractures may require anterior buttressing so that a firm endpoint is obtained for bone grafting and cup placement. Posterior column or transverse patterns may require posterior column plate fixation to allow for a stable cup, and some patterns may require fixation of both columns to gain stability for acetabular component placement. Another option is for the components of the acetabular reconstruction to help bridge the fracture gap and gain stability. Simultaneous ORIF and acute THA allows for early mobilization without weight bearing restriction.

Combined THA and fixation requires skilled surgeons in both advanced trauma and arthroplasty techniques. Depending on the specific center, this may require 2 specialists or 1 who is skilled in both of these complex surgical skills. This combination of surgeons may be difficult to obtain in smaller centers where both trauma and arthroplasty cases are not performed.

Indications for salvage arthroplasty following index ORIF include PTA, AVN, heterotopic ossification (HO), pain, and failed ORIF. In this cohort of patients, along with deconditioning secondary to limited weight bearing, a unique set of challenges is encountered and includes previous incisions and surgical scarring, retained hardware, the presence of subclinical indolent infection, and a propensity for HO[3,12,26,46] (Fig. 5). Complication rates in THA post-ORIF, including prosthetic joint infection, implant loosening, dislocation, HO, and neurovascular injury, are considerably higher than routine elective THA for primary OA.[11,13,47,48] Salvage THA after ORIF is associated with longer surgical times and higher estimated blood loss, however, required less bone grafting than the delayed THA after index non-operative management.[49] Proponents of salvage THA have reported acceptable midterm to long-term results of ORIF, initial restoration of bone stock with index surgery (with a lower usage rate of revision THA components), and excellent midterm to long-term outcomes of THA compared with THA for PTA in a nonoperatively treated cohort.[15,26,33,49,50]

Acute Versus Delayed Total Hip Arthroplasty

Few studies have directly compared acute THA and delayed THA as treatment of elderly AF. Sermon and colleagues[3] retrospectively analyzed 121 AFs undergoing "acute reconstruction" versus "delayed reconstruction." Average follow-up was 30.7 months. The mean age in the acute reconstruction group was significantly higher than in the delayed reconstruction group (78 years vs 53 years, respectively). There was no difference in primary and complex fracture patterns among the groups. Postoperative HHS were significantly better in the delayed reconstruction cohort, with 76% achieving an excellent or good score, whereas only 58% achieved an excellent or good result in the acute reconstruction group. There were fewer revisions in the acute reconstruction group (8% vs 22%, respectively).[3]

Nicol and colleagues[44] retrospectively analyzed 26 patients undergoing simultaneous acute ORIF and THA (N = 12) versus delayed THA post-ORIF (N = 14). Patient age was significantly higher in the ORIF and acute THA group (81 vs 76 years); however, Charlson Comorbidity Index, mechanism of injury, and fracture pattern did not differ between groups. Their results demonstrated that surgical time and length of stay were not different for the 2 groups (ORIF vs ORIF and THA).[44] The Oxford Hip Score (OHS) was significantly higher in the acute ORIF and THA group compared with the ORIF delayed THA group.[44] There was no difference in complication or reoperation rate between groups.

Prostheses and Implant Survivorship

Fixation constructs in acute simultaneous ORIF and THA can include plates and screws, closed reduction and percutaneous column screw fixation, and less commonly cable reconstruction.[10,43,45,46,51–53] The aim of ORIF in the setting of simultaneous acute THA is to restore stability of the acetabular columns and facilitate placement of a stable acetabular component as close to the native center of rotation as possible, while maintaining stability within physiologic range of motion.[14,40,43]

A variety of strategies have been used for immediate fixation of the acetabular component. These include cup-cage constructs with cemented liners, antiprotrusio cage with cemented dual mobility constructs, reinforcement rings, jumbo/screw-in coned cups, and press-fit revision components with tripolar screw fixation[3,40,42–44,54] (Fig. 6).

McMahon and Cusick[55] reported on a coned acetabular component, which allowed for stable fixation and early weight bearing in 6 cases of complex bicolumnar elderly AFs with a mean age of 75. A hemispherical multihole cup is attached to a partially hydroxyapatite coated pedestal, which bypasses the fracture, allowing fixation into the sciatic buttress. The cup allows

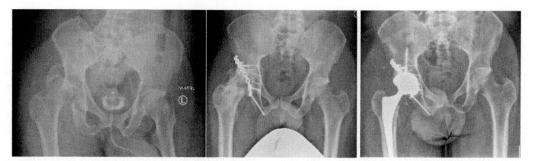

Fig. 5. A 44-year-old man who sustained a fracture dislocation of his right hip following a motor vehicle accident. (Left) The posterior wall fracture initially was treated with ORIF via a Kocher-Langenbeck approach. He subsequently went on to develop PTA and substantial HO. (Middle) At 18 months after the index injury he underwent débridement of HO, sciatic nerve neurolysis, and salvage THA using uncemented components and a dual mobility construct (Right).

for multipolar supplementary screw fixation and subsequent cemented cup/liner insertion. At 15 months, they reported no serious complications with 4 of 5 patients able to mobilize independently with a walking aid. Weight bearing was commenced on postoperative day 1 in 5 of the 6 cases.[55]

A systematic review by Makridis and colleagues[11] comparing acute THA and delayed THA reported that the acute THA group showed a cumulative revision rate of 7.5% for acetabular components and 4.6% for stems. Indications for revision in the acute group were dislocation in 46.1%, aseptic loosening in 38.5%, and infection in 15.4%. The delayed THA group had a cumulative revision rate of 9.6% for acetabular components and 8.2% for femoral stems. Indications for revision of uncemented cups in the delayed group was aseptic loosening in 88% and infection in 12%. Among revisions of cemented cups, 89% were indicated for aseptic loosening,

whereas dislocation and deep infection accounted for 5.3% each. The indication for revision of the femoral stem was aseptic loosening in 87% of cases.[11] The role of cemented cups in the setting of an acute fracture and the possibility of cement interdigitating the fracture site have yet to be elucidated.[56]

Kaplan-Meier survivorship analysis for loosening, osteolysis, and revision demonstrated a 10-year survival of 95% for the stems and 81% for the acetabular components in the acute THA group. In contrast, survivorship in the delayed THA group had an 85% survival rate of the stems and 76% survival rate of the acetabular components.[11]

Compared with THA for OA or AVN, delayed THA for PTA demonstrates significantly decreased implant survivorship.[57,58] It has been reported there is little difference in the revision rate of delayed THA where the index management of the AFs was nonoperative versus

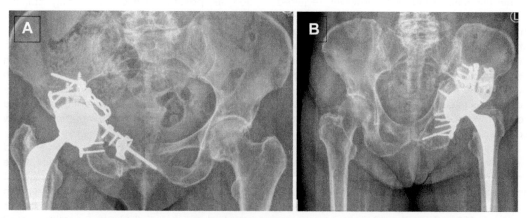

Fig. 6. Multiple acetabular fixation strategies for ORIF and acute THA, including (A) revision acetabular component with multiplanar screw fixation in addition to newer specific pelvic quadrilateral surface plates (to minimize medialization) and (B) cup-cage constructs with cemented liner.

ORIF.[57] Older studies have demonstrated that cemented components utilized for PTA had a 14% revision rate with 53% showing radiographic evidence of loosening.[59,60] Bellabarba and colleagues[49] showed that in delayed THA, survivorship for press fit components was 97% at 10 years, with 90% of patients reporting good or excellent outcomes.

Complications

A systematic review by Daurka and colleagues[10] compared ORIF with combined ORIF and THA. They found that surgical time was slightly less in the simultaneous ORIF and THA versus ORIF alone (208.6 vs 232.8 minutes, respectively); however, estimated blood loss was nearly double in the ORIF and THA group (1187.7 mL vs 664.2 mL, respectively).[10] Jauregui and colleagues[12] reported similar results. Herscovici and colleagues[45] reported on a series of 22 patients undergoing simultaneous ORIF and acute THA and have shown that those fracture patterns amenable to fixation and arthroplasty through a single approach demonstrate significantly less blood loss and lower transfusion rate than those where a dual approach was required. Delayed THA, especially after index ORIF, is associated with a higher rate of transfusion and longer surgical times compared with ORIF alone.[49,59]

Jauregui and colleagues[12] reported a 20% complication rate in 430 patients undergoing acute ORIF and THA in a systematic review of 21 studies. The most common complication was HO, with a prevalence rate of 19.5%; however, clinically significant Brooker class III and grade IV comprised only 6.8%. They reported a dislocation rate of 6.1%, deep venous thromboembolism rate of 4.1%, deep surgical site infection rate of 3.8%, neurologic complication rate of 1.9%, and revision rate of 4.3% at a mean of 44 months' follow-up.[12]

Makridis and colleagues[11] reported on the overall complication rates among 625 patients undergoing THA, either acute or delayed (acute defined as surgery within 4 weeks of fracture). The reported rates of HO were 30%, which was not significantly different between the acute THA and late THA groups.[11] Similarly, Sermon and colleagues,[3] who directly compared acute THA and delayed THA, reported an HO rate of 28% in the acute group and 41% in the delayed group. As expected, cumulative complications rates, including deep surgical site infection 2.1%, dislocation 4.4%, and nerve injury in 2.1%, all were higher than a primary THA for elective OA.[11] They reported an overall mortality rate of 5%.[11]

Patient-reported Outcome Measures

In their systematic review, Makridis and colleagues[11] demonstrated a mean HHS of 88, with 81% of patients reporting good to excellent results for their entire cohort of patients undergoing THA, both acute and delayed, after an AF. They did not separately report short-term patient-reported outcome measures (PROMs) or long-term PROMs.[11] Lin and colleagues[43] reported on 33 AFs treated with simultaneous ORIF and acute THA. In their case series with an average age of 66 years, 93% reported having good to excellent function at an average of 67 months' follow-up. They reported a 94% implant survival rate.[43] Jauregui and colleagues[12] performed a meta-analysis on 430 patients undergoing acute THA for AFs and the mean weighted HHS was 83.3 postoperatively.

Mears and Velyvis[41] reported on 57 patients undergoing simultaneous ORIF and acute THA with an average age of 69 and mean follow-up of 8.1 years. Their cohort of patients reported 79% good to excellent HHS which was inversely proportional to age, with a mean HHS of 87 in the eighth decade of life but only 75 in the ninth decade of life. The revision rate was higher in the younger group.[41] Sermon and colleagues[3] demonstrated a statistically significant difference in the mean HHS with good to excellent scores reported in 76% of patients undergoing delayed THA versus only 58% in the acute group despite a higher revision rate in the delayed THA group. The mean age in the acute group, however, was 25 years older than in the delayed THA group.

Nicol and colleagues[44] directly compared acute ORIF with acute THA and found a significantly better OHS score compared with delayed THA (40.1 vs 33.5, respectively).[44] They reported no difference in independent mobility status between groups; however, 4 of the 12 patients in the acute THA group and 3 of the 14 patients in the delayed THA group did not return to their baseline functional status.[44]

Tidermark and colleagues[61] reported on postoperative mobility, with a series of 10 patients who underwent acute ORIF and THA using an antiprotrusio cage and autologous femoral head bone grafting. All 10 patients mobilized independently at a mean follow-up of 38 months, with only 30% requiring a gait aid. Mears and Velyvis[42] demonstrated that 68% of patients walked normally, with 23% able to mobilize long distance using a single cane after acute ORIF and THA. Of their series, 9% of patients were unable to mobilize even with the use of a gait aid.[42]

Both Bellabarba and colleagues[49] and Ranawat and colleagues[50] demonstrated excellent PROMs in patients undergoing delayed THA for PTA following AF. Ranawat and colleagues[50] showed an average improvement in HHS from 28 to 82 post–delayed THA, with 81% of patients reporting good to excellent results. Similarly, Bellabarba and colleagues[49] indicated that 90% of patients achieved similar HHS scores, with a mean score of 88, following delayed THA at a follow-up range of 24 months to 140 months.

SUMMARY

Although the incidence of AFs in the elderly is on the rise, the optimal management of such fractures remains uncertain.[9] Given the complexity and multifactorial considerations, which influence management of AFs in the elderly, it is clear these injuries should be managed by surgeons with skills in both orthopedic trauma and reconstruction with a multidisciplinary approach to maximize patient outcomes and lower complications.[9,10,14]

Nonoperative management of AF is reserved for specific cases of fracture pattern, pre-morbid immobility and high risk acute or chronic medical conditions that preclude exposing patients to the considerable stress of an operative intervention.[10,11,25,32] ORIF remains a mainstay of treatment; however, several features specific to the elderly predispose patients to failure of ORIF and a high conversion rate to salvage THA.[11,16,41] Specific indications for acute THA as treatment of AF have been recognized.[16,41] These include preexisting OA, osteoporosis, fracture comminution and non-reconstructible fracture patterns, increased age, chondral injuries to the femoral head, and ipsilateral femoral head and neck fractures.[11,16,41] THA also may allow for earlier weight bearing, which is particularly important in the frail patient. In the absence of these factors, ORIF is a reasonable management option; however, it can carry an approximately 40% perioperative/postoperative complication rate.[10,18,20,41,62]

THA in the setting of AF is technically demanding. These challenges vary based on the timing of arthroplasty (acute vs delayed) and index treatment. When comparing acute THA and delayed THA, there is an increased revision rate in the delayed THA group.[3,11] Studies where cemented acetabular components were used showed considerable rates of radiographic loosening and component revision.[11,59,60,63] More recent data, using highly porous press fit acetabular components in delayed THA, have shown promising survivorship, which is comparable with acute THA.[11,44,49,50]

When compared with THA for OA, THA in the management of AF is associated with an increased rate of HO, dislocation, infection, neurovascular damage, and revision rates.[11,12,57] Irrespective of timing, a majority of patients treated with THA for AF report good to excellent PROMs and many can achieve independent mobility.[3,11,44,49,50]

There is a paucity of high-level prospective randomized evidence on the management of AFs in the elderly. Most studies are level III or level IV evidence, consisting mainly of retrospective cohort studies or case series.[11,12,14,26] Future research should focus on prospective randomized controlled studies to further elucidate the optimal management of AFs in the elderly patient population.

CLINICS CARE POINTS

- Incidence of AFs in the elderly is increasing, with a majority involving the anterior column.
- The goal of surgical intervention is to facilitate early mobilization and maintain functional independence.
- Nonoperative management is reserved for minimally displaced fracture patterns and/or secondary congruence and for medically unwell patients.
- ORIF is an acceptable treatment in fracture patterns with adequate bone stock in the absence of instability, osteochondral impaction injury to the femoral head and/or weight-bearing dome, and preexisting OA.
- Arthroplasty in the setting of AF is technically demanding, with a higher complication rate compared with primary THA for elective OA.
- Both acute THA and delayed THA can result in improved PROM scores and maintenance of independent mobility.
- Use of uncemented press fit acetabular components is associated with superior outcomes in both acute THA and delayed THA.
- Acute THA allows for early mobilization without restricted weight bearing but is complex surgery and best performed by a specialist with skill in both orthopedic traumatology and complex hip reconstruction.

DISCLOSURE

The authors have nothing to disclose.

REFERENCES

1. Cahueque M, Martinez M, Cobar A, et al. Early reduction of acetabular fractures decreases the risk of post-traumatic hip osteoarthritis? J Clin Orthop Trauma 2017;8(4):320–6.
2. Matta JM. Fractures of the acetabulum: accuracy of reduction and clinical results in patients managed operatively within three weeks after the injury. J Bone Joint Surg Am 1996;78(11):1632–45.
3. Sermon A, Broos P, Vanderschot P. Total hip replacement for acetabular fractures. Results in 121 patients operated between 1983 and 2003. Injury 2008;39(8):914–21.
4. Letournel E. Acetabulum fractures: classification and management. J Orthop Trauma 2019;33(Suppl 2):S1–2.
5. Ferguson TA, Patel R, Bhandari M, et al. Fractures of the acetabulum in patients aged 60 years and older: an epidemiological and radiological study. J Bone Joint Surg Br 2010;92(2):250–7.
6. Best MJ, Buller LT, Quinnan SM. Analysis of incidence and outcome predictors for patients admitted to US hospitals with acetabular fractures from 1990 to 2010. Am J Orthop (Belle Mead NJ) 2018;47(9).
7. Mears DC. Surgical treatment of acetabular fractures in elderly patients with osteoporotic bone. J Am Acad Orthop Surg 1999;7(2):128–41.
8. Mardian S, Rau D, Hinz P, et al. Acetabular fractures in an advanced age - current knowledge and treatment options. Acta Chir Orthop Traumatol Cech 2017;84(4):241–6.
9. Manson TT, Reider L, O'Toole RV, et al. Variation in treatment of displaced geriatric acetabular fractures among 15 level-I trauma centers. J Orthop Trauma 2016;30(9):457–62.
10. Daurka JS, Pastides PS, Lewis A, et al. Acetabular fractures in patients aged > 55 years: a systematic review of the literature. Bone Joint J 2014;96-B(2):157–63.
11. Makridis KG, Obakponowwe O, Bobak P, et al. Total hip arthroplasty after acetabular fracture: incidence of complications, reoperation rates and functional outcomes: evidence today. J Arthroplasty 2014;29(10):1983–90.
12. Jauregui JJ, Weir TB, Chen JF, et al. Acute total hip arthroplasty for older patients with acetabular fractures: a meta-analysis. J Clin Orthop Trauma 2020;11(6):976–82.
13. Boelch SP, Jordan MC, Meffert RH, et al. Comparison of open reduction and internal fixation and primary total hip replacement for osteoporotic acetabular fractures: a retrospective clinical study. Int Orthop 2017;41(9):1831–7.
14. Antell NB, Switzer JA, Schmidt AH. Management of acetabular fractures in the elderly. J Am Acad Orthop Surg 2017;25(8):577–85.
15. Henry PDG, Si-Hyeong Park S, Paterson JM, et al. Risk of hip arthroplasty after open reduction internal fixation of a fracture of the acetabulum: a matched cohort study. J Orthop Trauma 2018;32(3):134–40.
16. Tannast M, Najibi S, Matta JM. Two to twenty-year survivorship of the hip in 810 patients with operatively treated acetabular fractures. J Bone Joint Surg Am 2012;94(17):1559–67.
17. Mears DC, Velyvis JH, Chang CP. Displaced acetabular fractures managed operatively: indicators of outcome. Clin Orthop Relat Res 2003;407:173–86.
18. Bible JE, Wegner A, McClure DJ, et al. One-year mortality after acetabular fractures in elderly patients presenting to a level-1 trauma center. J Orthop Trauma 2014;28(3):154–9.
19. Khoshbin A, Atrey A, Chaudhry H, et al. Mortality rate of geriatric acetabular fractures is high compared with hip fractures. a matched cohort study. J Orthop Trauma 2020;34(8):424–8.
20. O'Toole RV, Hui E, Chandra A, et al. How often does open reduction and internal fixation of geriatric acetabular fractures lead to hip arthroplasty? J Orthop Trauma 2014;28(3):148–53.
21. Firoozabadi R, Cross WW, Krieg JC, et al. Acetabular fractures in the senior population- epidemiology, mortality and treatments. Arch Bone Jt Surg 2017;5(2):96–102.
22. Matta JM, Anderson LM, Epstein HC, et al. Fractures of the acetabulum. A retrospective analysis. Clin Orthop Relat Res 1986;(205):230–40.
23. Kammerlander C, Pfeufer D, Lisitano LA, et al. Inability of older adult patients with hip fracture to maintain postoperative weight-bearing restrictions. J Bone Joint Surg Am 2018;100(11):936–41.
24. Jain R, Basinski A, Kreder HJ. Nonoperative treatment of hip fractures. Int Orthop 2003;27(1):11–7.
25. Tornetta P 3rd. Displaced acetabular fractures: indications for operative and nonoperative management. J Am Acad Orthop Surg 2001;9(1):18–28.
26. Jauregui JJ, Clayton A, Kapadia BH, et al. Total hip arthroplasty for acute acetabular fractures: a review of the literature. Expert Rev Med Devices 2015;12(3):287–95.
27. Spencer RF. Acetabular fractures in older patients. J Bone Joint Surg Br 1989;71(5):774–6.
28. Peter RE. Open reduction and internal fixation of osteoporotic acetabular fractures through the ilioinguinal approach: use of buttress plates to control medial displacement of the quadrilateral surface. Injury 2015;46(Suppl 1):S2–7.

29. Baker G, McMahon SE, Warnock M, et al. Outcomes of conservatively managed complex acetabular fractures in the frail and elderly one year post injury. Injury 2020;51(2):347–51.

30. Ryan SP, Manson TT, Sciadini MF, et al. Functional outcomes of elderly patients with nonoperatively treated acetabular fractures that meet operative criteria. J Orthop Trauma 2017;31(12):644–9.

31. Walley KC, Appleton PT, Rodriguez EK. Comparison of outcomes of operative versus non-operative treatment of acetabular fractures in the elderly and severely comorbid patient. Eur J Orthop Surg Traumatol 2017;27(5):689–94.

32. Capone A, Peri M, Mastio M. Surgical treatment of acetabular fractures in the elderly: a systematic review of the results. EFORT Open Rev 2017;2(4):97–103.

33. Verbeek DO, van der List JP, Tissue CM, et al. Long-term patient reported outcomes following acetabular fracture fixation. Injury 2018;49(6):1131–6.

34. Starr AJ, Jones AL, Reinert CM, et al. Preliminary results and complications following limited open reduction and percutaneous screw fixation of displaced fractures of the acetabulum. Injury 2001;32(Suppl 1):SA45–50.

35. Gary JL, Lefaivre KA, Gerold F, et al. Survivorship of the native hip joint after percutaneous repair of acetabular fractures in the elderly. Injury 2011;42(10):1144–51.

36. Boudissa M, Francony F, Drevet S, et al. Operative versus non-operative treatment of displaced acetabular fractures in elderly patients. Aging Clin Exp Res 2020;32(4):571–7.

37. Navarre P, Gabbe BJ, Griffin XL, et al. Outcomes following operatively managed acetabular fractures in patients aged 60 years and older. Bone Joint J 2020;102-B(12):1735–42.

38. Anglen JO, Burd TA, Hendricks KJ, et al. The "Gull Sign": a harbinger of failure for internal fixation of geriatric acetabular fractures. J Orthop Trauma 2003;17(9):625–34.

39. Kreder HJ, Rozen N, Borkhoff CM, et al. Determinants of functional outcome after simple and complex acetabular fractures involving the posterior wall. J Bone Joint Surg Br 2006;88(6):776–82.

40. Butterwick D, Papp S, Gofton W, et al. Acetabular fractures in the elderly: evaluation and management. J Bone Joint Surg Am 2015;97(9):758–68.

41. Mears DC, Velyvis JH. Acute total hip arthroplasty for selected displaced acetabular fractures: two to twelve-year results. J Bone Joint Surg Am 2002;84(1):1–9.

42. Mears DC, Velyvis JH. Primary total hip arthroplasty after acetabular fracture. Instr Course Lect 2001;50:335–54.

43. Lin C, Caron J, Schmidt AH, et al. Functional outcomes after total hip arthroplasty for the acute management of acetabular fractures: 1- to 14-year follow-up. J Orthop Trauma 2015;29(3):151–9.

44. Nicol GM, Sanders EB, Kim PR, et al. Outcomes of total hip arthroplasty after acetabular open reduction and internal fixation in the elderly-acute vs delayed total hip arthroplasty. J Arthroplasty 2021;36(2):605–11.

45. Herscovici D Jr, Lindvall E, Bolhofner B, et al. The combined hip procedure: open reduction internal fixation combined with total hip arthroplasty for the management of acetabular fractures in the elderly. J Orthop Trauma 2010;24(5):291–6.

46. Rickman M, Young J, Bircher M, et al. The management of complex acetabular fractures in the elderly with fracture fixation and primary total hip replacement. Eur J Trauma Emerg Surg 2012;38(5):511–6.

47. Khurana S, Nobel TB, Merkow JS, et al. Total hip arthroplasty for posttraumatic osteoarthritis of the hip fares worse than THA for primary osteoarthritis. Am J Orthop (Belle Mead NJ) 2015;44(7):321–5.

48. Hamlin K, Lazaraviciute G, Koullouros M, et al. Should total hip arthroplasty be performed acutely in the treatment of acetabular fractures in elderly or used as a salvage procedure only? Indian J Orthop 2017;51(4):421–33.

49. Bellabarba C, Berger RA, Bentley CD, et al. Cementless acetabular reconstruction after acetabular fracture. J Bone Joint Surg Am 2001;83(6):868–76.

50. Ranawat A, Zelken J, Helfet D, et al. Total hip arthroplasty for posttraumatic arthritis after acetabular fracture. J Arthroplasty 2009;24(5):759–67.

51. Mouhsine E, Garofalo R, Borens O, et al. Cable fixation and early total hip arthroplasty in the treatment of acetabular fractures in elderly patients. J Arthroplasty 2004;19(3):344–8.

52. Borens O, Wettstein M, Garofalo R, et al. [Treatment of acetabular fractures in the elderly with primary total hip arthroplasty and modified cerclage. Early results]. Unfallchirurgie 2004;107(11):1050–6.

53. Mears DC, Shirahama M. Stabilization of an acetabular fracture with cables for acute total hip arthroplasty. J Arthroplasty 1998;13(1):104–7.

54. Beaule PE, Griffin DB, Matta JM. The Levine anterior approach for total hip replacement as the treatment for an acute acetabular fracture. J Orthop Trauma 2004;18(9):623–9.

55. McMahon SE, Cusick LA. Total hip replacement in complex acetabular fractures using a coned hemipelvic acetabular component. Eur J Orthop Surg Traumatol 2017;27(5):631–6.

56. Larsson S. Cement augmentation in fracture treatment. Scand J Surg 2006;95(2):111–8.

57. Morison Z, Moojen DJ, Nauth A, et al. Total hip arthroplasty after acetabular fracture is associated with lower survivorship and more complications. Clin Orthop Relat Res 2016;474(2):392–8.

58. Weaver MJ, Smith RM, Lhowe DW, et al. Does total hip arthroplasty reduce the risk of secondary surgery following the treatment of displaced acetabular fractures in the elderly compared to open reduction internal fixation? a pilot study. J Orthop Trauma 2018;32(Suppl 1):S40–5.

59. Weber M, Berry DJ, Harmsen WS. Total hip arthroplasty after operative treatment of an acetabular fracture. J Bone Joint Surg Am 1998;80(9):1295–305.

60. Romness DW, Lewallen DG. Total hip arthroplasty after fracture of the acetabulum. Long-term results. J Bone Joint Surg Br 1990;72(5):761–4.

61. Tidermark J, Blomfeldt R, Ponzer S, et al. Primary total hip arthroplasty with a Burch-Schneider antiprotrusion cage and autologous bone grafting for acetabular fractures in elderly patients. J Orthop Trauma 2003;17(3):193–7.

62. Jimenez ML, Tile M, Schenk RS. Total hip replacement after acetabular fracture. Orthop Clin North Am 1997;28(3):435–46.

63. von Roth P, Abdel MP, Harmsen WS, et al. Total hip arthroplasty after operatively treated acetabular fracture: a concise follow-up, at a mean of twenty years, of a previous report. J Bone Joint Surg Am 2015;97(4):288–91.

64. Stoppa RE. The treatment of complicated groin and incisional hernias. World J Surg 1989;13(5):545–54.

Treatment of B1 Distal Periprosthetic Femur Fractures

Gerard A. Sheridan, MD, FRCSI[a],*,
Aresh Sepehri, MD, MSc[a], Karl Stoffel, MD, PhD, FRACS[b],
Bassam A. Masri, MD, FRCSC[a]

KEYWORDS

- Periprosthetic fracture • Supracondylar fracture • Distal femur fracture • TKA • Vancouver B1
- Locking plate • IM nail • Distal femoral replacement

KEY POINTS

- The burden of periprosthetic distal femoral fractures is likely to increase accordingly with the increase in total knee arthroplasties (TKAs) globally in the future.
- Less invasive approaches for plating confer higher healing rates and reduced operative times when compared with open procedures.
- There is no clear consensus as to whether locking plates or nails are superior but the largest recent study comparing both methods demonstrate a significantly lower risk of complication and revision surgery with plating.
- Distal femoral replacement has comparable financial implications and is associated with lower revision rates when compared with open reduction internal fixation for B1 distal femoral periprosthetic fractures.
- Distal femoral replacement should only be performed by a specialist knee arthroplasty surgeon in order to avoid issues of patellar maltracking and femoral component malposition.

INTRODUCTION

Definition

Periprosthetic fractures of the distal femur around total knee arthroplasty (TKA) components have been classified and defined in numerous ways in the past.[1–3] The Rorabeck and Su classifications are in common use for distal femoral periprosthetic fractures. However, perhaps the most influential classification system to describe periprosthetic fractures in the modern orthopedic literature has been the Vancouver classification by Duncan and Masri in relation to periprosthetic fractures around total hip arthroplasty (THA) implants.[4] An expansion of this original classification uses the same nomenclature as the 1995 classification but has applied this now to all periprosthetic fractures, including periprosthetic fractures around TKA, in what is now known as the Unified Classification System.[5]

For the purposes of this review, the authors describe the treatment options available for B1 distal femur periprosthetic fractures around a TKA implant. B type fractures involve bone stock supporting or adjacent to an implant. B1 subtypes are B type fractures with a well-fixed implant.

Epidemiology, Incidence, and Risk

Epidemiology and incidence

Fractures of the native distal femur are known to have a bimodal distribution of age at the time of

---

[a] Department of Orthopaedics, University of British Columbia, Vancouver, British Columbia, Canada;
[b] Department of Orthopaedics and Traumatology, University Hospital Basel, Gellertstrasse 144, 4052 Basel, Switzerland
* Corresponding author.
E-mail address: sheridga@tcd.ie

Orthop Clin N Am 52 (2021) 335–346
https://doi.org/10.1016/j.ocl.2021.05.001
0030-5898/21/© 2021 Elsevier Inc. All rights reserved.

occurrence.[6] Traditionally this injury of the native femur has been associated with either high-energy sporting injuries in younger men or low-energy falls from a standing height in elderly women.[7] The epidemiologic features of periprosthetic distal femur fractures differ in that they do not involve the young male cohort associated with sporting injuries; this increases the mean age from the seventh decade of life to the nineth decade of life.[8] A study from Denmark in 2018 reported that the prevalence of distal femoral periprosthetic fractures was 2.4/100,000 per year,[9] which is a fraction of the prevalence of native distal femur fractures, which was reported as 8.7/100,000 per year in this same study. Projection models for TKA volumes globally confirm an anticipated increase in the numbers of TKAs performed in the future. With the global burden of TKA on a steady incline, one can expect the burden of periprosthetic distal femoral fractures to increase accordingly.[10]

Risk

Technical surgical errors, such as femoral notching, were thought to predispose to the development of these fracture types. Initial biomechanical analyses in cadaveric femora found that torsional load to failure was significantly reduced for femora that were notched anteriorly due to suboptimal positioned anterior cuts.[11] Subsequent clinical studies investigating 1289 TKAs concluded that there was in fact no relationship between anterior femoral notching and periprosthetic fracture development.[12,13] Other known risk factors for periprosthetic fracture development include increasing age, osteoporosis, diabetes, and malpositioned implants.[14]

The clinical sequelae of this injury are significant. Jennison and colleagues reviewed 60 distal femoral periprosthetic fractures up to 2 years follow-up and confirmed a 20% complication rate requiring revision surgery.[8] The mortality rate at 30 days was reported at 3.3%, which increased to a rate of 13.3% within 1 year following fracture. This specific cohort of patients with periprosthetic fractures seems to be significantly more vulnerable than patients presenting with similar injuries to the native femur, consistent with the substantially older age group of patients.

Guidelines

The Arbeitsgemeinschaft für Osteosynthesefragen guidance for the management of a periprosthetic fracture in the distal femur with a stable implant and good bone stock consists of internal fixation.[15] This guidance also recommends assessment of the TKA components to ensure that they are correctly positioned and sized before excluding revision arthroplasty as the treatment of choice. It is acknowledged that there may be difficulty in definitively deciding whether the implants are stable or not based on standard radiographic imaging. It may be the case that implant stability may only truly be confirmed intraoperatively or with higher order imaging such as computed tomography (Figs. 1 and 2).

DISCUSSION

Nonoperative Management

Nonoperative management for the treatment of B1 distal femoral periprosthetic fractures was used historically in common practice. Some early studies demonstrated superior mechanical alignment with nonoperative intervention when compared with operative intervention,[16] and this was in the era of internal fixation implants that did not afford much fixation into the distal femur distal to the fracture. This approach has since been superseded by operative intervention, due to the superiority of current internal fixation implants, and only has a limited role in modern practice for some clinical settings where nonoperative options may be appropriate (eg, extreme comorbidity or nonconsenting adult with capacity).

Plating

Biomechanics

Traditional management of these fractures included osteosynthesis with nonlocking plates through a large open approach with extensive periosteal stripping. With the introduction of fixed-angle locking plates, the problem of osteoporotic bone was addressed, and this new improved technology provided superior mechanical stability within the construct, which then conferred superior clinical outcomes in terms of healing and early functionality with an ability for immediate weight-bearing.[17] It is widely accepted that locking screws are the preferred method of fixation in the distal metaphyseal portion of the fixation construct.

Other biomechanical considerations arise in relation to the configuration of screws and cerclage cables used in the diaphyseal segment of the fixation construct. Hoffmann and colleagues set out to analyze 3 possible diaphyseal fixation configurations in synthetic femora for periprosthetic THA.[18] These results supported the use of bicortical screw fixation, as this achieved the highest load to failure and the highest torsional/sagittal bending stiffness in the diaphysis. Although no biomechanical studies have

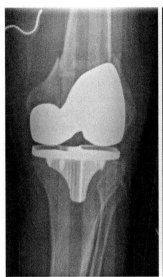
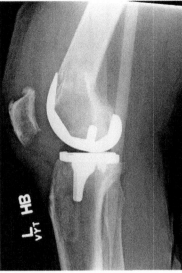

Fig. 1. Distal femoral periprosthetic fracture—implant appeared stable on radiographs.

assessed the optimal diaphyseal fixation in periprosthetic TKA fractures, it may be reasonable to consider bicortical screw fixation based on this study.

Biology

Biologically orientated improvements were also noted with the invention of the Less Invasive Skeletal Stabilization (LISS) plate. The concept underpinning the LISS plate was tissue preservation involving indirect reduction, preservation of the periosteum, and percutaneous screw insertion. Although more technically demanding, early reports demonstrated low infection rates and overall superiority over traditional plating methods with this less invasive approach.[19,20]

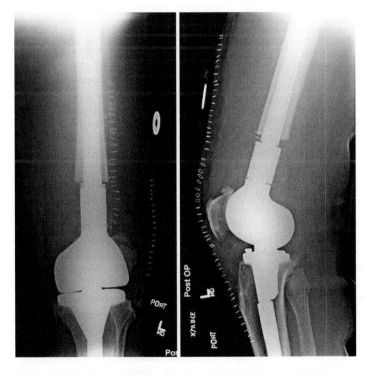

Fig. 2. Implant deemed loose on intraoperative inspection—distal femoral resection performed.

An early appreciation for soft tissue preservation when approaching these injuries led to excellent healing rates. From a cohort of 24 periprosthetic fractures around a well-fixed TKA implant, Ricci and colleagues demonstrated an 86% healing rate after initial treatment using minimally invasive plate insertion techniques.[17] Of the 3 patients who did not heal, 2 were infected and only 1 progressed to an aseptic nonunion. Of these 3 cases, all were obese and diabetic. More recent evidence by Hess and colleagues compared open techniques with less invasive techniques for approaching distal femoral periprosthetic fractures.[21] From a cohort of 46 fractures, less invasive approaches conferred a healing rate of 100% compared with a healing rate of 86% with open procedures. A significant reduction in operative time from 120 minutes in the open group to 73 minutes in the less invasive group was also reported. The approach to these fractures is evidently important, and the use of a submuscular approach with soft tissue preservation techniques has been shown to be positively associated with union rates in this cohort.[22]

Double plating

Double plating, or dual plating, techniques involve the stabilization of both medial and lateral cortices of the femur. The rationale behind this change in practice stemmed from the commonly observed failure of distal fixation with progression to a varus deformity and medial displacement of the distal fragment with pull-out of the locking screws from bone while remaining attached to the plate when a single lateral locking plate was used in certain fractures of the distal femur. This approach is more technically demanding, and numerous descriptive surgical techniques have been published recently.[23,24] The technique described by Beeres involves a supine position with bilateral limb draping, which allows contralateral intraoperative limb comparison. The knee is held in flexion to reduce the distal fragment, and a minimally invasive lateral approach is used to achieve reduction and fixation of the fracture fragments. Length, rotation, and alignment can be secured while referencing the normal limb, and the investigator recommends that the plate extends above the implant by at least 2 femoral diameters in order to reduce the risk of any stress riser formation. The medial plate is precontoured and then introduced in a submuscular epiperiosteal fashion using a subvastus approach; this is then fixed with bicortical locking screws, and unrestricted weight-bearing with crutches or a walker

is then allowed immediately. No loss of fixation or implant failure was seen in any of these patients at minimum 2-year follow-up.[23]

There are important anatomic considerations when implanting a medial plate. The femoral artery and profunda femoris may be injured if careful consideration of the local anatomy is not given. Kim and colleagues performed a radiological study to identify the safe zone of medial plate insertion in order to avoid injuring local vascular structures.[25] Thirty patients underwent computed tomography angiography, and it was concluded that there is a safe optimum position for minimally invasive medial plate insertion in distal femoral fractures. The anteromedial aspect of the distal half of the femur is the safe zone. A long medial plate can be positioned safely in this zone at the anterior aspect of the distal femur up to the level of 8 cm below the lesser trochanter, but this is almost never necessary, as a short plate medially will suffice. The use of a medial plate was found to induce minimal additional devascularization in the distal femur when added to a lateral plate construct.[26]

The reported clinical outcomes for this new fixation method are very promising. Park and colleagues report on a cohort of 21 Su type 3 periprosthetic fractures treated with this double-plating technique.[27] Twenty achieved union at an average of 14 weeks postoperatively, knee joint motion was comparable to the contralateral limb, and daily functioning returned to the premorbid status. Importantly, Park and colleagues also analyzed the postoperative mechanical lateral distal femoral angle (average 89°) and the mechanical posterior distal femoral angle (86°). These findings are very promising in support of double plating and its ability to maintain mechanical alignment, prevent distal fixation failure, and avoid mechanical failure in varus.

A recent systematic review analyzed 436 double platings in comparison to 64 single platings and 84 intramedullary (IM) nails.[28] Union rates achieved were 88.5% when double plating was used for periprosthetic fracture fixation. When compared with IM nails, double plating was associated with less hemorrhage, shorter surgery time, and reduced risk of malunion in polytraumatized patients. There was no significant difference in outcome when compared with single plating however. In our experience, distal femoral fractures with an obliquity medial superior to distal lateral have a tendency to displace and are best treated with double plating (**Fig. 3**). Medial comminution, severe osteoporosis, and revision surgery are also indications where double plating should be considered (**Fig. 4**).

Intramedullary Nailing

The use of retrograde nailing in the treatment of periprosthetic fractures showed good outcomes in early reports of small case series.[29] Contraindications include a closed box design of the femoral component, an intercondylar distance that is less than the IM nail diameter and an inability to flex the knee beyond 40° in order to gain access for the IM nail entry point.[30] The advantages of using an IM nail include smaller incisions, preservation of periosteal structures and associated vascular structures, and the ability to immediately weight-bear on the prosthesis. One of the main disadvantages of nails compared with plates include the need to navigate the nail past the femoral component of the TKA implant. Specifically, the femoral component may force a more posterior start point, resulting in an extension deformity, or depending on the lateral medial location of the femoral component, the entry point may force the nail into a more valgus position for the final construct.[31]

Technical implant compatibility considerations

Many investigators have given consideration to this issue. Service and colleagues developed the starting point ratio and a manufacturer-specific femoral component ratio that enabled the investigators to determine which specific TKA implants were at risk of an IM nail entry point posterior to Blumensaat line.[32] This study concluded that cruciate-retaining femoral component designs are at significantly higher risk of posterior IM nail entry points compared with posterior stabilized (PS) designs. **Figs. 5** and **6** illustrate a B1 fracture managed with an IM nail inserted using a posterior entry point, which leads to an extended distal fragment with a recurvatum malunion deformity of the femur in the sagittal plane. In 2016, Jones and colleagues designed a compatibility table detailing which TKA implants were compatible with which IM nail designs.[33] The only implant that was truly compatible with the 4 commonest IM nail implant types was the Biomet AGC Cruciate Retaining and Posterior Stabilized (PS) TKA designs, but these are old implants that are no longer in common use. All other implants required excess force for insertion, induced femoral component scratching, or required an entry point that was too posterior for optimal nail positioning. In order to circumvent the issue of IM nail entry, especially for PS TKA designs,

some investigators have described a technique of arthroscopically assisted retrograde IM nail insertion.[34] This technique has not transferred into contemporary orthopedic practice yet. Of note, in a case series of 30 patients with a minimum 10° hyperextension malunion following retrograde IM nail for B1 periprosthetic femur fracture, there were no significant deficits in functional outcomes measured by the Knee Society Score.[35]

Another consideration before IM nail fixation is the amount of bone stock available for stable distal interlocking fixation through the nail. The Su classification was developed to guide preoperative planning for periprosthetic femur fractures.[1] Su type 1 fractures, where the fracture line is proximal to the femoral component, are amenable to IM nailing. In Su type 2, where the fracture line originates at the proximal implant and extends proximally, IM nail should be used with caution. In these cases, IM nails that can accommodate multiplanar locking screws, or angular stable interlocking devices such as a spiral blade, can result in improved stability with minimal fixation points.[36] Additional stability can also be provided with the use of poller blocking screws or adding a plate construct (see "Combination nailing and plating").

Intramedullary nailing versus plating

Early biomechanical studies on synthetic femora demonstrated superior stability for retrograde IM nails under torsion and varus stress when compared with the LISS plate but the LISS plate was significantly more stable when valgus stress was applied.[37] In another biomechanical analysis of synthetic femora, 4 constructs were compared: (1) nonlocking plate; (2) polyaxial locking plate; (3) IM fibular strut allograft with polyaxial locking plate; and (4) a retrograde IM nail.[38] Results showed that IM nails were significantly less stiff than the other 3 constructs under cyclical torsional loading but had the highest axial stiffness under quasi-static axial loading to failure.

Clinical outcomes first emerged with conflicting results and no clear consensus as to the best surgical management option for these periprosthetic fractures. Hou and colleagues analyzed 34 plates and 18 IM nails for the treatment of distal femur periprosthetic fractures.[39] They found that union rates, time to union, intraoperative time, and intraoperative blood loss were comparable for both IM nails and locking plates. In 2013, Horneff and colleagues compared 35 nails with 28 locking plates for the treatment of Rorabeck

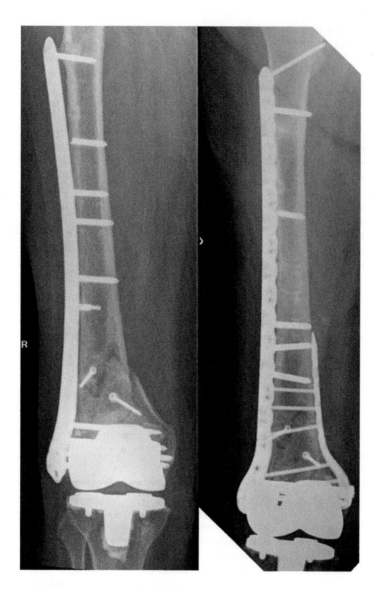

Fig. 3. Distal femoral fracture with obliquity medial superior to distal lateral—best treated with double plating.

type II distal femur periprosthetic fractures.[40] At 36 weeks postoperatively, the locking plate was reported to have superior rates of radiographic union and also had lower rates of reoperation. The locking plates did however have higher rates of perioperative transfusion when compared with the IM nails. Time to full weight-bearing was comparable for both groups in this study. In contrast, Meneghini and colleagues analyzed 29 nails and 66 locking plates, and their results confirmed a 9% nonunion rate with IM nails and a 19% nonunion rate with the locking plates[41]; this was statistically significant despite there being more screws in the distal aspect of the locking plates compared with the IM nails.

An early systematic review in 2014 analyzing 719 periprosthetic distal femur fractures concluded that locking plates and IM nails had similar radiographic rates of union and rates of revision surgery. This study does report a significantly greater risk of malunion with retrograde IM nails when compared with locking plates.[42] More recent reviews have been performed with most concluding that there are no significant differences between these 2 methods of fixation.[43,44] Shin and colleagues analyzed 8 studies comparing locking plates with retrograde IM nails for periprosthetic supracondylar femoral fractures and reported no significant difference in the rate of union or reoperation between both cohorts.[43] In a recent systematic

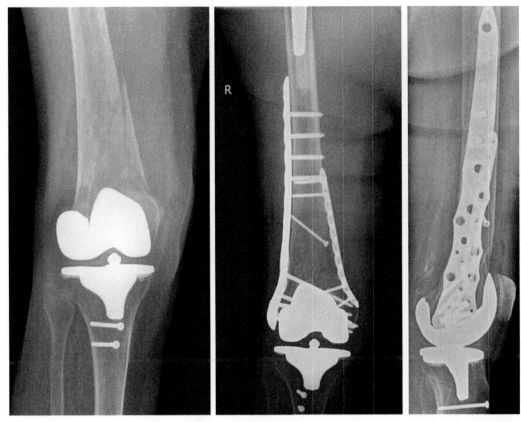

Fig. 4. Medial comminution requiring double-plating technique.

review and meta-analysis published by Magill and colleagues in 2021, 531 periprosthetic distal femoral fractures were reviewed and compared.[44] Outcomes including union rates, time to union, functional scores, and revision rates were comparable for both locking plates and IM nails. Shah and colleagues published their findings based on 1188 patients sustaining distal femoral periprosthetic fractures and reported similar union rates and time to union between the 2 groups.[45] Their findings did support the use of locking plates, as they were associated with lower risk of complication and revision surgery ($P < .003$). This study did report quicker times to full weight-bearing for the IM nails (7.6 weeks) when compared with locking plates (15.8 weeks). The differences in time to weight-bearing were not statistically significant but could be considered clinically relevant in this setting.

Alternative Techniques
Combination nailing and plating
The importance of immediate weight-bearing and early mobilization in this cohort is imperative for clinical and functional outcomes. New techniques involving concurrent plating and nailing may provide added mechanical stability, which will allow for immediate weight-bearing and superior clinical outcomes. Liporace and colleagues describe their surgical technique and rationale for this combination construct.[46] They recommend inserting a long lateral precontoured plate fixed with a linking screw distally that passes through both the plate and nail. The plate extends proximally to allow for prophylactic screw fixation of the femoral neck. A combination of bicortical diaphyseal screws and distal locking screws are used to achieve final fixation. Their results from a small cohort of 15 patients report 100% rates of healing from the 14 patients who survived to the time of review. Immediate weight-bearing was prescribed for all of these patients in the postoperative setting. Mirick Mueller describes a similar technique, using a midline incision through a lateral parapatellar approach and also recommending the "perfect circle" technique for insertion of distal locking screw through both plate and IM nail.[47] This technique uses a shorter plate and does not recommend prophylactic fixation of the femoral neck. For both techniques

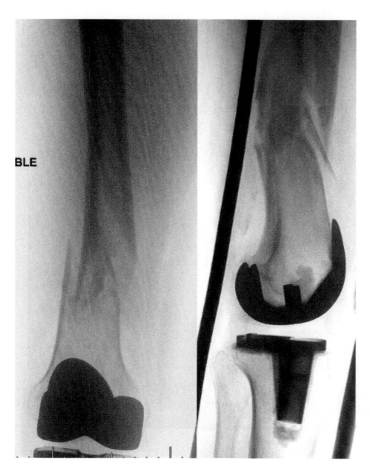

Fig. 5. B1 distal femoral periprosthetic fracture.

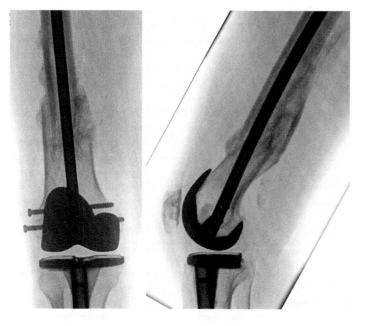

Fig. 6. Posterior entry point of IM nail resulting in distal fragment extension and a recurvatum malunion.

described, a significant disadvantage involves an increase in soft tissue trauma, prolonged operative times, increased risk of blood loss, and increased risk of infection due to increased hardware insertion.

Distal femoral replacement

Distal femoral replacement (DFR) is usually reserved for periprosthetic fractures with unstable implants.[48] For this reason, the authors have not explored this management option in extensive detail in this review. There may, however, be a role for DFR even in type B1 fractures with stable components. Darrith and colleagues analyzed 72 periprosthetic distal femoral fractures with stable components.[49] Fifty were treated with open reduction internal fixation (ORIF) and 22 with DFR. The only significant difference in outcome was related to the total revision rate, which was significantly higher in the ORIF group compared with the DFR group ($P < .001$). In the ORIF group, there were 3 revisions associated with infection and 3 for aseptic nonunion. In the DFR group there was 1 infection, 2 patellar maltrackings, and 1 femoral component malrotation requiring revision surgery. Many of the ORIF patients required subsequent revisions after their primary revision surgery, and in total there were more than twice as many revisions in the ORIF group when compared with the DFR group. DFR does require specialist training, however, in order to achieve good clinical and functional outcomes. Patellar tracking and accurate component positioning require diligent consideration, which is likely best performed by a trained knee arthroplasty surgeon. For this reason, DFR may not be suitable for all orthopedic surgeons to perform, and so the generalisability of this option is limited. Some studies have shown comparable financial costs between DFR and ORIF, meaning that it may be feasible to incorporate this option into the armamentarium for B1 periprosthetic fracture management from an economic perspective.[50]

External fixation

Although external fixation is not a commonly considered option in the management of this fracture type, Refaat and colleagues have shown that there may be a role in certain extenuating circumstances.[51] This report describes a patient who refused perioperative blood transfusion on religious grounds with a significant medical history including obesity, chronic osteoporosis, anemia, diabetes, and rheumatoid arthritis. In similar challenging clinical scenarios,

external fixation significantly may be useful, as it reduces blood loss due to less open incisions and may diminish the risk of significant infection that could complicate further management, and this has to be balanced with the risk of infection from the pin tracks and is not recommended as a mainstream surgical technique and is reserved only for very special circumstances.

SUMMARY

The burden of periprosthetic distal femoral fractures is projected to increase accordingly with the increase in TKAs performed globally in the future. Less invasive plating and IM nailing techniques still seem to provide similar outcomes based on current literature. Double-plating and combination techniques may prove to be beneficial in the future pending further large-scale studies but currently have not demonstrated superiority over single plating and IM nailing based on current evidence. Distal femoral replacement may provide a useful option for future treatment, provided it is performed by a trained knee arthroplasty surgeon.

CLINICS CARE POINTS

- One can expect the burden of periprosthetic distal femoral fractures to increase accordingly with the increase in TKAs globally in the future.

- Complications are common and mortality rates within 1 year following fracture may be as high as 13.3%.

- Less invasive approaches for plating confer higher healing rates and reduced operative times when compared with open procedures.

- When compared with IM nails, double plating is associated with less hemorrhage, shorter surgery time, and reduced risk of malunion in polytraumatized patients.

- No comparative studies have shown clinical superiority of double plating over single plating to date.

- When double plating, in order to avoid vascular injury, the anteromedial aspect of the distal half of the femur is considered to be the safe zone up to the level of 8 cm below the lesser trochanter.

- Contraindications to retrograde IM nailing include a closed box design of the femoral component, an intercondylar distance that is less than the IM nail diameter and an inability to flex the knee beyond 40° in order to gain access for the IM nail entry point.

- There is no clear consensus as to whether locking plates or nails are superior but the largest recent study comparing both methods demonstrate a significantly lower risk of complication and revision surgery with plating.
- Distal femoral replacement has comparable financial implications and is associated with lower revision rates when compared with ORIF for B1 distal femoral periprosthetic fractures.
- Distal femoral replacement should only be performed by a specialist knee arthroplasty surgeon in order to avoid issues of patellar maltracking and femoral component malposition.

DISCLOSURE

The authors have no commercial or financial conflicts of interest to disclose. There were no funding sources for any of the authors listed.

REFERENCES

1. Su ET, DeWal H, Di Cesare PE. Periprosthetic femoral fractures above total knee replacements. J Am Acad Orthop Surg 2004;12(1):12–20.
2. Rorabeck CH, Taylor JW. Periprosthetic fractures of the femur complicating total knee arthroplasty. Orthop Clin North Am 1999;30(2):265–77.
3. Fakler JKM, Pönick C, Edel M, et al. A new classification of TKA periprosthetic femur fractures considering the implant type. BMC Musculoskelet Disord 2017;18(1):490.
4. Duncan CP, Masri BA. Fractures of the femur after hip replacement. Instr Course Lect 1995;44:293–304.
5. Duncan CP, Haddad FS. The Unified Classification System (UCS): improving our understanding of periprosthetic fractures. Bone Joint J 2014;96-B(6):713–6.
6. Martinet O, Cordey J, Harder Y, et al. The epidemiology of fractures of the distal femur. Injury 2000;31(Suppl 3):C62–3.
7. Pietu G, Lebaron M, Flecher X, et al, SOFCOT. Epidemiology of distal femur fractures in France in 2011-12. Orthop Traumatol Surg Res 2014;100(5):545–8.
8. Jennison T, Yarlagadda R. A case series of mortality and morbidity in distal femoral periprosthetic fractures. J Orthop 2019;18:244–7.
9. Elsoe R, Ceccotti AA, Larsen P. Population-based epidemiology and incidence of distal femur fractures. Int Orthop 2018;42(1):191–6.
10. Rupp M, Lau E, Kurtz SM, et al. Projections of primary TKA and THA in Germany from 2016 through 2040. Clin Orthop Relat Res 2020;478(7):1622–33.
11. Shawen SB, Belmont PJ Jr, Klemme WR, et al. Osteoporosis and anterior femoral notching in periprosthetic supracondylar femoral fractures: a biomechanical analysis. J Bone Joint Surg Am 2003;85(1):115–21.
12. Gujarathi N, Putti AB, Abboud RJ, et al. Risk of periprosthetic fracture after anterior femoral notching. Acta Orthop 2009;80(5):553–6.
13. Ritter MA, Thong AE, Keating EM, et al. The effect of femoral notching during total knee arthroplasty on the prevalence of postoperative femoral fractures and on clinical outcome. J Bone Joint Surg Am 2005;87(11):2411–4.
14. Canton G, Ratti C, Fattori R, et al. Periprosthetic knee fractures. A review of epidemiology, risk factors, diagnosis, management and outcome. Acta Biomed 2017;88(2S):118–28.
15. Fracture around a stable femoral component with good bone stock AO surgery reference. Available at: https://surgeryreference.aofoundation.org/orthopedic-trauma/periprosthetic-fractures/knee/fracture-around-a-stable-femoral-component-with-good-bone-stock. Accessed March 1, 2021.
16. Cain PR, Rubash HE, Wissinger HA, et al. Periprosthetic femoral fractures following total knee arthroplasty. Clin Orthop Relat Res 1986;208:205–14.
17. Ricci WM, Loftus T, Cox C, et al. Locked plates combined with minimally invasive insertion technique for the treatment of periprosthetic supracondylar femur fractures above a total knee arthroplasty. J Orthop Trauma 2006;20(3):190–6.
18. Hoffmann MF, Burgers TA, Mason JJ, et al. Biomechanical evaluation of fracture fixation constructs using a variable-angle locked periprosthetic femur plate system. Injury 2014;45(7):1035–41.
19. Althausen PL, Lee MA, Finkemeier CG, et al. Operative stabilization of supracondylar femur fractures above total knee arthroplasty: a comparison of four treatment methods. J Arthroplasty 2003;18(7):834–9.
20. Fulkerson E, Tejwani N, Stuchin S, et al. Management of periprosthetic femur fractures with a first generation locking plate. Injury 2007;38(8):965–72.
21. Hess F, Knoth C, Welter J, et al. Polyaxial locking plate fixation in periprosthetic, peri-implant and distal shaft fractures of the femur : a comparison of open and less invasive surgical approaches. Acta Orthop Belg 2020;86(1):46–53.
22. Karam J, Campbell P, David M, et al. Comparison of outcomes and analysis of risk factors for nonunion in locked plating of closed periprosthetic

and non-periprosthetic distal femoral fractures in a retrospective cohort study. J Orthop Surg Res 2019;14(1):150.

23. Beeres FJP, Emmink BL, Lanter K, et al. Minimally invasive double-plating osteosynthesis of the distal femur. Minimal-invasive Doppelplattenosteosynthese des distalen Femurs. Oper Orthop Traumatol 2020;32(6):545–58.

24. Medda S, Kessler RB, Halvorson JJ, et al. Technical trick: dual plate fixation of periprosthetic distal femur fractures. J Orthop Trauma 2021;35(4):e148–52.

25. Kim JJ, Oh HK, Bae JY, et al. Radiological assessment of the safe zone for medial minimally invasive plate osteosynthesis in the distal femur with computed tomography angiography. Injury 2014; 45(12):1964–9.

26. Rollick NC, Gadinsky NE, Klinger CE, et al. The effects of dual plating on the vascularity of the distal femur. Bone Joint J 2020;102-B(4):530–8.

27. Park KH, Oh CW, Park KC, et al. Excellent outcomes after double-locked plating in very low periprosthetic distal femoral fractures. Arch Orthop Trauma Surg 2021;141(2):207–14.

28. Lodde MF, Raschke MJ, Stolberg-Stolberg J, et al. Union rates and functional outcome of double plating of the femur: systematic review of the literature. Arch Orthop Trauma Surg 2021. https://doi.org/10.1007/s00402-021-03767-6.

29. Weber D, Pomeroy DL, Schaper LA, et al. Supracondylar nailing of distal periprosthetic femoral fractures. Int Orthop 2000;24(1):33–5.

30. Biber R, Bail HJ. Retrograde Marknagelung bei periprothetischen Frakturen des distalen Femurs. [Retrograde intramedullary nailing for periprosthetic fractures of the distal femur]. Oper Orthop Traumatol 2014;26(5):438–54.

31. Wallace SS, Bechtold D, Sassoon A. Periprosthetic fractures of the distal femur after total knee arthroplasty: plate versus nail fixation. Orthop Traumatol Surg Res 2017;103(2):257–62.

32. Service BC, Kang W, Turnbull N, et al. Influence of femoral component design on retrograde femoral nail starting point. J Orthop Trauma 2015;29(10):e380–4.

33. Jones MD, Carpenter C, Mitchell SR, et al. Retrograde femoral nailing of periprosthetic fractures around total knee replacements. Injury 2016;47(2):460–4.

34. Udagawa K, Niki Y, Harato K, et al. Arthroscopically assisted retrograde intramedullary nailing for periprosthetic fracture of the femur after posterior-stabilized total knee arthroplasty. Case Rep Orthop 2018;2018:1805145.

35. Pelfort X, Torres-Claramunt R, Hinarejos P, et al. Extension malunion of the femoral component after retrograde nailing: no sequelae at 6 years. J Orthop Trauma 2013;27(3):158–61.

36. Chen SH, Tai CL, Yu TC, et al. Modified fixations for distal femur fractures following total knee arthroplasty: a biomechanical and clinical relevance study. Knee Surg Sports Traumatol Arthrosc 2016;24(10):3262–71.

37. Bong MR, Egol KA, Koval KJ, et al. Comparison of the LISS and a retrograde-inserted supracondylar intramedullary nail for fixation of a periprosthetic distal femur fracture proximal to a total knee arthroplasty. J Arthroplasty 2002;17(7):876–81.

38. Mäkinen TJ, Dhotar HS, Fichman SG, et al. Periprosthetic supracondylar femoral fractures following knee arthroplasty: a biomechanical comparison of four methods of fixation. Int Orthop 2015;39(9):1737–42.

39. Hou Z, Bowen TR, Irgit K, et al. Locked plating of periprosthetic femur fractures above total knee arthroplasty. J Orthop Trauma 2012;26(7):427–32.

40. Horneff JG 3rd, Scolaro JA, Jafari SM, et al. Intramedullary nailing versus locked plate for treating supracondylar periprosthetic femur fractures. Orthopedics 2013;36(5):e561–6.

41. Meneghini RM, Keyes BJ, Reddy KK, et al. Modern retrograde intramedullary nails versus periarticular locked plates for supracondylar femur fractures after total knee arthroplasty. J Arthroplasty 2014;29(7):1478–81.

42. Ristevski B, Nauth A, Williams DS, et al. Systematic review of the treatment of periprosthetic distal femur fractures. J Orthop Trauma 2014;28(5):307–12.

43. Shin YS, Kim HJ, Lee DH. Similar outcomes of locking compression plating and retrograde intramedullary nailing for periprosthetic supracondylar femoral fractures following total knee arthroplasty: a meta-analysis. Knee Surg Sports Traumatol Arthrosc 2017;25(9):2921–8.

44. Magill H, Ponugoti N, Selim A, et al. Locked compression plating versus retrograde intramedullary nailing in the treatment of periprosthetic supracondylar knee fractures: a systematic review and meta-analysis. J Orthop Surg Res 2021;16(1):78.

45. Shah JK, Szukics P, Gianakos AL, et al. Equivalent union rates between intramedullary nail and locked plate fixation for distal femur periprosthetic fractures - a systematic review. Injury 2020;51(4):1062–8.

46. Liporace FA, Yoon RS. Nail plate combination technique for native and periprosthetic distal femur fractures. J Orthop Trauma 2019;33(2):e64–8.

47. Mirick Mueller GE. Nail-plate constructs for periprosthetic distal femur fractures. J Knee Surg 2019;32(5):403–6.

48. Leino OK, Lempainen L, Virolainen P, et al. Operative results of periprosthetic fractures of the distal femur in a single academic unit. Scand J Surg 2015;104(3):200–7.

49. Darrith B, Bohl DD, Karadsheh MS, et al. Periprosthetic fractures of the distal femur: is open

reduction and internal fixation or distal femoral replacement superior? J Arthroplasty 2020;35(5): 1402–6.

50. Tandon T, Tadros BJ, Avasthi A, et al. Management of periprosthetic distal femur fractures using distal femoral arthroplasty and fixation - comparative study of outcomes and costs. J Clin Orthop Trauma 2020;11(1):160–4.

51. Refaat M, Coleman S, Meehan JP, et al. Periprosthetic supracondylar femur fracture treated with spanning external fixation. Am J Orthop (Belle Mead NJ) 2015;44(2):90–3.

Classification and Management of Periprosthetic Patella Fractures

Justin Deans, DO[a], Giles R. Scuderi, MD[b,c,*]

KEYWORDS

- Periprosthetic patella fracture • Resurfaced patella • Un-resurfaced patella
- Total knee arthroplasty • Patellectomy • Patelloplasty • Open reduction internal fixation

KEY POINTS

- Periprosthetic patella fractures are a relatively rare but challenging complication following total knee arthroplasty.
- The Ortiguera and Berry classification is the mostly widely used classification system and helps to guide treatment.
- Because of risks of surgical complication, nonoperative management is often used if the extensor mechanism is intact and the patellar component is well fixed.
- Surgery is indicated if the extensor mechanism is disrupted or the patellar component is loose.
- Quality and thickness of the remaining patellar bone stock will help guide between patellar component revision and partial or complete patellectomy.

INTRODUCTION

Periprosthetic patella fractures are relatively rare but are the second most common periprosthetic knee fracture, behind periprosthetic femur fractures.[1] Historically, they have an incidence between 0.2% to 21% after total knee arthroplasty (TKA) with a resurfaced patella.[1–5] A series of patellar fractures after TKA from the Mayo Clinic found a 0.68% incidence.[6] The incidence of patella fractures after revision TKA has been reported higher than the incidence following primary TKA.[4] A periprosthetic fracture in an un-resurfaced patella is exceedingly rare, with reported incidence of 0.05%.[3] However, with increasing life expectancy combined with the increased incidence of TKA in the United States, this difficult problem is being encountered more frequently. Approximately 50% of the reported cases are not associated with a traumatic event and are found on routine follow-up within 2 years of TKA.[6,7] In more than 50% of the cases, a loose patellar component further complicates management.[7] These technically complex cases are often made more difficult in that they frequently occur in patients with advanced age, osteoporosis, and a previously disrupted soft tissue envelope, which puts them at greater risk for postoperative complications. There has long been debate regarding the optimum management of periprosthetic patella fractures. The management goal of these fractures is to provide a stable knee that is pain free, well aligned, and functional. Complications after nonoperative management include nonunion, malunion, extensor lag, and continued pain. Complications after surgical intervention include loss of fixation, nonunion, prosthetic loosening, extensor lag, continued pain, and wound complications. One of the first studies of surgically treated periprosthetic patellar fractures observed a 100%

[a] Department of Orthopaedic Surgery, Lenox Hill Hospital, 130 East 77th Street, 11th Floor Black Hall, New York, NY 10075, USA; [b] Zucker School of Medicine at Hofstra, 500 Hofstra Blvd, Hempstead, NY 11549, USA; [c] Northwell Orthopaedic Institute, 130 East 77th Street, Black Hall, 7th Floor, New York, NY 10075, USA
* Corresponding author.
E-mail address: gscuderi@northwell.edu

Orthop Clin N Am 52 (2021) 347–355
https://doi.org/10.1016/j.ocl.2021.05.003

nonunion rate and an extensor lag of 10° or greater in 7/12 cases.[8] Because of the historically poor outcomes with surgical intervention, a better understanding of periprosthetic patella fractures and when and how to intervene surgically is of critical importance. The purpose of this article is to review the current literature to best understand the risk factors for periprosthetic patella fractures to help prevent future occurrence and to identify the best course of management of these fractures in order to optimize outcomes.

RISK FACTORS FOR FRACTURE

Numerous risk factors have been identified to influence the incidence of periprosthetic patella fractures and can be categorized as patient factors, surgical factors, and implant factors (Table 1). Understanding these factors can help avoid this complication.[9]

Patient Risk Factors
Patient-specific risk factors that have been identified include obesity,[10] high activity level,[11–13] and excessive or rapid knee flexion.[14,15] Patella fractures occur more commonly in men (1.01%) than in women (0.4%),[6] unlike periprosthetic femur and tibia fractures. This common occurrence in men is thought to relate to increased activity level, force generated through the extensor mechanism, and weight of the patient. Trauma, often caused by direct impact on the patella during a fall, is responsible for approximately 50% of periprosthetic patella fractures.[6] Rheumatoid arthritis also has been associated with increased risk of periprosthetic patella fracture,[16] which may be due to rheumatoid patients taking steroids and having more osteopenic bone.[2,17]

Surgical Risk Factors
Surgical factors also play a role in risk of periprosthetic patella fractures. Osteonecrosis of the patella can occur after primary TKA if the blood supply to the patella is compromised. Typically, with the standard medial parapatellar arthrotomy, the medial blood flow to the patella is compromised. Often, the inferior lateral geniculate artery is also compromised during removal of the fat pad and lateral meniscus. This makes the superior lateral geniculate artery (SLGA) extremely important to maintain patella vascularity. A lateral retinacular release to improve patellar tracking may disrupt the SLGA, contributing to further devascularization of the patella, increasing the risk of periprosthetic patella fracture.[4,18,19] Osteonecrosis can also occur from the heat generated by bone cement

polymerization and compression forces generated during repeated knee flexion of ≥95°.[5,6]

Another technical risk factor for fracture is overresection of the patella, leading to decreased mechanical strength of the patella and subsequent fracture during high-stress movements, such as rapid hyperflexion of the knee.[15,20,21] Multiple studies have discussed how the thickness of the patella correlates with fracture risk. Patellae with a thickness of less than 12 to 14 mm have a substantially increased strain in the anterior patella region and increased risk of fracture.[22,23] Asymmetric resection of the patella also increases mechanical strain on the patella, especially when the subchondral bone of the lateral articular surface is included in the resection, leading to increased risk of fracture.[24]

Overstuffing the patellofemoral joint by more than 2 mm can lead to patellofemoral maltracking, increased patellofemoral contact and compression pressures, decreased range of movement, anterior knee pain, and increased shear forces leading to loosening and failure of the patella component.[25] When dealing with a native patella less than 20 mm thick and using a typical 8-mm-thick patellar component, the surgeon often has to make a decision whether to (1) cut the patella to less than 12 mm thick, risking fracture, but avoiding overstuffing the joint; (2) cut the patella to 12 mm thick, decreasing the risk of fracture but risking complications related to overstuffing the joint; or (3) leaving the patella un-resurfaced but risking late development of anterior knee pain.

Malalignment of the lower limb or the prosthesis has also been identified as a risk factor for periprosthetic patella fractures. Malalignment of the femoral component leads to an increased eccentric load on the tibiofemoral joint, causing subluxation of the patella, which can cause fracture.[26] Malposition or malrotation of the femoral component and or tibial component will impact the alignment of the extensor mechanism.[27] Extensor mechanism malalignment can affect patella function and possibly lead to fracture. In addition, selecting an oversized femoral component or anteriorizing the femoral component will overstuff the patellofemoral joint, increase the joint reaction forces, and potentially lead to a patella fracture.[28]

During exposure of the knee joint, excessive patellar eversion has been associated with intraoperative inferior pole fractures or rupture of the patellar tendon. For that reason, it is preferable to sublux the patella laterally rather than

Table 1
Risk factors influence the chance of periprosthetic patella fracture

Influencing Factors	Specific Conditions
Patient factors	Obesity
	Osteopenia
	Thin patella
	Male
	Excessive knee flexion
	High activity
	Prior surgery
	Trauma
Surgical factors	Femoral component malposition
	Tibial component malposition
	Asymmetric patella resection
	Overresection of the patella
	Patella maltracking
	Lateral retinacular release
	Devascularization of the patella
	Revision surgery
Implant factors	Resurfaced patella
	Large single central lug
	Inset patella
	Uncemented patella
	Metal-backed patella

everting it or performing a more extensile approach, like the quadriceps snip.[29]

Implant Risk Factors

Implant-related factors may also play a role in patella fracture. Occurrence of a fracture in an unsurfaced patella is exceedingly rare, with nearly all fractures occurring after resurfacing.[10,30,31] Implant design has been implicated. Patella components with a large central peg have been associated with an increased risk of fracture because of the creation of a large central bone defect and increased anterior patella strain.[3,10,18,19,28,32] Modern patella components typically are fixed using 3 small pegs to help decrease this risk by reducing the anterior

strain.[31] Metal-backed patellae have also been associated with increased risk of fracture.[33]

CLASSIFICATION

Several different classification systems have been created to help organize periprosthetic patella fractures, but the most widely used is the Ortiguera and Berry classification (Box 1). The main features of the classification are the integrity of the extensor mechanism, the stability of the patellar component, and the quality of the residual bone. A type 1 fracture has an intact extensor mechanism and a stable patella component. Type 2 has a disrupted extensor mechanism and either a stable or loose patellar component. A type 3 has an intact extensor mechanism and loose patellar component, and then is further subdivided based on remaining bone stock. Type 3A has reasonable bone stock with a patellar thickness greater than 10 mm, and a type 3B has poor bone stock with less than 10 mm thickness or comminution of the patella.

TREATMENT

There are numerous reports on the management of periprosthetic patella fractures. Nonoperative treatment is preferred for patients with an intact extensor mechanism and a stable patella component (type 1). Surgical repair or reconstruction for type 2 or 3 fractures is based on fracture displacement, quality of the residual bone and extensor mechanism, and patella component fixation (Box 2). Un-resurfaced patella fractures are treated like any typical traumatic patella fracture.

TYPE 1 FRACTURES

Periprosthetic patellar fractures with an intact extensor mechanism and a stable patellar component can be managed nonoperatively.[18] Many patients with type 1 fractures present with no or mild pain and thus are often discovered incidentally on routine follow-up radiographs, and 6 to 10 weeks of knee immobilization in extension typically yield optimal results.[3,6,34] Operative treatment is usually not warranted because the clinical results of nonoperative treatment are comparable to operative treatment without the risk of postoperative complications.[15,32] Although nonoperative treatment has been able to restore knee function, radiographic evaluation has demonstrated fibrous union or asymptomatic nonunion in many cases.[6] The complication rate of operative treatment with internal fixation for mild displacement without component loosening can be as high as 50%.[6]

Authors' Preferred Treatment

It is the authors' preference to treat type 1 fractures nonoperatively with immobilization and activity modification. The period of immobilization is determined by the fracture pattern. Nondisplaced transverse (**Fig. 1**) or comminuted fractures are immobilized in extension for 6 to 8 weeks, followed by gradual resumption of motion in a control dial hinged knee brace. Initial immobilization in a long leg cast or hinged knee brace locked in extension depends on the likelihood of patient compliance with bracing.

Nondisplaced longitudinal fractures of the patella can be treated with a short period of immobilization followed by gradual resumption of knee flexion (**Fig. 2**).

TYPE 2 FRACTURES

Type 2 periprosthetic patella fractures typically require open reduction internal fixation (ORIF) because of displacement of the patella fracture and disruption of the extensor mechanism.[34] Treatment is determined by the quality of the bone and fixation of the patella component. If the patella component is stable, ORIF can be done with various known patella fracture techniques based on the quality and comminution of the residual bone; however, no fixation method has shown superiority. In highly comminuted fractures, it may be preferable to perform partial patellectomy of small fragments with fixation of the quadriceps or patellar tendon to remaining bone.[6,34] If the patella component is

loose, it will need to be removed, followed by ORIF of fracture or partial patellectomy with repair of the extensor mechanism.

Knowing that surgical management has a high complication rate, as high as 50%, it may be preferred to accept some extensor lag or consider nonoperative management of a severely comminuted patella fracture. In the Mayo Clinic series, 12 patients had type 2 fractures. Surgical intervention was performed in 11 cases, and 6 developed complications with 5 requiring reoperation (45%).[6] In a more contemporary series, 3 type 2 fractures were managed with ORIF using tension band wiring, and all went on to radiographic union at 21 weeks with an average extensor lag of 5°.[35] Another recent series of 5 patella fractures managed operatively reported overall poor functional outcomes with a 20% incidence of implant failure and reoperation.[36] A complete patellectomy can be considered in highly comminuted fractures with fragments too small to support fixation or as a salvage procedure for failure of prior treatment. Chang and colleagues[37] reported 9 patients treated with patellectomy after sustaining periprosthetic patella fractures, observing an extensor lag of less than 10° in 8 cases and an average range of motion of 104°.

Authors' Preferred Treatment

Treatment of type 2 fractures is based on the location and displacement of the patella fracture, as well as the fixation of the patella component. Avulsion fractures of the inferior or superior pole of the patella, with a stable patella component, are managed with a partial patellectomy and repair of either the patella tendon or the quadriceps tendon to the residual large fragment of patella bone (**Fig. 3A, B**). The repair is usually performed with number 5 FiberWire with a Krackow stitch in the respective tendon and secured to the patella through interosseous drill holes. Postoperatively, the knee is immobilized in extension for 6 to 8 weeks, followed by gradual resumption of motion in a control dial hinged knee brace.

Larger displaced transverse fractures with a stable patella component are managed with either partial patellectomy and repair of the detached tendon or ORIF of the large fragments. The means of fixation is dependent on the quality and thickness of the residual patella bone. Although it is important to achieve stable fixation, the least elaborate construct is preferred.

In cases with a displaced fracture and loose patella component, the patella component is

Box 2
The treatment options based on the classification of periprosthetic patella fracture

Type 1

  Extensor mechanism intact

  Stable patella component

    Nonoperative treatment

    • Knee brace in extension

    • Cylinder cast

Type 2

  Extensor mechanism disrupted

  Operative repair or reconstruction of the extensor mechanism

    Stable patella component

    • Partial patellectomy and repair of tendon

    • Open reduction and internal fixation of fracture

    Loose patella component with adequate bone

    • Revision of patella component with partial patellectomy and repair of tendon

    • Revision of patella component with open reduction and internal fixation of fracture

    Loose patella component with inadequate bone

    • Removal of loose component with partial patellectomy and repair of tendon

    • Removal of loose component and complete patellectomy

    • Reconstruction of the extensor mechanism with extensor allograft or Marlex mesh

Type 3

  Intact extensor mechanism

  Loose patella component

    Asymptomatic with nondisplaced patella component

    • Knee braced in extension

    • Cylinder cast

    Asymptomatic with displaced patellar component

    • Removal of loose patella component, then knee braced or casted in extension

    Symptomatic with displaced patella component

    • Removal and revision of loose patella component if adequate bone for secure component fixation

    • Removal of loose component and consider alternatives, such as patelloplasty, marsupialization with bone graft, and trabecular metal patella augmentation

removed, and the fracture is repaired with techniques similar to that described above. If there is a large fragment of patella bone that can support a patella component and track appropriately, then placement of a new patella component may be considered. However, it has been the authors' experience that in these cases the bone is usually comminuted, is of poor quality, and will not support a new component. In these situations, it may be preferable to perform a partial or total patellectomy and repair the extensor mechanism. Mild to moderate anterior knee pain can be expected in up to one-third of these patients.[38] In situations with a chronic patella fracture or nonunion with a symptomatic extensor lag, it may be necessary to perform an extensor mechanism reconstruction with allograft or Marlex mesh.[39–41]

TYPE 3 FRACTURES

Type 3 fractures have an intact extensor mechanism and a loose patellar component. With a loose patellar component, the patient will either

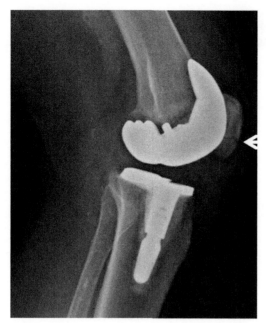

Fig. 1. Lateral radiograph demonstrating a nondisplaced patella fracture of the inferior pole (*arrow*) at 2 years following TKA.

require a patellar resection arthroplasty (patelloplasty) or a patellar component revision. That treatment decision is based on the quality of the patella bone stock. With less than 10 mm of remaining bone stock, it may be preferred to perform a resection arthroplasty, leaving the shell of patella bone fragments. Other options, such as a trabecular metal patella, augment, or cancellous impaction bone grafting, can be considered based on the quality of the residual bone fragments.

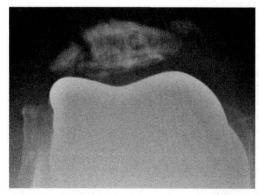

Fig. 2. Radiographic Merchant view demonstrating a minimally displaced longitudinal patella fracture with a stable patella component.

Historically, type 3 fractures have a high complication rate. In the Mayo Clinic series, 28 type 3 fractures were identified, and 20 were treated operatively. Complications developed in 9 out of 20 knees (45%) with 4 knees (20%) requiring reoperation. Even with appropriate management, this fracture pattern is associated with poor outcomes with 57% of patients symptomatic at follow-up.[6]

Authors' Preferred Technique

In type 3 fractures, the extensor mechanism is intact, and treatment is based on fixation of the patella component. In patients with an asymptomatic loose patella component with no displacement, it may be preferable to initiate nonoperatively, allowing the patella fracture to heal. The patella component may become encapsulated with a fibrous membrane and remain asymptomatic. If it displaces after the fracture heals, it can then be removed. However, if the patient initially presents with a loose and displaced patella component, it should be removed. The patella fracture then can be treated nonoperatively with immobilization in extension, as detailed above.

In patients who are symptomatic with a loose patella component, the patella component should be removed, and if there is adequate bone, then a new patella component may be implanted. If there is inadequate bone to cement a patella component, then other alternatives need to be considered, such as patelloplasty, marsupialization with impaction bone graft, or trabecular metal augmentation (Fig. 4A–D).

POSTOPERATIVE MANAGEMENT

After ORIF of the patella fracture, the leg is placed in a compression dressing with a hinged knee brace locked in 0 to 5 degrees of flexion. The wound is checked at 48 hours, and the patient is either kept in the hinged knee brace or changed to a long leg cylinder cast for 6 to 10 weeks. If there is concern over patient compliance with the brace and keeping the leg in extension, a well-padded, long leg cylinder cast is typically chosen. If casting is needed, there should be frequent skin checks to make sure of adequate wound healing, and this can be done through bivalving the cast or cast changes every 2 weeks. A wound complication at this time can be catastrophic to the surgical outcome. At 6 to 10 weeks, the hinged knee brace is unlocked to allow gradual controlled flexion over the following weeks. Throughout

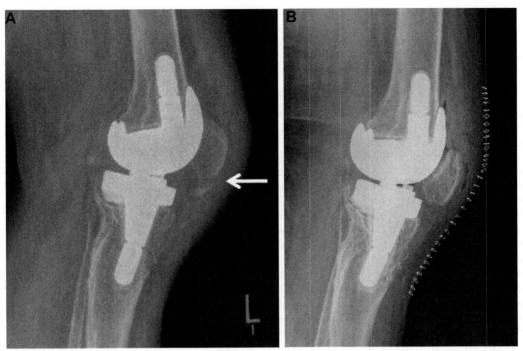

Fig. 3. (A) Lateral radiograph of a total knee replacement with a displaced comminuted fracture of the inferior pole of the patella (arrow). (B) Postoperative lateral radiograph following partial patellectomy and repair of the patella tendon. Note the patella infera.

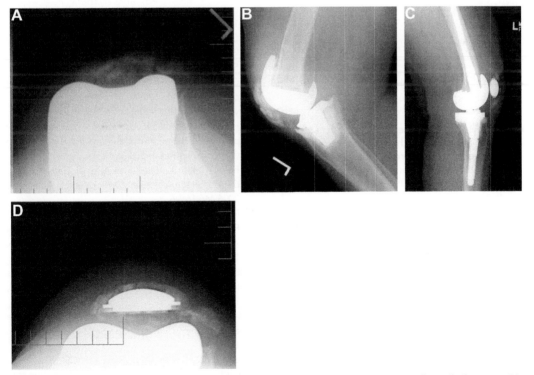

Fig. 4. (A–D) Lateral radiograph (A) and Merchant view (B) demonstrating a comminuted patella fracture with a loose patella component. Postoperative lateral radiograph (C) and Merchant view (D) show treatment of the patella fracture with a trabecular metal patella augment during revision TKA.

rehabilitation, the patient can be weight-bearing as tolerated with an assistive device, such as a cane or crutches, depending on the patient's stability.

SUMMARY

Periprosthetic patella fractures continue to be a challenging problem for surgeons, with complication rates approaching 50%, many of which will require reoperation. Knowledge of these fractures continues to evolve, and numerous risk factors related to the patient, implant, and surgical technique have been identified. This knowledge allows us to educate our patients and our surgical team in order to decrease the incidence and improve the management of these difficult fractures. To achieve optimal outcomes, it is recommended that the fracture be classified based on the integrity of the extensor mechanism, quality of the bone, and stability of the patella component. Using the above-mentioned classification system, a treatment plan can be determined. It is critical to thoroughly assess the risks and benefits of surgical intervention before proceeding because of the high rate of postoperative complications.[8,42]

CLINICS CARE POINTS

- The Ortiguera and Berry classification system is useful for classification and to guide management.

- Determine whether the extensor mechanism is intact and whether the patellar component is loose through clinical examination and imaging. If not intact or the component is loose, surgery is typically indicated.

- If nonoperative management is chosen, either a well-padded long leg cast or a hinged knee brace locked in extension for 6 to 10 weeks is used.

- If operative intervention is indicated for extensor mechanism disruption, initial reports recommended avoiding tension band or cerclage wiring, if possible, because of a roughly 90% complication rate[7]; however, more contemporary studies have found no superiority of any 1 technique.

- Consider fragment excision (partial patellectomy) if not amenable to surgical fixation.

- Total patellectomy should be used as last resort if other techniques fail or in highly comminuted fractures.

- Recommend a hinged knee brace locked in extension for 6 to 10 weeks after open reduction internal fixation before beginning physical therapy to regain range of motion.

DISCLOSURE

The authors report no disclosures directly related to the article.

REFERENCES

1. Berry DJ. Epidemiology: hip and knee. Orthop Clin North Am 1999;30:183–90.
2. Parvizi J, Jain N, Schmidt AH. Periprosthetic knee fractures. J Orthop Trauma 2008;22:663–71.
3. Goldberg CM, Figgie HE 3rd, Inglis AE, et al. Patellar fracture type and prognosis in condylar total knee arthroplasty. Clin Orthop Relat Res 1988;236L115–22.
4. Grace JN, Sim FH. Fracture of the patella after total knee arthroplasty. Clin Orthop Relat Res 1988;230: 168–75.
5. Windsor RE, Scuderi GR, Insall JN. Patellar fractures in total knee arthroplasty. J Arthroplasty 1989;4(Suppl):S63–7.
6. Ortiguera CJ, Berry DJ. Patellar fracture after total knee arthroplasty. J Bone Join Surg Am 2002;84: 532–40.
7. Chalidis B, Tsiridis E, Tragas A, et al. Management of periprosthetic patellar fractures. A systematic review of literature. Injury 2007;38:714–24.
8. Hozack WJ, Goll SR, Lotke PA. The treatment of patellar fractures after total knee arthroplasty. Clin Orthop Relat Res 1988;236:123–7.
9. Parvizi J, Kim K, Oliashirazi A, et al. Periprosthetic patellar fractures. Clin Orthopaedics Relat Res 2006;446:161–6.
10. Rosenberg AG, Andriacchi TP, Barden R, et al. Patellar component failure in cementless total knee arthroplasty. Clin Orthop Relat Res 1988;236: 106–14.
11. Doolittle KH II, Turner RH. Patellofemoral problems following total knee arthroplasty. Orthop Rev 1988; 17:696–702.
12. Insall JN, Dethmers DA. Revision of total knee arthroplasty. Clin Orthop Relat Res 1982;170: 123–30.
13. Insall JN, Scott WN, Ranawat CS. The total condylar knee prosthesis. A report of two hundred and twenty cases. J Bone Joint Surg Am 1979;61: 173–80.

14. Aglietti P, Buzzi R, Gaudenzi A. Patellofemoral functional results and complications with the posterior stabilized total condylar knee prosthesis. J Arthroplasty 1988;3:17–25.

15. Scott RD, Turoff N, Ewald EC. Stress fracture of the patella following duopatellar total knee arthroplasty with patellar resurfacing. Clin Orthop Relat Res 1982;170:147–51.

16. Lynch AF, Rorabeck CH, Bourne RB. Extensor mechanism complications following total knee arthroplasty. J Arthroplasty 1987;2:135–40.

17. Le Ax, Cameron HU, Otsuka NY, et al. Fracture of the patella following total knee arthroplasty. Orthopedics 1999;22:395–8.

18. Boyd AD Jr, Ewald FC, Thomas WH, et al. Long-term complications after total knee arthroplasty with or without resurfacing of the patella. J Bone Joint Surg Am 1993;75:674–81.

19. Ritter MA, Herbst SA, Keating EM, et al. Patellofemoral complications following total knee arthroplasty. Effect of a lateral release and sacrifice of the superior lateral geniculate artery. J Arthroplasty 1996;11:368–72.

20. Calyton ML, Thirupathi R. Patellar complications after total condylar arthroplasty. Clin Orthop Relat Res 1982;170:152–5.

21. Cameron HU, Fedorkow DM. The patella in total knee arthroplasty. Clin Orthop Relat Res 1982;165:197–9.

22. Reuben JD, McDonald CL, Woodard PL, et al. Effect of patella thickness on patella strain following total knee arthroplasty. J Arthroplasty 1991;6:251–8.

23. Lee QJ, Yeung ST, Wong YC, et al. Effect of patellar thickness on early results of total knee replacement with patellar resurfacing. Knee Surg Sports Traumatol Arthrosc 2014 Dec;22(12):3093–9.

24. Yoo JD, Kim NK. Periprosthetic fractures following total knee arthroplasty. Knee Surg Relat Res 2015;27(1):1–9.

25. Abolghasemian M, Samiezadeh S, Sternheim A, et al. Effect of patellar thickness on knee flexion in total knee arthroplasty: a biomechanical and experimental study. J Arthroplasty 2014;29(1):80–4.

26. Huberti HH, Hayes WC. Patellofemoral contact pressures. The influence of q-angle and tendofemoral contact. J Bone Joint Surg Am 1984;66:715–24.

27. Berger RA, Crossett LS, Jacobs JJ, et al. Malrotation causing patellofemoral complications after total knee arthroplasty. Clin Orthop Relat Res 1998 Nov;(356):144–53.

28. Stulberg SD, Stulberg BN, Hamati Y, et al. Failure mechanisms of metal backed patellar components. Clin Orthop Relat Res 1988;236:88–105.

29. Garvin KL, Scuderi G, Insall JN. Evolution of the quadriceps snip. Clin Orthop Relat Res 1995 Dec;(321):131–7.

30. Bourne RB. Fracture of the patella after total knee replacement. Orthop Clin North Am 1999;30:287–91.

31. Goldstein SA, Coale E, Weiss AP, et al. Patella surface strain. J Orthop Res 1986;4:372–7.

32. Keating EM, Hass G, Meding JB. Patella fracture after post total knee replacements. Clin Orthop Relat Res 1988;229:221–7.

33. Roffman M, Hirsh DM, Mendes DG. Fracture of the resurfaced patella in total knee replacement. Clin Orthop Relat Res 1980;148:112–6.

34. Dennis DA. Periprosthetic fractures following total knee arthroplasty. Instr Course Lect 2001;50:379–89.

35. Agarwal S, Sharma RK, Jain JK. Periprosthetic fractures after total knee arthroplasty. J Orthop Surg (Hong Kong) 2014;22:24–9.

36. Nagwadia H, Joshi P. Outcome of osteosynthesis for periprosthetic fractures after total knee arthroplasty: a retrospective study. Eur J Orthop Surg Traumatol 2018;28(4):683–90.

37. Chang MA, Rand JA, Trousdale RT. Patellectomy after total knee arthroplasty. Clin Orthop Relat Res 2005;440:175–7.

38. Pagnano MW, Scuderi FR, Insall JN. Patellar component resection in revision and reimplantation total knee arthroplasty. Clin Orthop Relat Res 1998;356:134–8.

39. Brown NM, Murray T, Sporer SM, et al. Extensor mechanism allograft reconstruction for extensor mechanism failure following total knee arthroplasty. J Bone Joint Surg Am 2015;97:279–83.

40. Lim CT, Amanatullah DF, Huddleston JI 3rd, et al. Reconstruction of disrupted extensor mechanism after total knee arthroplasty. J Arthroplasty 2017;32(10):3134–40.

41. Ricciardi BF, Oi K, Trivellas M, et al. Survivorship of extensor mechanism allograft reconstruction after total knee arthroplasty. J Arthroplasty 2017;32(1):183–8.

42. Keating EM, Haas G, Meding JB. Patella fracture after post total knee replacements. Clin Orthop Relat Res 2003;416:93–7.

A Review of Periprosthetic Tibial Fractures
Diagnosis and Treatment

Samantha A. Mohler, MS, Jeffery B. Stambough, MD,
Simon C. Mears, MD, PhD, Charles Lowry Barnes, MD,
Benjamin M. Stronach, MD, MS*

KEYWORDS

- Periprosthetic tibia • Tibial fracture • Total knee arthroplasty • ORIF • Revision TKA

KEY POINTS

- Bone quality, prosthetic component configuration and malalignment, arthroplasty technique, and revision arthroplasty contribute to risk of periprosthetic tibial fracture.
- Several strategies have been documented for management of periprosthetic tibial fractures including nonoperative management, internal fixation, external fixation, and revision arthroplasty.
- Few studies have examined outcomes based on fracture type. More research needs to be conducted to establish best practice standards.

INTRODUCTION

Periprosthetic fractures (PPFxs) related to total knee arthroplasty (TKA) are commonly defined as fractures of the femur, patella, or tibia that occur within 15 cm of the joint or within 5 cm of the prosthetic's intramedullary stem.[1–3] PPFx during or after TKA is a rare complication and poses significant challenges to the surgeon and the patient. Tibial PPFxs occur less commonly than femoral PPFxs, limiting the available guidance for evidence-based management. Literature concerning periprosthetic tibial fractures is sparse.

We seek to provide readers with an overview of the epidemiology, risk factors, fracture classification, and management recommendations for periprosthetic tibial fractures. In addition, we emphasize the need for high-quality research on this topic and identify gaps in the literature that need further exploration.

EPIDEMIOLOGY

TKA is one of the most common elective surgical procedures. An estimated 680,150 primary TKAs were performed in the United States during 2014 with 1.5 million anticipated by 2030.[4,5] The demand for TKA is expected to grow as life expectancy and factors contributing to the development of osteoarthritis, such as obesity, continue to increase. Significant strides have been made to improve outcomes and streamline recovery protocols for TKA, but the potential for complications still exists. It is anticipated that complications associated with TKA will increase proportionally with procedural volume unless fundamental improvements in treatment are implemented. Concurrent osteoporosis is present in at least one-third of patients undergoing TKA, and so the future number of PPFxs may increase at an even higher rate.[6,7]

Fracture occurring during or after TKA presents a significant treatment challenge. There is

---

Department of Orthopaedic Surgery, University of Arkansas for Medical Sciences, 4301 W Markham St, Mail Slot # 531, Little Rock, AR 72205, USA
* Corresponding author.
E-mail address: bstronach@uams.edu

Orthop Clin N Am 52 (2021) 357–368
https://doi.org/10.1016/j.ocl.2021.05.006

significant associated morbidity with high rates of nonunion (23.7%, at 6 months), and many patients (31.6%) require a second operation.[8] Intraoperative fractures occur in approximately 0.2% to 4.4% of cases.[9–11] Likewise, approximately 2.5% of patients undergoing TKA will have a postoperative fracture.[12] It is estimated that periprosthetic tibial fractures occur in 0.4% to 1.7% of primary TKA and 0.9% of revision TKA.[12–15] Although seemingly uncommon, the occurrence of these fracture is likely underreported.[9,13,16]

RISK FACTORS

Risk factors for periprosthetic TKA fractures are not well established in the literature. Nevertheless, several factors and management strategies have been proposed and documented in case reports or case series. Most of the literature on this topic is composed of systematic reviews and meta-analysis.

Risk factors reported in the broader literature on periprosthetic and fragility fractures should also increase the risk of periprosthetic tibial fractures. This risk factors include conditions that compromise bone quality such as osteopenia/osteoporosis, diabetes,[17] female sex,[18–20] older age, prolonged steroid use,[21] rheumatologic diseases,[22] and other metabolic derangements.[17,18] It has been reported that females are 2.3 to 4.4 times more likely than males to sustain PPFxs during or after TKA.[18–20] Increasing age is also a nonmodifiable risk factor for fracture because of a higher probability of poor bone quality and a higher susceptibility for falls. Meek and colleagues[18] reported that individuals older than 70 years are 1.6 times more likely to have a PPFx when compared with their younger counterparts. In contrast, Singh and colleagues[16] found that individuals younger than 60 years and older than 80 years were at increased risk when compared with individuals outside of these age ranges. The investigators hypothesized that the younger cohort was at risk of fracture owing to higher rates of trauma.[16] About one-third of patients undergoing total knee replacement are thought to have osteoporosis at the time of knee replacement.[6,7] Until now, knee replacement has not been a trigger for an osteoporotic workup. Some have suggested that evaluation of patients with a screening tool and subsequent laboratory workup, dual-energy X-ray absorptiometry scan, and Fracture Risk Assessment Tool (FRAX) evaluation may be conducted so that patients with osteoporosis can be treated before arthroplasty.[7] Surgical

techniques may change if a diagnosis of osteoporosis is recognized.[23] Osteoporosis may be a modifiable risk factor for surgery that can be improved. Efforts to improve our diagnosis and treatment of osteoporosis may be able to decrease rates of PPFx.

Risk factors specific to tibial PPFxs include component stem length and baseplate size, revision TKA, malalignment, instability, atypical tibial anatomy, tibial tuberosity elevation, and type of fixation.[5,18,24,25] Stress shielding of the proximal tibia can occur after TKA due to tibial baseplate rigidity.[26] This stress shielding can then lead to proximal bone loss beneath the tibial tray with subsequent increased strain immediately distal to the implant keel in an uncemented TKA.[27,28] Wolff's law likely accounts for these findings, and there may be associated pain that can occur at the distal tip of the tibial component.[29] The type of tibial baseplate material has also been noted to play a role in periprosthetic bone remodeling.[28,30] Efforts are ongoing to optimize prosthesis design to create more biocompatible materials that avoid bone reabsorption and decrease the risks of component-loosening PPFx.

Long press-fit-type stems have been associated with increased risk of fracture. Long press-fit stem designs have greater contact with the diaphysis,[31] and fractures can occur intraoperatively due to overly aggressive insertion or anatomic/prosthetic mismatch.[27,31,32] Smaller-sized primary components are at risk of abutting metaphyseal cortical bone, and keel/plate mismatch is associated with increased risk of fracture[24,33]; this is due to the larger size of the stem/keel within the bone compared with a larger-sized prosthesis with the same sized keel and stem.[24,33]

Malalignment of TKA components at the time of implantation introduces risk of abnormal wear and contact forces at the prosthesis-bone interface. Factors that are associated with malalignment include poor surgical technique, anatomic variability, and implant design. Correction of tibial coronal deformity with TKA is associated with risk of fracture due to the bone resection extending beyond the subchondral surface that is most supportive of the implant.[20,34] It has been recommended that surgeons consider the use of short cemented stem extensions to protect against fracture in this setting.[34,35]

Many studies report that revision TKA has a higher risk of tibial PPFx when compared with primary TKA.[18,25,36] Many of the revision TKA fracture risks are associated with underlying poor bone stock and the need for implant and/

or cement removal, iatrogenically creating weaker bone. The tibial tubercle osteotomy technique is a helpful tool to improve exposure in difficult revision TKA surgeries but may be associated with intraoperative fracture.[9,24,37] This technique may introduce microfractures in the cortex, and specific precautions have been proposed to decrease fracture.[37]

Unicompartmental and computer- and robot-guided knee arthroplasty are associated with particular risk for PPFxs. Intraoperative tibial PPFx after unicompartmental replacement may be associated with tibial cortex violation during bone preparation. Tibial cortex pin holes (inserted to attach the cutting guide) may create stress risers that lead to fracture with component impaction.[38–42] Likewise, fractures reported with computer- and robot-guided arthroplasty have been associated with tracking pin holes.[43–46] Pin diameter and placement (bicortical, unicortical, transcortical) have been scrutinized.[46] Finite element analysis indicates that pin holes placed close to the medial edge of the proximal tibia yield the highest stress values and are at increased risk of fracture.[47]

CLASSIFICATION

In 1996, the Arbeitsgemeinschaft für Osteosynthesefragen Trauma (AO) International Board and the Orthopedic Trauma Association (OTA) developed the AO/OTA Fracture and Dislocation Classification Compendium to standardize the description of fracture patterns and was most recently updated in 2018.[11] This system provides an alphanumeric system that systematically describes fractures based on bone (tibia: 4), fracture location (1, proximal; 2, mid shaft; 3, distal), fracture pattern (A, simple; B, wedge; C, multifragmented), subgroups (for articular fractures), and universal modifiers (to be placed in square brackets).[11]

The Unified Classification System for Periprosthetic Fractures (UCPF) is a system developed to use in conjunction with the AO/OTA classification that provides nomenclature specific for PPFx. The UCPF code is placed in square brackets following the AO/OTA code and identifies the joint involved [knee, V]. This code further delineates the fracture type based on its relation to the prosthesis and implant stability.[48] This approach has been adopted from the Vancouver classification system for periprosthetic hip fractures and provides a principle-based guide to management and diagnosis.[12,49]

The Felix classification system is specific to periprosthetic tibia fractures and is the most referenced classification in the literature (Fig. 1). Felix and colleagues[14] have reported on the largest cohort study of periprosthetic tibial fractures and proposed management strategies specific to the classification subtypes they established. This system groups fracture types based on 3 distinct factors: location, timing (intraoperative vs postoperative) and component stability. Type is determined by location: type I, tibial plateau; type II, involves the component stem; type III, distal to stem; type IV, tibial tubercle. Subtype is determined by stability and timing: subtype A, component is well fixed; subtype B, component is loose; subtype C, fracture occurs intraoperatively. This classification groups fractures based on treatment options, which in turn provides guidance for the surgeon and allows standardization for further research.

MANAGEMENT

Best practice guidelines have not been established for the management of periprosthetic tibial fractures due to the limited availability of high-quality literature on the topic and the high variability in fracture location, pattern, and underlying component fixation. Despite these shortcomings, it is important for surgeons to assess implant stability, alignment, bone quality, and bone loss when choosing a management strategy.[12] Potential strategies include nonoperative management, fixation with screws and/or plate(s), intramedullary nailing, cerclage cables, external fixation, and revision TKA. Intraoperative fractures have been independently assessed with unique strategies proposed for assessment and management of these complications.[10,50,51]

Nonoperative Management

Nonoperative management is an option in patients who are not surgical candidates and for PPFxs that are nondisplaced or stable when reduced with a well-fixed tibial implant (Fig. 2).[12–14] The treatment algorithm proposed by Felix and colleagues[14] recommends 6 to 8 weeks of protected non–weight bearing with brace or cast for a stable tibial plateau, nondisplaced fractures involving the implant stem, and nondisplaced fractures distal to the stem.[13,52,53] It is important that implants remain well fixed and alignment is maintained throughout the healing process for a successful outcome with conservative management. Healing and alignment are best monitored using close follow-up with serial imaging.[53] Although nonoperative treatment may avoid the risks associated with surgery, this strategy comes at

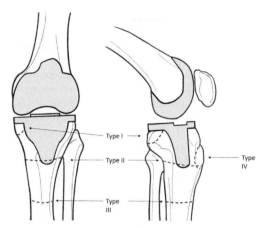

Fig. 1. The Felix classification system for PPFx. Type I, tibial plateau; type II, involves the component stem; type III, distal to stem; type IV, tibial tubercle. Subtype A, component is well fixed; subtype B, component is loose; subtype C, fracture occurs intraoperatively. (*Adapted from* Felix NA, Stuart MJ, Hanssen D. Periprosthetic tibial fractures associated with total knee arthroplasty. Clin Orthop Relat Res 1997;345:113–24; with permission.)

the cost of a delay in the return of ambulatory function (typically 6–12 weeks) and risks associated with immobilization such as pressure sores and deep vein thrombosis.[54,55] It is important to avoid bed rest, even in the short term, because this can cause significant declines in muscle mass and muscle strength with increased morbidity and mortality.[19,56,57]

Plate Fixation

Plate fixation is a common method used for fracture management with a variety of available plate shapes and lengths that can be used to obtain fracture stabilization. Plate fixation can typically allow the surgeon to meet the AO principles for successful fixation to include anatomic restoration of the anatomy, attainment of fracture stability, preservation of blood supply for healing, and rapid postoperative mobility.[58]

The locking compression plate has proved to be an effective fixation tool for the management of tibial PPFx in the setting of a stable underlying TKA implant (**Fig. 3**).[12,51,53] Nagwadia and Prateek[36] colleagues recommend using a minimum of 3 locking screws in proximal tibia fractures to attain fracture stability when using a singular plate construct. The most difficult part of plate fixation is getting purchase in the proximal tibia around the tibial implant. Fractures distal to the arthroplasty stem have been successfully treated with either locking or nonlocking plate techniques.[36,59] Locking attachment plates are useful

to gain fixation around revision stems. Verma and colleagues[59] have recommended minimally invasive techniques with locked compression plating in an effort to preserve soft tissue integrity and blood flow for optimal healing. Anatomic reduction is very important especially in less-comminuted fractures, and the surgeon should not hesitate to open the fracture for reduction purposes (**Fig. 4**).

The surgeon may choose to use single- or double-plate fixation to maintain alignment and provide immediate stabilization based on fracture characteristics. Dual plating may be a better option for proximal tibial fractures in proximity to pre-existing tibial implants, whereas single plating constructs can often provide adequate fixation for fractures distal to the implant stem (**Fig. 5**).[8] Other factors such as comminution, soft tissue trauma, bone quality, and segmental fracture patterns can influence the surgical decision for single versus dual plating.

Intramedullary Fixation

Despite adequate evidence for the use of locking plates in the setting of periprosthetic tibia fracture, intramedullary nail fixation is an option for the treatment of fractures distal to the tibial implant.[60] Intramedullary nailing frequently allows for immediate weight bearing, which may not be advocated in the setting of plate fixation. Surgeons are typically comfortable with antegrade intramedullary nailing because it is frequently the preferred approach for tibial shaft fractures, but the presence of prosthetic implants complicates the surgical approach because the existing implant interferes with the standard starting point.[60,61] This surgical fixation option is typically reserved for the subset of TKA PPFxs with more distal fracture patterns where there is sufficient space proximally for nail insertion to avoid the implant with the required starting point.[60] Intramedullary nail may be an option in patients with PPFxs associated with unicompartmental knee arthroplasty, because the natural anatomy of the proximal tibia is better preserved and more accessible.[62]

Several variations of cerclage wiring and cable fixation have been described in case studies for the management of periprosthetic tibial fractures.[13,41,51] These techniques are useful in comminuted or avulsed proximal tibial fractures.[63] Banim and colleagues[64] described using a Dall-Miles (Stryker, Mahwah, NJ, USA) plate and cable fixation strategy for a proximal fracture. Cables must be carefully passed to avoid neurovascular damage.[64] Although a few studies

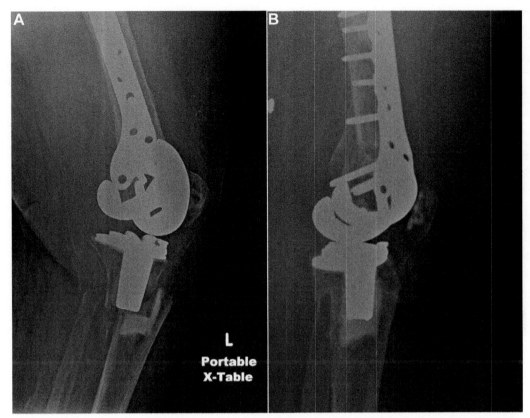

Fig. 2. Lateral view of PPFx of the left knee. (*A*) The fracture is a type IIa with Felix classification. The tibial component seems to be fixed proximally, but the fracture has gone through the cement mantle with anterior translation of the distal piece. (*B*) A lateral radiograph at 6-month follow-up is shown. The fracture was reduced using closed technique and treated with a cast for 6 weeks and then a knee brace. The fracture healed radiographically, and the patient began walking at 3 months after injury.

have analyzed this treatment strategy, wires and cables may have additional utility as a supplemental fixation tool in the management of complex PPFxs with otherwise limited bone surface area for plate or screw fixation.

External Fixation
External fixation is a minimally invasive approach to periprosthetic tibia fracture management. This strategy can provide patients the opportunity to weight bear quicker when compared with nonoperative management because relative stability is provided by spanning the fracture and the knee joint. Circular ring fixation has the additional advantage of allowing for gradual multiplanar correction following the initial reduction obtained at the time of fixation placement surgery.[65] Despite these potential advantages, there are significant potential risks associated with using external fixation as a definitive treatment in the setting of a retained TKA. Risks include decreased mobility from the fixator

device, the potential for joint stiffness due to knee immobilization, and increased risk of prosthetic joint infection due to the proximity of the pin sites to the joint and knee replacement implant.[66]

Revision Total Knee Arthroplasty
Revision TKA is the standard of care for PPFxs associated with component loosening or implant instability.[14,19,67] Revision TKA should also be considered if the fracture is associated with uncorrectable malalignment or prior failure of fixation.[63] A stemmed component that extends beyond the fracture should be used when possible to provide appropriate stability and fixation.[51] Literature involving periprosthetic hip fracture management suggests that the stemmed component should bypass the fracture site by at least 2 cortical diameters; however, this has not been established in tibial literature.[68,69] Fractures that cannot be adequately treated with revision arthroplasty alone may

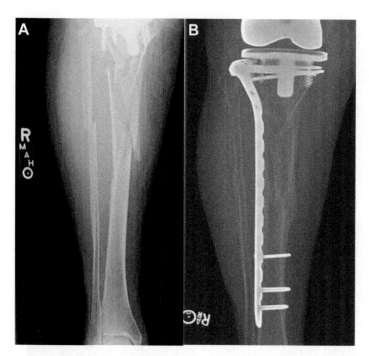

Fig. 3. Anteroposterior view of PPFx of the right knee. (A) The injury films show a type IIa with Felix classification. The fracture is below a well-fixed uncemented tibial implant and has considerable comminution. The fracture extends to the middiaphysis of the tibia. (B) Six-month postoperative fracture radiograph. A locking plate was placed using bridging technique, and the fracture is radiographically healed.

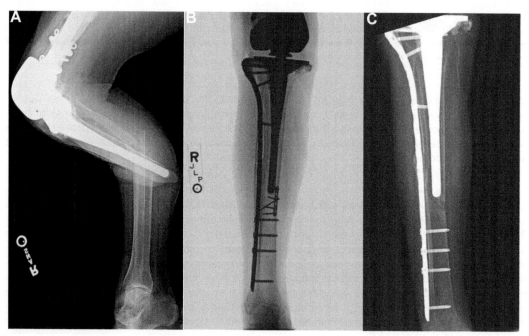

Fig. 4. Periprosthetic fracture of right knee. (A) Lateral injury view. This fracture is a type IIa with Felix classification. Revision implants are in place, and the fracture is at the tip of a well-fixed long revision stem. (B) Intraoperative anterior/posterior view fixed with lateral bridging plate. The fracture was opened and directly reduced and held with an initial 2.7-mm plate. The lateral plate was then placed for fixation. (C) Anteroposterior view of PPFx 6 months postoperatively. The 2.7-mm plate was removed at 6 weeks due to a traumatic open wound. Fracture and wound healed without infection.

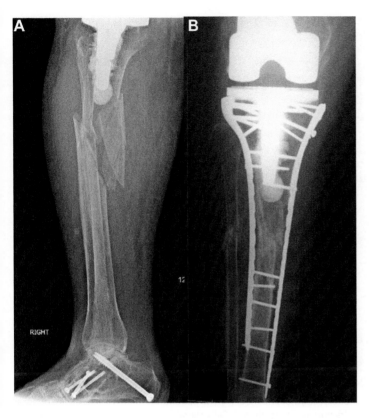

Fig. 5. Radiological views of a PPFx of the right knee. (A) Injury lateral view shows a well-fixed cemented tibial component with small stem. This fracture is a Felix IIa classification with extensive comminution and a large posterior fracture fragment. (B) Anteroposterior view at 6 months after fracture. Dual plating was used for fixation due to the extensive comminution. Radiographic healing is shown.

require supplemental fracture fixation.[51] Patients with massive bone loss or severely comminuted fractures may require bone grafts, bone cement, or secondary stabilization with metaphyseal cones, augments, or screws to secure the revised implant.[52,70] Proximal tibial replacement with megaprosthesis may provide a viable option for patients who have previously undergone several revisions or have a type Ib Felix fracture (Fig. 6).[71] Care should be taken during fixation to leave the tibial tubercle in place to maintain the extensor mechanism. If the extensor mechanism cannot be maintained, alternatives include extensor mechanism reconstruction, modular knee fusion, or above-knee amputation.[72]

Special Considerations

Patients with polytrauma with a periprosthetic tibial fracture may need special consideration when planning surgical management. It is important for the surgeon to prioritize life-threatening injuries while also minimizing the risk of infection. A staged approach may be necessary in these rare cases.[73] Open fractures with exposed or communicating arthroplasty components present a significant risk for infection. Few case reports of

open PPFxs have been published.[61,73–75] All documented reports have been associated with high-energy injuries. If arthroplasty components are not grossly contaminated, stable implants may be retained, but thorough irrigation, debridement, and antibiotic prophylaxis should precede wound closure.[61,73,75,76] The surgeon must also be aware of the potential for pre-existing prosthetic TKA infection with resultant bone loss and implant loosening that can lead to fracture. Treatment can be challenging in this setting of underlying prosthetic infection with PPFxs because surgical management must seek to promote fracture healing while treating the infection.[77] Surgical management frequently necessitates removal of the infected implant. Consideration should be given for placement of an articulating versus static spacer when viable, along with fixation of the fracture.[78,79] Antibiotic cement-coated plates or nails can be used to address this unique challenge.

Intraoperative Management

Patients who sustain an intraoperative fracture at the time of TKA have a higher subsequent rate of revision when compared with patients without fracture.[9,10,25] It is important to recognize this

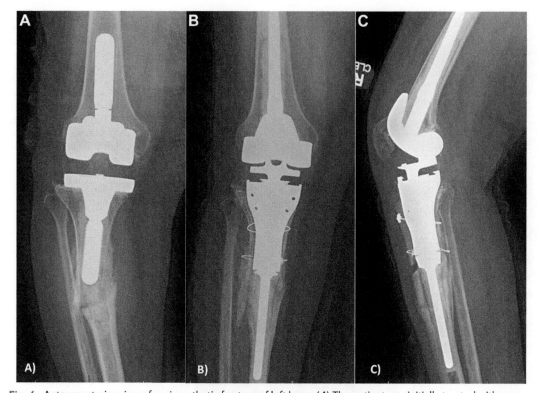

Fig. 6. Anteroposterior view of periprosthetic fracture of left knee. (*A*) The patient was initially treated with nonoperative management without healing. This fracture is a type IIIa with Felix classification. The fracture is through the cement mantle at the tip of a well-fixed revision stem. (*B*) Anteroposterior view 6 months postoperatively. (*C*) Lateral view 6 months postoperatively. Revision surgery was chosen because of the chronic nature of the nonunion. The proximal tibia further fractured when removing the cement and well-fixed prosthesis. The implants were revised with a proximal tibia replacement megaprosthesis and cerclage wires. The new stem bypasses the previous nonunion.

complication when it occurs to avoid a delay in treatment or need for return to the operating room. Several different fixation methods have been described for intraoperative tibial fractures at the time of TKA. Surgical fixation using partially threaded 3.5-mm cancellous screws that are inserted while the bone cement is still setting has been described for vertical fractures of the medial plateau anterior cortex.[50] In another study of intraoperative tibial PPFxs, 77.7% (42 of 54) were treated without intervention, whereas 16.7% (9 of 54) required screws and/or plate fixation and the remaining 5.5% (3 of 54) of fractures were managed using a combination of bone cement, cables, plates, and screws.[51] Other options include bridging the fracture site with a longer-stemmed tibial component or supplemental plate fixation.[10]

OUTCOMES

Periprosthetic tibial fractures encompass a small proportion of TKA-related complications, but these injuries can pose a significant challenge. Missed or untreated fractures can cause early component failure.[29] Even when these fractures are appropriately detected and managed early, there is a high nonunion rate (23.7%; [9 of 38]) with many patients requiring a second operation (31.6%; [12 of 38]).[8] A study examining early and late outcomes of periprosthetic tibial fractures found that Felix type II fractures are at the highest risk of nonunion when compared with type I and III. In this same cohort, readmission rates for all Felix PPFxs exceeded 50%.[80]

SUMMARY

It is hard to draw conclusions in regard to the best practice for the treatment of periprosthetic tibial fractures because this injury occurs infrequently and with a high variability of presentation. The surgeon has many treatment options as we have described, and we recommend that surgeons use AO principles when selecting the optimal fixation or revision strategy based on a comprehensive evaluation of the patient and fracture pattern. The treatment of periprosthetic tibial fractures remains an area of orthopedic surgery ripe for further study. A well-conducted consortium study would be an appropriate next step for further standardizing the treatment of this rare but potentially devastating injury.

CLINICS CARE POINTS

- Periprosthetic tibial fractures are rare.
- Several strategies can be used to manage periprosthetic fractures.
- Assessing the stability of the pre-existing prosthesis is essential for choosing proper management.
- Fracture pattern, alignment, and bone quality are important to consider when choosing fixation technique.

DISCLOSURE

C. Lowry Barnes receives royalties from DJO, Medtronic, and Zimmer; is a paid consultant for Health Trust, Medtronic, and Responsive Risk Solutions; receives research support from ConforMIS; and receives other financial/material support from Corin-Non-PI. The authors have no other disclosures to report.

ACKNOWLEDGMENTS

Special thanks to Dr Matt Graves, Professor of Orthopedic Surgery, University of Mississippi Medical Center, for contribution of many associated images.

REFERENCES

1. Doo Yoo J, Kim NK. Periprosthetic Fractures Following Total Knee Arthroplasty. Knee Surg Relat Res 2015;27:1–9.
2. Cordeiro E, Costa R, Carazzato J, et al. Periprosthetic Fractures in Patients With Total Knee Arthroplasties. Clin Orthop Relat Res 1990;252:182–9.
3. Dennis DA. Periprosthetic fractures following total knee arthroplasty. Tech Orthop 1999;14:138–43.
4. Sloan M, Premkumar A, Sheth NP. Projected volume of primary total joint arthroplasty in the u.s., 2014 to 2030. J Bone Joint Surg Am 2018;100: 1455–60.
5. Kurtz S, Ong K, Lau E, et al. Projections of Primary and Revision Hip and Knee Arthroplasty in the United States from 2005 to 2030. J Bone Jt Surg 2007;89:780–5.
6. Chang CB, Kim TK, Kang YG, et al. Prevalence of Osteoporosis in Female Patients with Advanced Knee Osteoarthritis Undergoing Total Knee Arthroplasty. J Korean Med Sci 2014;29:1425–31.
7. Bernatz JT, Krueger DC, Squire MW, et al. Unrecognized Osteoporosis Is Common in Patients With a Well-Functioning Total Knee Arthroplasty. J Arthroplasty 2019;34:2347–50.
8. Morwood MP, Gebhart SS, Zamith N, et al. Outcomes of fixation for periprosthetic tibia fractures around and below total knee arthroplasty. Injury 2019. https://doi.org/10.1016/j.injury.2019.03.014.
9. Purudappa PP, Ramanan SP, Tripathy SK, et al. Intra-operative fractures in primary total knee arthroplasty - a systematic review. Knee Surg Relat Res 2020;32:1–13.
10. Alden KJ, Duncan WH, Trousdale RT, et al. Intraoperative fracture during primary total knee arthroplasty. Clin Orthop Relat Res 2010;468:90–5.
11. Meinberg E, Agel J, Roberts C, et al. Fracture and Dislocation Classification Compendium—2018. J Orthop Trauma 2018;32:S1–10.
12. Konan S, Sandiford N, Unno F, et al. Periprosthetic fractures associated with total knee arthroplasty an update. Bone Joint J 2016;98-B:1489–96.
13. Benkovich V, Klassov Y, Mazilis B, et al. Periprosthetic fractures of the knee: a comprehensive review. Eur J Orthop Surg Traumatol 2020;30:387–99.
14. Felix NA, Stuart MJ, Hanssen AD. Periprosthetic fractures of the tibia associated with total knee arthroplasty. Clin Orthop Relat Res 1997;113–24. https://doi.org/10.1097/00003086-199712000-00016.
15. Rand JA, Coventry MB. Stress fractures after total knee arthroplasty. J Bone Joint Surg Am 1980;62: 226–33.
16. Singh JA, Jensen M, Lewallen D. Predictors of periprosthetic fracture after total knee replacement: An analysis of 21,723 cases. Acta Orthop 2013;84:170–7.
17. Ricci WM, Loftus T, Cox C, et al. Locked plates combined with minimally invasive insertion technique for the treatment of periprosthetic supracondylar femur fractures above a total knee arthroplasty. J Orthop Trauma 2006;20:190–6.
18. Meek RMD, Norwood T, Smith R, et al. The risk of peri-prosthetic fracture after primary and revision total hip and knee replacement. J Bone Joint Surg Br 2011;93 B:96–101.
19. Sarmah SS, Patel S, Reading G, et al. Periprosthetic fractures around total knee arthroplasty. Ann R Coll Surg Engl 2012;94:302–7.
20. Delasotta LA, Orozco F, Miller AG, et al. Distal femoral fracture during primary total knee arthroplasty. J Orthop Surg (Hong Kong) 2015;23:202–4.

21. Van Staa TP, Leufkens HGM, Abenhaim L, et al. Use of Oral Corticosteroids and Risk of Fractures. J Bone Miner Res 2000;15(6):993–1000.

22. Xue A-L, Wu S-Y, Jiang L, et al. Bone fracture risk in patients with rheumatoid arthritis. Medicine (Baltimore) 2017;96:e6983.

23. Huang C-C, Jiang C-C, Hsieh C-H, et al. Local bone quality affects the outcome of prosthetic total knee arthroplasty; Local bone quality affects the outcome of prosthetic total knee arthroplasty. J Orthop Res 2015. https://doi.org/10.1002/jor.23003.

24. Pinaroli A, Piedade SR, Servien E, et al. Intraoperative fractures and ligament tears during total knee arthroplasty. A 1795 posterostabilized TKA continuous series. Orthop Traumatol Surg Res 2009;95:183–9.

25. Sassoon AA, Wyles CC, Morales GAN, et al. Intraoperative Fracture During Aseptic Revision Total Knee Arthroplasty. J Arthroplasty 2014;29:2187–91.

26. Small SR, Ritter MA, Merchun JG, et al. Changes in tibial bone density measured from standard radiographs in cemented and uncemented total knee replacements after ten years' follow-up. Bone Joint J 2013;95 B:911–6.

27. Thompson NW, McAlinden MG, Breslin E, et al. Periprosthetic tibial fractures after cementless low contact stress total knee arthroplasty. J Arthroplasty 2001;16:984–90.

28. Rathsach Andersen M, Winther N, Lind T, et al. Bone remodeling of the proximal tibia after uncemented total knee arthroplasty: secondary endpoints analyzed from a randomized trial comparing monoblock and modular tibia trays-2 year follow-up of 53 cases. Acta Orthop 2019;90:479–83.

29. Completo A, Fonseca F, Simões JAS. Strain shielding in proximal tibia of stemmed knee prosthesis: Experimental study. J Biomech 2008;41:560–6.

30. Martin JR, Watts CD, Levy DL, et al. Medial Tibial Stress Shielding: A Limitation of Cobalt Chromium Tibial Baseplates. J Arthroplasty 2017;32:558–62.

31. Cipriano CA, Brown NM, Della Valle CJ, et al. Intraoperative periprosthetic fractures associated with press fit stems in revision total knee arthroplasty: Incidence, management, and outcomes. J Arthroplasty 2013;28:1310–3.

32. Agarwala S, Bajwa S, Vijayvargiya M. Intra- operative fractures in primary Total Knee Arthroplasty. J Clin Orthop Trauma 2019;10:571–5.

33. Charng JR, Chen ACY, Chan YS, et al. Proximal tibial morphology and risk of posterior tibial cortex impingement in patients with AA-sized Oxford unicompartmental knee arthroplasty tibial implants. J Orthop Surg Res 2020;15. https://doi.org/10.1186/s13018-020-01900-6.

34. Perillo-Marcone A, Taylor M. Effect of varus/valgus malalignment on bone strains in the proximal tibia after TKR: An explicit finite element study. J Biomech Eng 2007;129:1–11.

35. Hegde V, Bracey DN, Brady AC, et al. A Prophylactic Tibial Stem Reduces Rates of Early Aseptic Loosening in Patients with Severe Preoperative Varus Deformity in Primary Total Knee Arthroplasty. J Arthroplasty 2021. https://doi.org/10.1016/j.arth.2021.01.049.

36. Nagwadia H, Prateek J. Outcome of osteosynthesis for periprosthetic fractures after total knee arthroplasty: a retrospective study. Eur J Orthop Surg Traumatol 2018;28:683–90.

37. Ritter MA, Carr K, Keating EM, et al. Tibial shaft fracture following tibial tubercle osteotomy. J Arthroplasty 1996;11:117–9.

38. Lu C, Ye G, Liu W, et al. Tibial plateau fracture related to unicompartmental knee arthroplasty Two case reports and literature review. Medicine (Baltimore) 2019. https://doi.org/10.1097/MD.0000000000017338.

39. Yang KY, Yeo SJ, Lo NN. Stress fracture of the medial tibial plateau after minimally invasive unicompartmental knee arthroplasty: A report of 2 cases. J Arthroplasty 2003;18:801–3.

40. Hung YW, Chi-Ho Fan J, Ka-Bon Kwok C, et al. Delayed tibial-platform periprosthetic stress fracture after unicompartmental knee arthroplasty: Uncommon and devastating complication. J Orthop Trauma Rehabil 2018;25:29–33.

41. Kumar A, Chambers I, Wong P. Periprosthetic Fracture of the Proximal Tibia After Lateral Unicompartmental Knee Arthroplasty. J Arthroplasty 2008;23:615–8.

42. Sloper PJH, Hing CB, Donell ST, et al. Intra-operative tibial plateau fracture during unicompartmental knee replacement: A case report. Knee 2003;10:367–9.

43. Hoke D, Jafari SM, Orozco F, et al. Tibial Shaft Stress Fractures Resulting from Placement of Navigation Tracker Pins. J Arthroplasty 2011;26:504.e5-8.

44. Brown MJ, Matthews JR, Bayers-Thering MT, et al. Low Incidence of Postoperative Complications With Navigated Total Knee Arthroplasty. J Arthroplasty 2017;32:2120–6.

45. Khakha RS, Chowdhry M, Norris M, et al. Low incidence of complications in computer assisted total knee arthroplasty-A retrospective review of 1596 cases. Knee 2015;22:416–8.

46. Smith TJ, Siddiqi A, Forte SA, et al. Periprosthetic Fractures Through Tracking Pin Sites Following Computer Navigated and Robotic Total and Unicompartmental Knee Arthroplasty. JBJS Rev 2021;9. e20.00091.

47. Chun-sing Chui E, Chun-man Lau L, Ka-bon Kwok C, et al. Tibial cutting guide (resector) holding pins position and subsequent risks of periprosthetic fracture in unicompartmental knee arthroplasty: a finite element analysis study. J Orthop Surg Res 2021. https://doi.org/10.1186/s13018-021-02308-6.

48. Unified Classification System for Periprosthetic Fractures (UCPF). J Orthop Trauma 2018;32:S141–4.

49. Duncan C, Masri B. Fractures of the Femur After Hip Replacement. Instr Course Lect 1995;44:293–304.

50. Pun AHF, Pun WK, Storey P. Intra-operative fracture in posterior-stabilised total knee arthroplasty. J Orthop Surg 2015;23:205–8.

51. Ebraheim NA, Ray JR, Wandtke ME, et al. Systematic review of periprosthetic tibia fracture after total knee arthroplasties. World J Orthop 2015;6:649–54.

52. Hanssen AD, Stuart MJ. Treatment of periprosthetic tibial fractures. Clin Orthop Relat Res 2000;91–8. https://doi.org/10.1097/00003086-200011000-00013.

53. Agarwal S, Sharma RK, Jain JK. Periprosthetic fractures after total knee arthroplasty. J Orthop Surg 2014;22:24–9.

54. Dennis DA. Periprosthetic Fractures Following Total Knee Arthroplasty. J Bone Jt Surg 2001;83:120–30.

55. Culp R, Schmidt R, Hanks G, et al. Supracondylar fracture of the femur following prosthetic knee arthroplasty. Clin Orthop Relat Res 1987;(222):212–22.

56. Dirks ML, Wall BT, Van De Valk B, et al. One week of bed rest leads to substantial muscle atrophy and induces whole-body insulin resistance in the absence of skeletal muscle lipid accumulation. Diabetes 2016;65:2862–75.

57. Prado CM, Purcell SA, Alish C, et al. Implications of low muscle mass across the continuum of care: a narrative review. Ann Med 2018;50:675–93.

58. Buckley R, Moran C, Apivatthakakul T, editors. AO principles of fracture management. Thieme. Stuttgart, Germany: Theime; 2018. https://doi.org/10.1055/b-006-149767.

59. Verma N, Jain A, Pal C, et al. Management of periprosthetic fracture following total knee arthroplasty-a retrospective study to decide when to fix or when to revise? J Clin Orthop Trauma 2020. https://doi.org/10.1016/j.jcot.2019.10.005.

60. Haller JM, Kubiak EN, Spiguel A, et al. Intramedullary nailing of tibial shaft fractures distal to total knee arthroplasty. J Orthop Trauma 2014;28:e296–300.

61. Greco N, Goyal K, Tarkin I. Intragrade intramedullary nailing of an open tibial shaft fracture in a patient with concomitant ipsilateral total knee arthroplasty. Am J Orthop (Belle Mead Nj) 2015;44:E81–6.

62. Born CT, Gil JA, Johnson JP. Periprosthetic tibial fractures. J Am Acad Orthop Surg 2018;26:e167–72.

63. Kuzyk PRT, Watts E, Backstein D. Revision Total Knee Arthroplasty for the Management of Periprosthetic Fractures. J Am Acad Orthop Surg 2017;25:624–33.

64. Banim RH, Fletcher M, Warren P. Use of a Dall-Miles plate and cables for the fixation of a periprosthetic tibial fracture. J Arthroplasty 2000;15:131–3.

65. Assayag MJ, Bor N, Rubin G, et al. Circular hexapod external fixation for periprosthetic tibial fracture. Arthroplast Today 2018;4:192–9.

66. Nozaka K, Miyakoshi N, Hongo M, et al. Effectiveness of circular external fixator in periprosthetic fractures around the knee. BMC Musculoskelet Disord 2020;21:1–9.

67. Haidukewych GJ, Langford JR, Liporace FA. Revision for periprosthetic fractures of the hip and knee. Instr Course Lect 2013;62:333–40.

68. Larson JE, Chao EYS, Fitzgerald RH. Bypassing femoral cortical defects with cemented intramedullary stems. J Orthop Res 1991;9:414–21.

69. Fleischman AN, Chen AF. Periprosthetic fractures around the femoral stem: overcoming challenges and avoiding pitfalls. Ann Transl Med 2015;3:234.

70. Ghazavi MT, Stockley I, Yee G, et al. Reconstruction of massive bone defects with allograft in revision total knee arthroplasty. J Bone Joint Surg Am 1997;79:17–25.

71. Windhager R, Schreiner M, Staats K, et al. Megaprostheses in the treatment of periprosthetic fractures of the knee joint: indication, technique, results and review of literature. Int Orthop 2016;40:935–43.

72. Mayes WH, Severin AC, Mannen EM, et al. Management of Periprosthetic Joint Infection and Extensor Mechanism Disruption With Modular Knee Fusion: Clinical and Biomechanical Outcomes. Arthroplast Today 2021;8:46–52.

73. Raglan K, Cherney SM, Stambough JB, et al. Open Periprosthetic Knee Fracture: A Case Report and Review of the Literature. Geriatr Orthop Surg Rehabil 2020;11. https://doi.org/10.1177/2151459320939547.

74. Devendra A, Gupta NP, Zackariya Jaffrulah M, et al. Management of Tibial Shaft Fractures Distal to TKA Prosthesis by Intramedullary Nail: A Report of Three Cases. Indian J Orthop 2020;54:901–8.

75. Gulotta LV, Gardner MJ, Rose HA, et al. Periprosthetic patellar fracture after an open knee dislocation. Clin Orthop Relat Res 2005;265–9. https://doi.org/10.1097/01.blo.0000162999.01156.d1.

76. Masmoudi K, Grissa Y, Benzarti S, et al. Open Periprosthetic Patellar Fracture after Total Knee Replacement. J Orthop Case Rep 2016;6:89–91.

77. Lazic I, Scheele C, Pohlig F, et al. Treatment options in PJI – is two-stage still gold standard? J Orthop 2021;23:180–4.

78. Kapadia BH, Berg RA, Daley JA, et al. Periprosthetic joint infection. Lancet 2016;387:386–94.

79. Puhto A-P, Puhto TM, Niinimäki TT, et al. Two-Stage Revision for Prosthetic Joint Infection: Outcome and Role of Reimplantation Microbiology in 107 Cases. J Arthroplasty 2014. https://doi.org/10.1016/j.arth.2013.12.027.

80. Pannu TS, Villa JM, Cohen EM, et al. Periprosthetic Tibial Fractures After Total Knee Arthroplasty: Early and Long-Term Clinical Outcomes. J Arthroplasty 2021;36:1429–36.

Shoulder and Elbow

Decision-Making and Management of Proximal Humerus Nonunions

David Clayton Tapscott, MD, Edward Scott Paxton, MD*

KEYWORDS

- Allograft • Proximal humerus nonunion • Revision proximal humerus fracture

---

KEY POINTS

- Proximal humerus fracture nonunions are a heterogenous group of injuries that require an individualized treatment plan.
- Understanding the residual bone stock allows for better patient management and choice of treatment.
- Open reduction internal fixation, intramedullary nailing, and reverse arthroplasty are all reasonable treatment choices in the correct patient.
- Demineralized bone matrix, cortical strut allograft, and synthetic bone graft substitute should be given strong consideration when considering open reduction internal fixation of a proximal humerus nonunion.
- Reverse shoulder arthroplasty for proximal humerus nonunion is a viable choice; the tuberosity fragments should be maintained whenever possible to augment stability.

INTRODUCTION/BACKGROUND/PREVALENCE

Proximal humerus fractures are a very common injury in the elderly population in the United States and abroad. Multiple studies have looked at the incidence of this injury. Launonen and colleagues retrospectively studied patient records from a region in Finland between 2006 and 2010. In that study the incidence was 82/100,000 person years.[1] They also demonstrated a clear seasonal variation in the timing of the fractures. Court-Brown and colleagues performed a 5-year prospective study and found 2-part proximal humerus fractures having a mean age of 72 years.[2] They also demonstrated a unimodal age distribution with no patient younger than 50 years having this fracture. Roux and colleagues report an odds ratio of 2:1 for female to male for proximal humerus fractures.[3] They reported risk factors for osteoporosis and falls being main predictors. Incidence

of nonunion of these fractures has been reported as about 1.4% in a large database review study.

Definition of Proximal Humerus Nonunion

In literature, there has not been a single consistent definition of the time required to diagnose a nonunion after a proximal humerus fracture. Norris and colleagues defined the time period required as 3 months and began treating patients after that point as a nonunion.[4] Other investigators have used a time period of 1 year without radiologic signs of a union in their definitions. A large Medicare database study by Klement and colleagues showed an increasing number of patients being diagnosed as having a nonunion at the 3-month, 6-month, and 12-month time point; this implies that there is no universally agreed on definition, and it can be inferred that treating surgeons used different time thresholds to make the diagnosis as the time from injury lengthened.

Brown University, 1 Kettle Point Avenue, East Providence, RI 02914, USA
* Corresponding author.
E-mail address: espaxton@universityorthopedics.com

Orthop Clin N Am 52 (2021) 369–379
https://doi.org/10.1016/j.ocl.2021.05.008

We use 6 months from injury or fixation (if treated operatively) without radiographic union as our definition.

Proximal Humerus Nonunion Classification

In 2000, Checchia and colleagues devised a classification scheme for nonunions of the proximal humerus based on 21 shoulders in 20 patients from their institution over 6-year period as well as a review of the available literature at the time.

Checchia classification

- Group 1—high, 2-part nonunion (Fig. 1)
  - Fracture at the anatomic neck with very small proximal fragment
  - Includes 3-part factures if the tuberosity fragment has now consolidated in a position displaced less than 5 mm
- Group 2—low, 2-part nonunion (Fig. 2)
  - Two-part fracture of the surgical neck
  - Includes consolidated lesser tuberosity fragments if displaced less than 5 mm
- Group 3—complex nonunion (Fig. 3)
  - Nonunion secondary to 3-part, 4-part, or head-split fractures
  - Residual displacement of the tuberosities greater than 5 mm, even if consolidated
- Group 4—lost fragment nonunion (Fig. 4)
  - Usually occurs after open fracture and/or posttraumatic osteomyelitis of the proximal humerus
  - Defined as a missing segment of bone

The investigators noted that the differentiation between Group 1 and Group 2 is with respect to the proximal fragment. They noted that a very small proximal fragment with significant cavitation into the metaphyseal cancellous bone of the head may necessitate a different surgical treatment option. They noted that often in type 1 there would be very limited bone stock for fixation and healing based on previous reported results.[4]

Proximal Humerus Nonunion Predictors

In 2016, Klement and colleagues used the Pearl Diver database to evaluate more than 300,000 proximal humerus fractures. Arthritis of the shoulder was a predictor of nonunion with a 2.97% rate of nonunion in patients with osteoarthritis and a 3.17% rate of nonunion with rheumatoid arthritis of the shoulder, which is compared with a nonunion rate of 1.36% at 12 months in patients without either of these diagnoses.

In 2008, Court-Brown and colleagues retrospectively reported on 1027 consecutive proximal humerus fractures with complete data on 995 cases. Of these fractures, 89.1% were treated nonoperatively. Eleven (1.1%) fractures failed to unite in this cohort. In subgroup analysis, they report that the rate of nonunion in their 520 displaced proximal humerus fractures was 1.7% whereas only 0.4% in 507 minimally displaced fractures. These data were able to offer some insight into certain fracture patterns with a higher rate of nonunion.

Court-Brown nonunion rates by OTA classification:

- 3.8% of translated surgical neck fractures (A3.2)
- 4.3% of comminuted surgical neck fractures (A3.3)
- 4.2% of bifocal fractures with head rotation (B2.2)
- 33.3% of comminuted bifocal fractures (B2.3)
- 8.3% of displaced articular fractures (C2.3)

Hanson and colleagues prospectively followed 124 proximal humerus fractures out to 1 year of treatment. At 1 year, 93% of the patients had a union by radiographic evaluation with the median time to union of 14 weeks. They reported a statistically significant risk factor of smoking for nonunion, with 20.8% of their smokers going on to nonunion versus 4.5% of the nonsmoking patients.[5]

In a systematic review of the literature, Cagle evaluated 508 patients who were surgically treated for the diagnosis of proximal humerus fracture nonunion. In that group, 64% of the patients had sustained a 2-part fracture, whereas 12.6% had 4-part fractures, although the prevalence of the fracture types of the demographics is unknown.

From the studies, several risk factors for nonunion can be concluded. These risk factors included displaced 2-part proximal humerus fracture, smoking, preexisting glenohumeral osteoarthritis or rheumatoid arthritis, OTA B2.3 and C2.3 fractures, and metaphyseal comminution.

PATIENT EVALUATION

Biological Considerations in Nonunion

In addition to mechanical factors, a treating surgeon must consider the biological factors that can contribute to a nonunion of any fracture site. It is reasonable to work up these patients

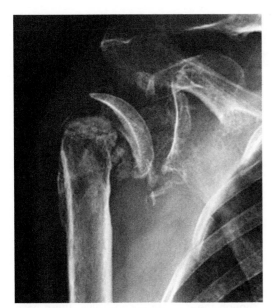

Fig. 1. Group 1 head type fragment with very thin residual bone stock present beneath the articular segment.

for possible biological or infectious causes of their nonunion. Certainly, in patients who have been previously operated on, it is prudent to rule out infectious causes of the nonunions. In 2020, Brinker and colleagues reported on 204 subjects with 211 nonunions who were older than 18 years and had a nonunion requiring surgery. Of the reported 211 nonunions, 62 were

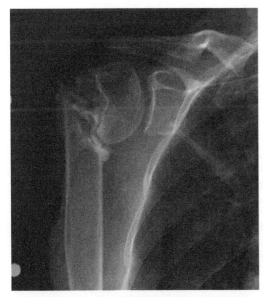

Fig. 2. Group 2 fracture with excellent residual bone stock available in the head fragment.

open fractures, 141 were closed fractures, and the initial injury status was unknown in 8 of the cases. Eighty-nine percent of these nonunions as evaluated by this team had undergone 1 or more previous operative procedures.[6]

The research team directly sampled medullary canal tissue from all 211 nonunion sites. They then compared these gold-standard culture base diagnoses against preoperative laboratories including a white blood cell count, erythrocyte sedimentation rate, and C-reactive protein (CRP) before surgery. This study found that when treating all comers for nonunion, these preoperative laboratories were not predictive in any statistically significant way.[6]

Conversely, Stucken and colleagues reported on 93 patients with 95 nonunions in 2013. They reported that 30 of the 95 nonunions were ultimately diagnosed as being infected. They determined that an elevated CRP at the time of initial evaluation had an odds ratio of 4.2 for infection, whereas an elevated erythrocyte sedimentation rate (ESR) had an odds ratio of 5.2 for infection. Both of these findings reached statistical significance in their study.[7] The white blood cell count alone or the indium scan alone did not have any statistically significant positive predictive value in their study. This study team defined an elevated CRP, ESR, or white blood cell count as a positive finding and developed a model for predicting infection based on the number of positives for each patient. They determined 18.3%, 23.5%, 50%, and 85.7% probability of infection based on having 0, 1, 2, or 3 positives for the patient, respectively.[7]

Based on these and other studies, it is reasonable to obtain inflammatory markers before surgical intervention if there is any concern for infection, particularly on a patient who had been previously treated surgically. However, in the complex clinical picture of infection, especially in the setting of less virulent organisms such as *cutibacterium acnes*, we conclude that positive or negative inflammatory markers in isolation are not sufficient to include or exclude the possibility of an infected nonunion. Further evaluation with intraoperative cultures or dedicated biopsy may be reasonable, and indeed prudent, in clinical settings where there is a high suspicion of infection. More study is needed in this field to be able to offer definitive recommendations.

Endocrine-Specific Nonunion Considerations

Endocrine abnormalities can contribute to nonunion in both operatively and nonoperatively treated proximal humerus fractures, especially in

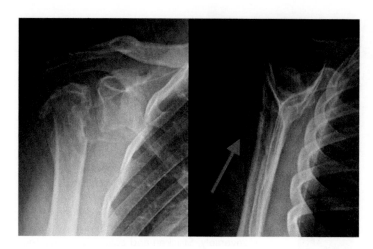

Fig. 3. Group 3 nonunion after a proximal humerus fracture dislocation; the red arrow indicates the residual head fragment in a chronically dislocated position.

the setting of oligotrophic nonunions. In 2007, Brinker and colleagues reported on metabolic findings of nonunion and recommended a laboratory panel including 25 hydroxycholecalciferol, ionized calcium, parathyroid hormone, alkaline phosphatase, phosphorus, thyroid stimulating hormone, and/or free testosterone be ordered if endocrine drivers for nonunion are of concern. Although the data are inconclusive, there have been studies to suggest that low levels of vitamin D, and low levels of calcium may contribute to the development of nonunions.[8] Anabolic agents, including hormone analogues such as teriparatide, have shown promise in small off-label studies to facilitate fracture union[9] but have yet to be proved safe and effective as a standard adjunct in the setting of nonunion.

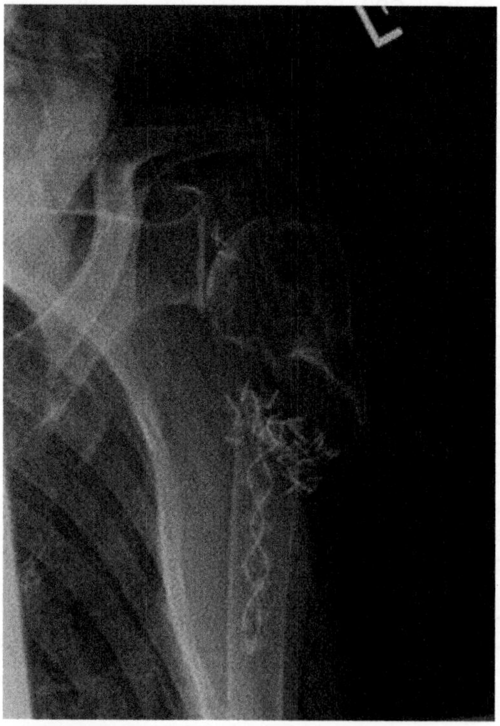

If there is concern for any metabolic abnormality, a basic metabolic workup should be obtained. Treating physicians should have a very low threshold to perform this evaluation. The investigators recommend initial endocrine laboratory evaluations of the following:

- 25-hydroxycholecalciferol
- Ionized calcium
- Parathyroid hormone
- Alkaline phosphatase
- Phosphorus
- Thyroid stimulating hormone
- Free testosterone

In addition, as smoking has been associated with nonunion, tobacco cessation should be implemented. In the setting of suspected metabolic nonunions, early involvement of an endocrine specialist may be prudent.

Radiographic Evaluation

Plain radiographs are often sufficient for diagnosis, including 4 views of the affected shoulder (anteroposterior, Grashey view, outlet view, and axillary lateral). Fine-cut computed tomography scan will allow for evaluation of any cavitary defects or bone loss that may not be appreciated

Fig. 4. Group 4 nonunion after debridement with large missing calcar segment after aggressive debridement and placement of antibiotic beads for fracture osteomyelitis.

on the radiographs. Furthermore, 3-dimensional imaging allows for better understanding of fragment position and fracture morphology and is beneficial in preoperative planning. Occasionally, computed tomography may be necessary for the diagnosis of nonunion, especially if hypertrophic or in fibrous nonunions. MRI is rarely needed, but if rotator cuff pathology is suspected, this study is useful.

TREATMENT

Nonoperative Treatment of Proximal Humerus Nonunion

Every proximal humerus nonunion must be given consideration for nonoperative management. Although the patient may continue to have suboptimal function of the shoulder, the risks of surgery may be too great in certain populations. Consideration must also be given to the overall instability of the nonunion. Certain fibrous nonunions may be stable enough for function in low-demand individuals. Frank conversations about the expectations and probability/possibility of improvement should be had with every patient before considering surgical intervention for a proximal humerus nonunion. If a patient is not medically, mentally, or situationally ready to proceed with intervention, nonoperative management should be undertaken.

Bone stimulators, including stimulation with low-intensity pulsed ultrasound, may be a reasonable option in patients who are being considered for nonoperative treatment. There have been multiple studies regarding the application of these devices in the upper extremity. Mahr and colleagues retrospectively reviewed 933 delayed unions and 366 nonunions, reporting a mean fracture age of 150 days at the time of treatment. They reported a 76% success rate in the group of "humerus" patients. Although these data are not specific to proximal humerus fractures, it does suggest some viability in treating a patient with a bone stimulator.[10] Other studies have also demonstrated generally favorable outcomes in the setting of nonunion, with multiple studies reporting greater than 50% rate of union in nonunions in the upper extremity.[11]

Other investigators have called into question the reliability of some of the studies,[11] considering conflicts of interest of the investigators and possible industry bias. Given the minimal risk, we recommend considering bone stimulation in the setting of an early proximal humerus nonunion or in a patient who is not a good candidate for operative intervention.

Open Reduction and Internal Fixation for Proximal Humerus Nonunion

Open reduction and internal fixation of the fracture using a plate and screw construct has been described to treat certain proximal humeral nonunions with success. In the meta-data reported by Cagle and colleagues, it was found that fixed angle plating of the nonunion went on to union in 97% of patients at an average time of 5.7 months.[12] Interestingly, they found a nearly 95% rate of union in reports using nonlocked plates to treat these fractures. It is worth noting that a significant portion of the data in the nonlocked plating group may have been from a time before locked plating was considered a standard treatment and that fixed angle blades and current locked plating technology may be grouped in some reports.

Badman and colleagues reported on 18 metadiaphyseal proximal humerus fracture nonunions, 12 of which had initially been treated nonoperatively, and successfully attained union in 17 of 18 cases.[13] Prior operative treatments included proximal humerus open reduction and internal fixation as well as intramedullary nailing. They reported the use of fixed angle plating and an intramedullary cortical strut allograft as the surgical technique of choice with additional morselized bone graft in these patients. They were able to obtain union at an average of 5.4 months. The patients' ASES scores improved from 40 preoperatively to 81 postoperatively.

Rollo and colleagues reported on 16 proximal humerus nonunions, with 13 being either 3- or 4-part fractures, that were all initially treated nonoperatively. The patients underwent open reduction and internal fixation supplemented with an extramedullary cortical strut medially and allograft cancellous chip grafting of the fractures. They reported an average time to union of 126 days (4.2 months) and reported meaningful improvements in the patient-reported outcomes. They reported no cases of hardware failure, avascular necrosis, or infection.[14]

These studies suggest that open reduction internal fixation of a nonunited proximal humerus fracture may provide reliably good results for most of the patients treated. Furthermore, both of these papers used allograft cortical strut reinforcement of the calcar, one in intramedullary fashion and the other in an extramedullary fashion. Both used the use of cancellous allograft as well. Based on the aforementioned findings, it may be reasonable to consider some type of cortical strut as well as cancellous allograft chips in these cases. Important considerations for selecting open reduction internal fixation are adequate bone stock, particularly of the head fragment, viability of the tuberosity fragments, and a concentric articular surface on both the humeral and glenoid sides (**Fig. 5**). Group 2 fractures and some Group 4 fractures may be best suited for open reduction and internal fixation. Significant glenohumeral arthrosis is a relative contraindication to this treatment.

Intramedullary Nailing of a Proximal Humeral Nonunion

Cagle and colleagues compiled from the literature 50 nonunions treated by intramedullary nailing, 47 of those went on to unite at an average of 5 months.[12] Yanmane and colleagues reported on 13 patients with symptomatic proximal humerus nonunions being treated with a straight intramedullary nail. All but one of the cases were 2-part proximal humerus fractures, and most of these 2-part fractures were initially treated conservatively. Iliac crest cancellous autograft was used to fill the defect in 10 of the cases, and in the remaining cases a small defect was addressed using tricalcium phosphate paste. All proximal humerus fractures went on to union with no cases of avascular necrosis. Two patients required reoperation to remove proximal interlocking screws, which had backed out. Excellent results were reported in 4 shoulders, 7 reported good results, and 2 reported only fair results.[15] For 2-part fractures, intramedullary nailing is a viable option and should be supplemented with a bone graft or bone graft substitute, and the investigators recommend compressing across the fracture, with reverse nail impaction or other methods, before proximal locking to ensure good cortical contact. Group 2 fractures may be strong candidates for this technique. Further augmentation with demineralized bone matrix and/or cancellous chips may augment the biology and be advisable in some cases.

Hemiarthroplasty or Total Shoulder Arthroplasty

When joint preservation is not possible, shoulder arthroplasty is the surgical treatment of choice, with either anatomic or reverse shoulder arthroplasty. Boileau and colleagues originally reported on his fracture sequelae patients in 2001, including 6 patients with a type 3 sequelae (surgical neck nonunion). A greater tuberosity osteotomy was made in all 6 patients, as is necessary to treat a surgical neck nonunion with a hemiarthroplasty. They reported their worst results of all fracture sequalae treatment

with hemiarthroplasty in this patient group and recommended against arthroplasty to treat surgical neck nonunions, as they had poor healing of the greater tuberosity with poor outcomes.

The largest report on unconstrained anatomic shoulder arthroplasty for the treatment of proximal humerus nonunions was published by Duquin and colleagues in 2012. They reported on 67 patients in the Mayo Health System from 1976 to 2007 treated with either hemiarthroplasty or total shoulder arthroplasty for a proximal humerus nonunion. The arthroplasty was performed on a heterogenous group of nonunions. They reported a mean visual analogue scale pain score improvement from 8.3 preoperatively to 4.1 at the most recent follow-up. However, the mean patient's satisfaction score was only 5.7 on a 10-point scale, and only 33 of the 67 patients had a satisfactory or excellent result by the Neer result rating. They concluded that this was not a reliable way to provide a predictably beneficial outcome in the treatment of proximal humeral nonunions. They also found that tuberosity healing was inconsistent and significantly influences the functional outcome of these patients.[16] With these findings in mind, we can only recommend anatomic arthroplasty in the setting of well-positioned, united tuberosities and an intact cuff or in extenuating circumstances or the very young.

Reverse Shoulder Arthroplasty

Reverse shoulder arthroplasty has the benefit of less reliance on tuberosity healing compared with anatomic arthroplasty; however, reported complications rates are concerning. Cagle and colleagues found a 16% rate of prosthetic dislocation and a 4% rate of infection.[12] These figures far outpaces the average overall rate of instability in reverse total shoulder arthroplasty, including for acute fracture management. Importantly, they reported a 5-fold increase in the rate of prosthetic dislocation in patients who had a tuberosity resection at the time of reverse shoulder arthroplasty; this means that most of the instability was in the setting of complete metaphyseal excision.

Raiss and colleagues reported on 32 patients who were treated with reverse shoulder arthroplasty as a treatment of a nonunion of a proximal humerus fracture. The initial treatment of these fractures included nails, plates, and conservative management. These patients were reported to have mean increases in their constant scores from 14 to 46 points, as well as an increased forward flexion from 42° to 109°. However, they reported a remarkably high complication rate of

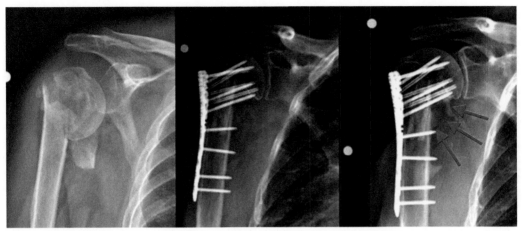

Fig. 5. Proximal humerus nonunion treated with ORIF, fibular strut allograft, and demineralized matrix placement. The red arrows denote the neocalcar formation at 1-year post op.

41%. Furthermore, they had a revision rate of 28%. The most common complication was dislocation, which occurred in 11 patients. They reported that 10 of the 11 dislocations occurred in patients in whom the tuberosity fragments as well as the head fragments were excised at the time of reverse shoulder arthroplasty. They could find no difference in the outcomes of reverse shoulder arthroplasty for the groups treated initially operatively versus nonoperatively. Tuberosity excision is not recommended.[17]

In 2016, Hattrup and colleagues reported on a variety of reverse total shoulders for posttraumatic sequelae of a proximal humerus fracture, including a group of patients reported on for a "type 3" sequelae, the description of a proximal humerus nonunion in the Boileau classification system.[18] They reported on 6 of these patients and demonstrated unsatisfactory outcomes based on their data collection in 3 of the patients due to unsatisfactory Neer scores in 2 and a dislocation with brachial plexopathy requiring revision surgery in the third.[18]

It should be noted that early reports of reverse shoulder arthroplasty revealed much higher complication rates than are currently seen with modern techniques. In 2020, Kuhlmann and colleagues reported mid-term results on 140 patients. One hundred two patients underwent acute reverse shoulder arthroplasty for fracture, whereas 38 underwent reverse shoulder arthroplasty after at least a 4-week trial of nonoperative treatment due to worsening displacement of the fracture. In these groups the tuberosity was repaired according to the attending surgeon's preference. They found no differences between the 2 groups with regard to complication rate or final outcome on midterm follow-up.[19]

Although concerns about stability persist, modernized implant designs and tuberosity retaining techniques can generate reproducible and reliable results with reverse shoulder arthroplasty. We recommend for reverse shoulder arthroplasty as a treatment of proximal humerus nonunions, particularly in the setting of cuff/tuberosity deficiency and/or inadequate bone stock of the humeral head fragment for fixation. We also recommend reverse shoulder arthroplasty in the cases of nonunion of preexisting shoulder arthritis (Fig. 6) or when there is concern about the viability of the head fragment. We strongly recommend maintaining and repairing any remnant tuberosities and being diligent in tensioning/balancing when performing reverse shoulder arthroplasty in the nonunion setting.

Biological Augmentation and Bone Grafting

The treatment of nonunions generally involves biological augmentation, especially in the setting of atrophic nonunions. Several grafting options can be considered in the treatment of a proximal humerus fracture nonunion. Autograft bones has many benefits; however, harvesting of iliac crest or other bone graft is not without its morbidity. Significant donor site morbidities associated with iliac crest harvest and complication rates have been reported from between 2.8% and nearly 38%. The complications can include persistent donor site pain, superficial sensory nerve damage, hematoma, infection, incisional hernia, donor site fracture, or vascular

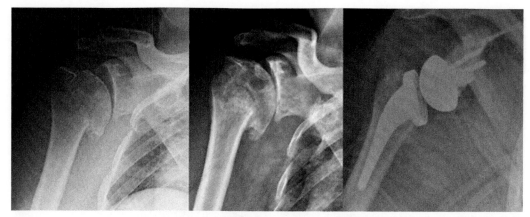

Fig. 6. Group II proximal humerus fracture that went on to nonunion immediately after injury, 1 year after nonsurgical treatment, and after conversion to reverse shoulder arthroplasty with tuberosity retention. Note the preexisting osteoarthritis.

injury.[20] Autograft, however, may yet have a role in the treatment of some segmental defects in which a viable, structural bone stock is needed.

Structural allografts, including fibular strut allograft as reported on by Badman and colleagues,[13] have been reported on with excellent results in proximal humerus fractures in both the primary and nonunion setting. These struts have the unique benefit of providing immediate mechanical support without donor site morbidity. Potential downsides include prolonged incorporation time, failure of incorporation, cost, difficulty if later arthroplasty revision is required along with standard graft risks of infection, and disease transmission. These grafts are osteoconductive but not osteoinductive or osteogenic.[21] The reports of their successful and safe use in both the proximal humerus as well as other sites in the upper and lower extremity make them an attractive option in the setting of proximal humerus nonunion treatment with open reduction internal fixation.

Demineralized bone matrix is generated by acid extraction of allograft bone material. It contains collagen as well as growth factors and proteins without the structural allograft bone. By containing these osteoinductive factors, demineralized bone matrix helps to encourage the formation of bone as well as provide increased surface area as an osteoconductive material. A more recent form of demineralized bone matrix is a cellular bone allograft, which includes viable bone matrices. Most reports to date on this group of graft substitutes have been positive, showing equivalent levels of fusion or higher levels of fusion when compared with autograft.[21] They also reported no decrease in efficacy when mixed in a 1:1 or 2:1 ratio with cancellous allograft. In a retrospective review of 78 humeral

shaft nonunions, a 97% rate of union was found in the demineralized bone matrix group and 100% rate in the autologous bone graft group with similar times to union of just over 4 months. In that study 44% of the autologous bone graft recipient had donor site morbidity with 1 requiring reoperation.[22]

Synthetic bone graft substitutes including calcium phosphate and tricalcium phosphate have been used reliably in the setting of osteoporotic proximal humerus fracture. Although we were unable to identify comparative studies of synthetic bone graft substitutes in proximal humerus fracture nonunions, we can translate data from the primary fracture treatment setting. In a study of 92 acute proximal humerus fractures treated with calcium phosphate cement during open reduction internal fixation, Egol and colleagues evaluated calcium phosphate against cancellous chips as well as no augmentation. They found the least settling of the fractures in the calcium phosphate group when compared with either cancellous chips or no augmentation. Furthermore, there were no intraarticular screw penetration in the calcium phosphate group but there was a 16% rate in the cancellous chips group and a 24% rate in the no augmentation group. They concluded that calcium phosphate was excellent as an adjunct[23] during open reduction internal fixation of osteoporotic proximal humerus fractures.

With these facts in mind, we recommend careful scrutiny of the commercially available grafting options before harvesting for cancellous autograft due to comparable outcomes with demineralized bone matrix without donor site morbidity. The evidence would suggest the use of demineralized bone matrix with or without cancellous

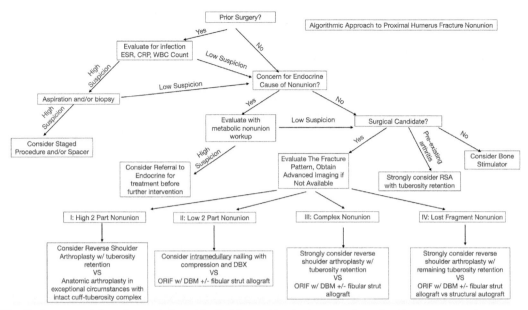

Fig. 7. A proposed flow chart to help guide decision-making in the care of proximal humerus nonunions.

chips as an augmentation to fracture healing. We recommend the use of fibular struts as an adjunct to support to the medial head fragment as needed. A recommendation cannot be made based on evidence regarding use of synthetic bone graft substitute in the setting of nonunion, but they likely have benefits of decreased screw penetration in the setting of limited bone stock in the humeral head fragment. We recommend reserving the use of cortical strut autograft for only otherwise unreconstructable Checchia Group IV nonunions.

SUMMARY

Proximal humerus fractures are a common injury, especially in the elderly population. Mechanical and biological factors are important to consider in the initial treatment of one of these fractures, as there are certain factors that can increase the risk of fracture nonunion. Appropriate infection workup should be performed in patients with failed operative fixation, and endocrine workup should be considered in most patients regardless of prior operative intervention. When operative intervention is used to treat these nonunions, open reduction and internal fixation (ORIF) with either a plate and screws or intramedullary nail has shown the best results in the small reported series.

Hemiarthroplasty or anatomic total shoulder arthroplasty is not recommended as treatment of a proximal humerus nonunion, except in rare circumstances. The literature to date does not demonstrate reliably favorable outcomes, and therefore anatomic reconstruction should be avoided, if possible. Although reverse total shoulder arthroplasty is a durable and reliable tool to treat unrepairable proximal humerus fractures, in the nonunion group it seems that the complication rate is slightly less favorable. Although there may be many situations where reverse shoulder arthroplasty is the most reasonable option, such as in the setting of preexisting arthritis, it is the recommendation of the investigators that great emphasis is placed on ORIF with either a plate and screws or intramedullary nail supplemented with bone graft. When joint salvage is not feasible, reverse shoulder replacement should be performed with the retention and repair of the tuberosity fragments whenever possible. Furthermore, we recommend counseling the patient on the increased risk of prosthetic instability. With a careful planning and consideration, proximal humerus fracture nonunions can be managed with a relatively high rate of success. See **Fig. 7** for a recommended flow chart to aid in the decision-making of proximal humerus nonunion care.

CLINICS CARE POINTS

• Proximal humerus fracture nonunions are relatively uncommon complication of proximal humerus fractures, regardless of management.

- Understanding the residual bone stock, the initial fracture pattern, and the outcomes of treatment is critical to planning an appropriate intervention.
- Open reduction internal fixation or intramedullary nailing of a nonunited 2-part proximal humerus fracture can provide a reliably excellent result.
- Do not excise the tuberosity fragments when performing reverse shoulder arthroplasty in the setting of a proximal humerus nonunion.
- Fibular strut allograft as well as demineralized bone matrix are excellent adjuncts when performing open reduction internal fixation of a proximal humerus fracture nonunion.

CONCLUSION

Proximal humerus nonunion is an uncommon but serious complication after both surgical and nonsurgical treatment of proximal humerus fractures. A better understanding of the anatomy of the nonunion, as well as the factors that led to it, will allow for better surgical planning. Factors such as the anatomic location/locations of the nonunion, prior treatment, the biological status of the patient, and the available bone stock should be considered. With appropriately planned and indicated surgical intervention, a high rate of successful outcomes can be achieved.

DISCLOSURE

D.C. Tapscott: No Disclosures. E.S. Paxton: Consultant: Miami Device Solutions and Wright Tornier; Research/Fellowship Support: Arthrex and American Society of Shoulder and Elbow Surgeons.

REFERENCES

1. Launonen AP, Lepola V, Saranko A, et al. Epidemiology of proximal humerus fractures. Arch Osteoporos 2015;10:209.
2. Court-Brown CM, Garg A, McQueen MM. The translated two-part fracture of the proximal humerus. Epidemiology and outcome in the older patient. J Bone Joint Surg Br 2001;83(6):799–804.
3. Roux A, Decroocq L, El Batti S, et al. Epidemiology of proximal humerus fractures managed in a trauma center. Orthop Traumatol Surg Res 2012; 98(6):715–9.
4. Rose AG, Park SJ, Bank AJ, et al. Partial aortic valve fusion induced by left ventricular assist device. Ann Thorac Surg 2000;70(4):1270–4.
5. Hanson B, Neidenbach P, de Boer P, et al. Functional outcomes after nonoperative management of fractures of the proximal humerus. J Shoulder Elbow Surg 2009;18(4):612–21.
6. Brinker MR, Macek J, Laughlin M, et al. Utility of common biomarkers for diagnosing infection in nonunion. J Orthop Trauma 2021;35(3):121–7.
7. Stucken C, Olszewski DC, Creevy WR, et al. Preoperative diagnosis of infection in patients with nonunions. J Bone Joint Surg Am 2013;95(15):1409–12.
8. Nino S, Soin SP, Avilucea FR. Vitamin d and metabolic supplementation in orthopedic trauma. Orthop Clin North Am 2019;50(2):171–9.
9. Canintika AF, Dilogo IH. Teriparatide for treating delayed union and nonunion: A systematic review. J Clin Orthop Trauma 2020;11(Suppl 1):S107–12.
10. Mayr E, Frankel V, Rüter A. Ultrasound–an alternative healing method for nonunions? Arch Orthop Trauma Surg 2000;120(1–2):1–8.
11. Riboh JC, Leversedge FJ. The use of low-intensity pulsed ultrasound bone stimulators for fractures of the hand and upper extremity. J Hand Surg Am 2012;37(7):1456–61.
12. Zastrow RK, Patterson DC, Cagle PJ. Operative management of proximal humerus nonunions in adults: a systematic review. J Orthop Trauma 2020;34(9):492–502.
13. Badman BL, Mighell M, Kalandiak SP, et al. Proximal humeral nonunions treated with fixed-angle locked plating and an intramedullary strut allograft. J Orthop Trauma 2009;23(3):173–9.
14. Rollo G, Rotini R, Pichierri P, et al. Grafting and fixation of proximal humeral aseptic non union: a prospective case series. Clin Cases Miner Bone Metab 2017;14(3):298–304.
15. Yamane S, Suenaga N, Oizumi N, et al. Interlocking intramedullary nailing for nonunion of the proximal humerus with the straight nail system. J Shoulder Elbow Surg 2008;17(5):755–9.
16. Duquin TR, Jacobson JA, Sanchez-Sotelo J, et al. Unconstrained shoulder arthroplasty for treatment of proximal humeral nonunions. J Bone Joint Surg Am 2012;94(17):1610–7.
17. Raiss P, Edwards TB, da Silva MR, et al. Reverse shoulder arthroplasty for the treatment of nonunions of the surgical neck of the proximal part of the humerus (type-3 fracture sequelae). J Bone Joint Surg Am 2014;96(24):2070–6.
18. Hattrup SJ, Waldrop R, Sanchez-Sotelo J. Reverse total shoulder arthroplasty for posttraumatic sequelae. J Orthop Trauma 2016;30(2):e41–7.
19. Kuhlmann N, Taylor A, Roche C, et al. Acute vs delayed reverse total shoulder arthroplasty for

proximal humerus fractures in the elderly, mid-term Outcomes. Semin Arthroplasty 2020;30(2):89–95.

20. De Long WG, Einhorn TA, Koval K, et al. Bone grafts and bone graft substitutes in orthopaedic trauma surgery. A critical analysis. J Bone Joint Surg Am 2007;89(3):649–58.

21. Baldwin P, Li DJ, Auston DA, et al. Autograft, allograft, and bone graft substitutes: clinical evidence and indications for use in the setting of orthopaedic trauma surgery. J Orthop Trauma 2019;33(4):203–13.

22. Hierholzer C, Sama D, Toro JB, et al. Plate fixation of ununited humeral shaft fractures: effect of type of bone graft on healing. J Bone Joint Surg Am 2006;88(7):1442–7.

23. Egol KA, Sugi MT, Ong CC, et al. Fracture site augmentation with calcium phosphate cement reduces screw penetration after open reduction-internal fixation of proximal humeral fractures. J Shoulder Elbow Surg 2012;21(6):741–8.

Management of Geriatric Elbow Injury

Naoko Onizuka, MD, PhD, MPH[a,b], Julie Switzer, MD[a,b], Chad Myeroff, MD[c,*]

KEYWORDS

- Geriatric trauma • Elderly • Elbow trauma • Distal humerus fracture • Olecranon fracture
- Elbow dislocation • Terrible triad injury • Radial head fracture

KEY POINTS

- Approximately 4.1% of all fractures in the elderly involve the elbow.
- Most elbow injuries in geriatric patients occur as the result of low-energy mechanisms such as falls from standing height.
- Elbow injuries in elderly patients present complex challenges because of insufficient bone quality, comminution, articular fragmentation, and preexisting conditions, such as arthritis.
- Medical comorbidities and baseline level of function must be heavily considered in surgical decision making.

MANAGEMENT OF GERIATRIC ELBOW TRAUMA

Introduction

Approximately 4.1% of fractures in the elderly involve the elbow.[1] Elderly patients are at risk for elbow injuries following low-energy falls. Such injuries occur secondary to deconditioning, muscle weakness, gait and balance deficits, poor vision, and concomitant osteopenia or osteoporosis.[2] In 1 study of 287 patients, it was determined that nearly 70% of patients who sustain an elbow fracture fall directory onto their elbow because they cannot break the fall with an outstretched arm.[3] Older patients with elbow trauma tend to be more fit than those with proximal humerus fractures but less fit than those with distal radius fractures.[3] Regardless of a patient's underlying state of health or age, elbow injuries in the elderly can impact mobility, function, and ultimately, independence.

DISTAL HUMERUS FRACTURE

Epidemiology

Distal humerus fractures comprise approximately 2% of all fractures but represent one-third of elbow fractures.[1] Distal humeral fractures have an estimated incidence of 5.7 per 100,000 persons per year.[4] Most distal humerus fractures in geriatric patients occur from low-energy injuries, such as falling from standing height.[5] They have a bimodal age distribution, with peak incidences between 12 and 19 years and those aged 80 years and older.[6]

Clinical Assessment

It is imperative to understand the patient's medical and physical frailty and level of independence, including gait assistance, living situation, and level of function. The physical evaluation includes assessing the ipsilateral shoulder and wrist. Skin needs to be carefully examined for abrasions, fracture blisters, skin tenting, and open wounds.[7] Open elbow injuries are common and should be treated with standard open fracture protocols that involve removing gross contamination, soft tissue coverage, splinting, early antibiotics, and timely surgical irrigation and debridement.[7–9] Neurologic examinations must be performed and accurately documented preoperatively and postoperatively. Incomplete

ᵃ Department of Orthopaedic Surgery, University of Minnesota, 2512 South 7th Street, Suite R200, Minneapolis, MN 55455, USA; ᵇ Department of Orthopaedic Surgery, Methodist Hospital, 6500 Excelsior Boulevard, Saint Louis Park, MN 55426, USA; ᶜ TRIA Orthopedic Center, 155 Radio Drive, Woodbury, MN 55125, USA
* Corresponding author.
E-mail address: Chad.M.Myeroff@healthpartners.com

ulnar neuropathy is present in 26% of patients with Arbeitsgemeinschaft für Osteosynthesefragen/Orthopaedic Trauma Association (AO/OTA) type C distal humerus fractures at the time of presentation.[10] Vascular injuries should be ruled out by examining the distal pulses, capillary refill, and color.[7,10]

Imaging

Standard anteroposterior and lateral radiographs of the elbow are necessary for diagnosis, classification, and surgical templating. Radiographs of the joints above and below are essential as concomitant distal radius fractures are not uncommon (case 2, see **Fig. 5**; case 3, see **Fig. 10**).[11] In elderly patients who have highly comminuted fractures, a computed tomographic (CT) scan is helpful to identify and visualize fracture patterns.[10,12]

Classifications

There are several classification systems, but the AO/OTA classification is used most frequently (**Fig. 1**).[13,14] Type A fractures are extra-articular and may involve the epicondyles or occur at the distal humerus metaphyseal level. Type B fractures are partial articular and include unicondylar fractures or fractures of the articular surface involving the capitellum, trochlea, or both. Type C fractures are complete articular fractures. In type C fractures, there is no continuity between the articular segments and the humeral shaft.

Treatment

The treatment of distal humerus fractures in older patients can be challenging.[15,16] High degrees of comminution, insufficient bone stock, underlying osteoarthritis, and preexisting medical comorbidities weigh heavily on treatment decision making.

Nonoperative treatment

Nonoperative treatment is generally reserved for patients who are medically unfit to undergo surgery. In patients for whom anesthesia or surgery-related risks are too high, conservative treatment is considered to be appropriate.[17,18] Low-demand patients with severe osteoporosis, patients with poor-quality skin, or patients with nondisplaced fractures may also be managed with nonoperative management (case 1, see **Fig. 1**; **Figs. 2** and **3**).[17] They can be managed with immobilization for 2 to 3 weeks followed by early mobilization.[17]

Open reduction and internal fixation

In the active patient, nonoperative treatment often results in loss of function and disability because of prolonged immobilization.[7,19–21] Nauth and colleagues[19] demonstrated that patients treated nonoperatively have almost 3 times the risk of an unacceptable result (relative risk = 2.8, 95% confidence interval, 1.78–4.4). In a study of 497 patients, Obert and colleagues[20] reported the conservative treatment group's complication rates were 60%. In this analysis, the main complication was malunion. Thus, anatomic reduction and rigid internal fixation with early physiologic motion is considered the gold standard for most fractures of the distal humerus (case 2, **Figs. 4–7**).[6,19–30]

Good to excellent outcomes of open reduction and internal fixation (ORIF) for distal humerus fractures in elderly patients have been reported. A retrospective cohort study of distal humerus fractures in patients older than 70 years of age reported an average flexion arc of 20.9° to 127°, average pronation and supination of 68.3° and 75.3, respectively, and a mean Mayo Elbow Performance Score (MEPS) of 88.7.[31] Similarly, Ducrot and colleagues[32] retrospectively studied 43 elderly patients (mean age of 80) who were treated with locking plate fixation. They reported a mean flexion arc of 23° to 127° and satisfactory functional recovery, with 95% good and excellent results. Clavert and colleagues[33] reported satisfactory results with a mean MEPS of 87 in elderly patients with ORIF. Complication rates were reported in a wide range (19% to 53%) and included neuropathies, mechanical failure, elbow stiffness, nonunions, deep infections, or wound dehiscence.[20,33–38]

An olecranon osteotomy is commonly used for AO/OTA type C fractures, as it allows visualization of the distal humerus articular surface.[39] The complications associated with an osteotomy include nonunion/malunion (3.3%) and hardware irritation (10%–82%).[40,41] Kaiser and colleagues[42] reported a limited columnar fixation and olecranon-sparing approach for intraarticular fractures in an elderly population as a valid treatment option with similar elbow motion, function, and pain relief when compared with ORIF with an osteotomy. This approach may be used in geriatric patients who are medically unwell or who have such poor bone quality that anatomic reduction with an olecranon osteotomy would be challenging. Avoiding an osteotomy may allow not only more aggressive rehabilitation but also arthroplasty as an intraoperative fallback.

OTA / AO Classification

Fig. 1. The AO/OTA classification of distal humerus fractures.

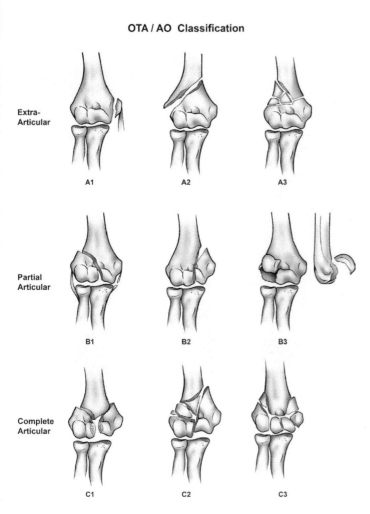

Fig. 1. The AO/OTA classification of distal humerus fractures.

Total elbow arthroplasty

Distal humerus fractures present complex challenges in the elderly patient because of osteopenia, comminution, articular fragmentation, and preexisting conditions of the elbow, such as osteoarthritis or rheumatoid arthritis. In those patients with these common diagnoses, rigid internal fixation and early mobilization can be challenging. In certain low, transcolumnar or coronal shear fractures in older patients with severe osteopenia, comminution, or preexisting arthritis, total elbow arthroplasty (TEA) has become a recognized alternative treatment. However, it is imperative to choose only low-demand patients for this intervention to minimize risk of failures, such as loosening, polyethylene wear, and periprosthetic fracture. The evidence for patient selection, complications, and functional outcomes is still conflicting.[15,43–49]

As a principle, it is recommended to perform ORIF on all adult patients fit for surgery with a reconstructible fracture pattern to reserve TEA for low-demand patients with unreconstructible fractures (case 3, Figs. 8–12). Several studies have compared ORIF and TEA for distal humerus fractures. However, sample sizes in these studies were limited, and inconsistent results have been reported. Egol and colleagues[46] reported good outcomes with either TEA or ORIF with no significant difference in functional outcomes, whereas McKee and colleagues[50] and Morrey[51] reported TEA had improved functional outcomes based on the MEPS and concluded TEA is a preferred alternative in elderly patients with complex distal humeral fractures. Varecka and Myeroff[52] reported that the outcomes of TEA for distal humerus fracture in the elderly included a physiologic range of motion (ROM; 26°–125°), adequate function (average MEPS, 87), and an acceptable implant survival rate of 94% at an average of 38.5 months. Although it has been reported that patients who undergo ORIF have a

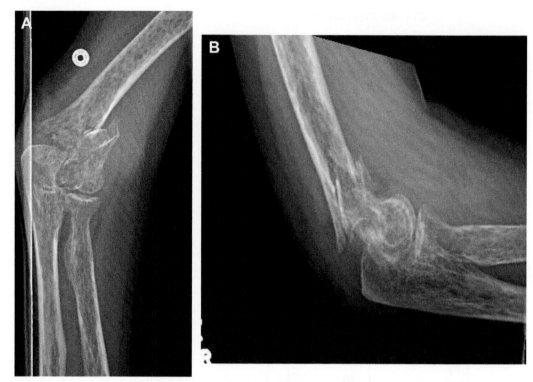

Fig. 2. Case 1: a 60-year-old woman with a past medical history of cerebrovascular disease with diminished right upper-extremity function sustained a low-energy fall. She had an extra-articular right distal humerus fracture (see Fig. 2). Originally, surgery was planned, but the soft tissue was not suitable with perceived high risk of deep infection. The patient's bone quality was poor, and the reliability of fixation was a concern. She underwent nonsurgical treatment with 3 weeks of splint and then a removable brace for another 3 weeks.

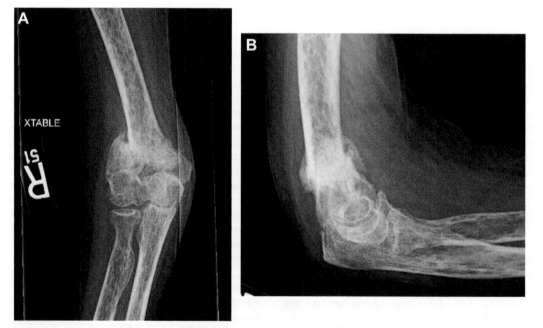

Fig. 3. Case 1: A 60-year-old woman with radiographs at 3-month visit. Elbow ROM was 10° to 95°, supination 20°, pronation 90° at the 3-month visit.

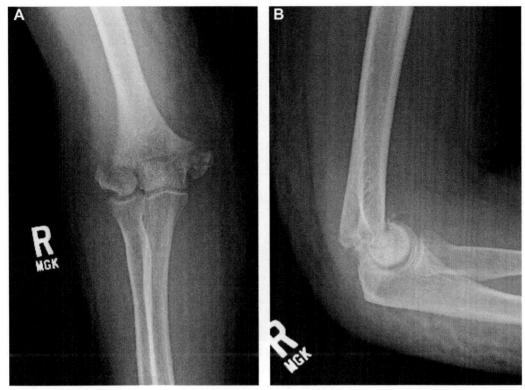

Fig. 4. Case 2: A 59-year-old woman who presented 6 days after a fall on ice, in which she sustained a right elbow injury. The radiograph revealed a right distal humerus intraarticular fracture (see Fig. 4) and right distal radius fracture (see **Fig. 5**). She underwent distal humerus ORIF with dual plating and olecranon osteotomy (see **Fig. 6**) and distal radius ORIF (see **Fig. 7**). She had an anterior subcutaneous transposition of the ulnar nerve but required a transfer of her anterior interosseous nerve to her right ulnar motor nerve for ulnar neuropathy.

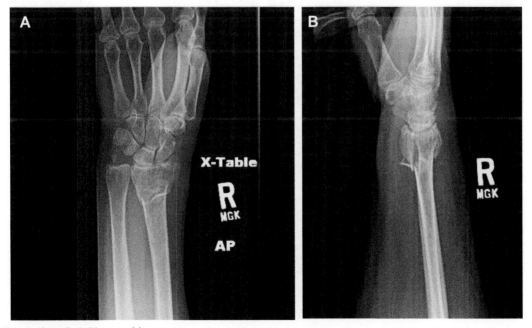

Fig. 5. Case 2: A 59-year-old woman.

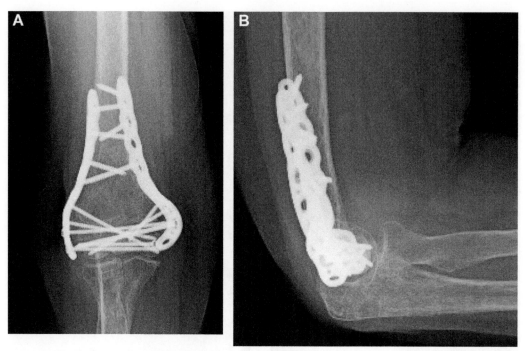

Fig. 6. Case 2: A 59-year-old woman with elbow ROM of 26° to 132°, supination 90°, pronation 90° at 10 months postoperatively.

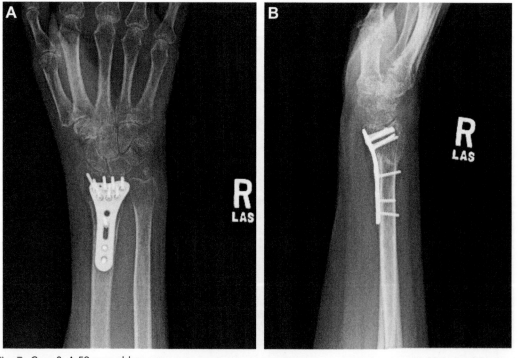

Fig. 7. Case 2: A 59-year-old woman.

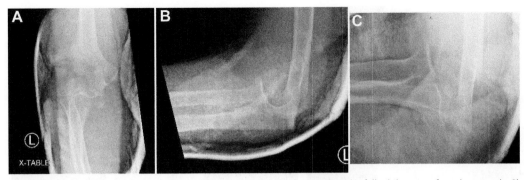

Fig. 8. Case 3: An 88-year-old right-hand–dominant woman, who sustained a fall while rising from her couch. She sustained a left elbow fracture-dislocation (see Fig. 8; Fig. 9) and ipsilateral distal radius fracture (see Fig. 10). She underwent a left TEA (see Fig. 11), left ulnar nerve decompression and transposition, and distal radius dorsal spanning bridge/ORIF (see Fig. 12). Left elbow ROM was 0° to 140° at 6 months postoperatively.

higher risk of complications compared with TEA, complications with TEA are often more severe.[20,52] The complications with TEA include periprosthetic fracture (1%), implant fracture (1%), and deep wound infection (2%).[52]

Thus, although TEA may provide improved early function and similar overall outcomes when compared with ORIF in appropriately selected patients, it can cause devastating complications, and appropriate hosts must be carefully selected.[52]

OLECRANON FRACTURES
Epidemiology
Fractures of the olecranon account for 20% of all proximal forearm fractures and 10% of all upper-extremity fractures.[53,54] The common mechanism is a direct fall onto the elbow.[54] For isolated fractures of the olecranon, the Mayo classification (Fig. 13) is preferred.[55]

Management
Nonoperative treatment
Closed treatment is the gold standard in elderly, low-demand patients with displaced and nondisplaced, isolated olecranon fractures. Several studies have reported excellent functional results and championed nonoperative management of displaced olecranon fractures as a viable treatment option for lower-demand patients with multiple comorbidities.[56–58] Duckworth and colleagues[57] conducted a retrospective cohort study of 43 elderly patients with isolated Mayo-2 olecranon fracture (mean displacement, 10 mm) who underwent nonoperative treatment. They showed nonoperative management of displaced olecranon fractures to be a viable treatment option for lower-demand patients with multiple comorbidities with a flexion arc of 18° to 126°, Disabilities of the Arm, Shoulder, and Hand (DASH) 2.9, 91% satisfaction, 17% push-off weakness despite an 88% nonunion (or fibrous union) rate.[57] In a similar

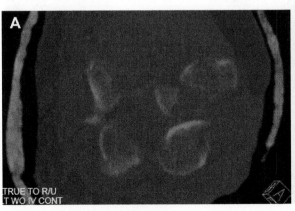
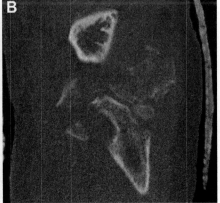

Fig. 9. Case 3: An 88-year-old woman.

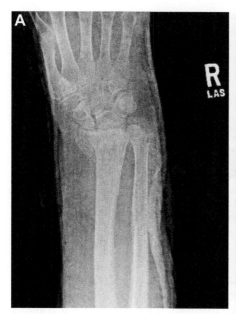
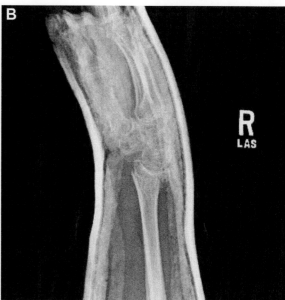

Fig. 10. Case 3: An 88-year-old woman.

study, Gallucci and colleagues[58] reported 4/5 push-off weakness with nonoperative care. Subsequently, Duckworth and colleagues[59] conducted a randomized trial of 19 olecranon fractures in the elderly (aged ≥ 75 years) to compare nonoperative versus operative management (either tension-band wiring [TBW] or fixation with a nonlocking plate) and reported no difference in the mean DASH scores between the groups at all times, although the trial was stopped prematurely

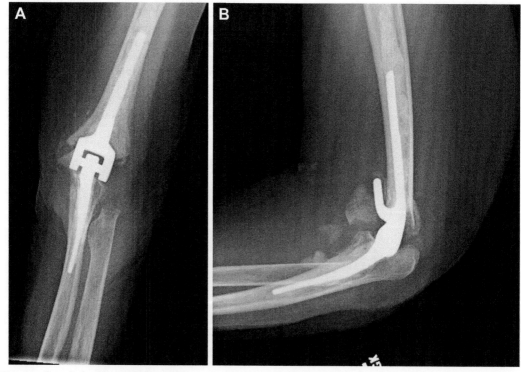

Fig. 11. Case 3: An 88-year-old woman.

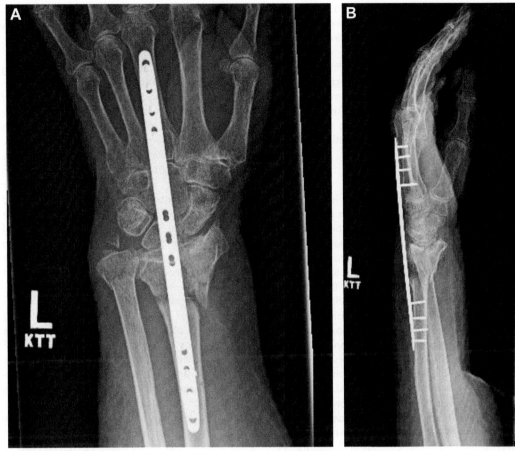

Fig. 12. Case 3: An 88-year-old woman.

➤ **Mayo type I**
Undisplaced

➤ **Mayo type II**
Displaced
A-Noncomminuted
B-Comminuted

➤ **Mayo type III**
Accompanying lesions-Instability
A-Noncomminuted
B-Comminuted

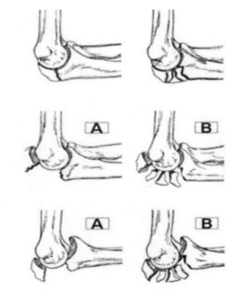

Fig. 13. The Mayo classification for olecranon fracture.

as the rate of complications (9/11%, 81.8%; 6 patients had loss of reduction, 3 patients required removal of hardware, 1 patient required excision of draining sinus) in the operative group was considered to be unacceptable.[59] It should be noted that no locking plate technology was used in the treatment of these short, metaphyseal fractures in the elderly despite the known unacceptable failure rate of TBW in this setting, reported previously by the same investigators and others.[59]

Operative treatment

The goal in surgical management is anatomic reconstruction of the sigmoid notch in order to enable early functional rehabilitation of the elbow and thereby inhibit posttraumatic stiffness and optimize extension strength (case 4, **Figs. 14** and **15**). TBW or plate fixation is frequently used for stable displaced fractures (Mayo type II). However, there have been conflicting findings regarding the outcomes and complications after operative fixation of olecranon fractures in elderly patients. The TBW technique is an acceptable option in simple transverse fractures with an intact dorsal cortex in young patients with good bone (Mayo type IA–IIA). However, the biomechanical limitations become evident in comminuted fractures, and in osteoporotic bone. Umer and colleagues[60] reviewed 79 operatively treated elderly olecranon fractures, in which TBW was used in 87%. They reported

the following adverse outcomes, including 14% wound problems, 16% persistent pain, 44% hardware problems (19% hardware removal), and 75% stiffness.[60] Duckworth and colleagues[61] performed a randomized clinical trial comparing plate fixation to TBW in 67 patients. Despite being biased toward younger patients in the TBW group, TBW was associated with twice the complication rate (63% vs 38%; $P = .042$), twice the hardware removal rate (50% vs 22%; $P = .021$), and twice the loss of reduction (27% vs 13%; $P = .206$). In a systematic review, Ren and colleagues[62] found more complications for TBW when compared with plate fixation and therefore recommended olecranon fracture plating as the contemporary treatment of choice. Higher rates of prominent hardware with the need for removal following TBW were found in several studies over the last decade.[63,64]

The management of comminuted and unstable fractures (Mayo IIb–IIIb) using locking compression plates via the dorsal approach has been well established in recent studies.[65–68] Wise and colleagues[68] reported low failure and complication rates using modern fixation principles and locked plating. They reported an 11% (4/36) major complication rate with only 3 mechanical failures, an 88% union rate (all patients who did not have a major complication went onto union), and a 120 flexion-extension arc of motion in their retrospective review of elderly

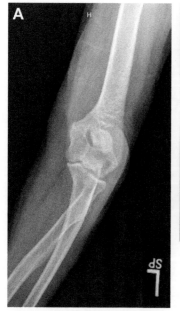
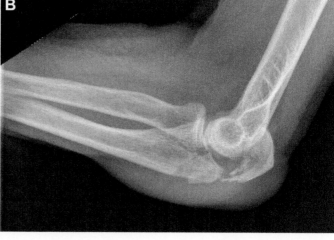

Fig. 14. Case 4: A 74-year-old woman with osteoporosis, diabetes, and hypothyroidism sustained a ground level fall resulting in a Mayo IIb olecranon fracture. She underwent ORIF with a triceps detensioning suture adjunct.

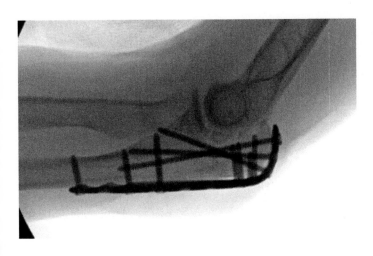

Fig. 15. Case 4: A 74-year-old woman.

patients greater than 75 years old treated with locked plating and early motion. Interestingly, upper-extremity gait dependence was associated with failures. Although not the "gold standard," precontoured locked plating and early mobilization is an effective and safe treatment for comminuted olecranon fractures in select geriatric patients, who are safe for surgery and comply with restrictions.[66–68]

In addition, especially for small tip fractures and/or in highly comminuted osteoporotic bone in the elderly, the use of an "off-loading triceps suture" (eg, with a nonabsorbable, high-tensile suture) has been shown to neutralize the distraction forces caused by the extensor mechanism and to decrease the risk of fixation failure.[69]

Most surgical complications are implant related because of soft tissue irritation. Complications such as ulnar neuropathy, deep infection, implant failure, or delayed/nonunion are relatively rarely reported. However, an uneven reconstruction of the articular surface can cause sequelae such as limited elbow ROM and post-traumatic arthritis.[70]

RADIAL HEAD FRACTURES

Epidemiology
Radial head fractures are the most common fractures of the elbow, with most fractures occurring in women older than 50 years of age. They constitute approximately one-third of all elbow fractures and approximately 2.5 to 2.8 per 10,000 people per year.[71–74] Over the last decades, the radial head is increasingly recognized as an essential stabilizer of the elbow.[75] Most radial head and neck fractures are minimally displaced and are isolated injuries. These fractures

typically have a good functional outcome with nonsurgical treatment. More displaced and comminuted fractures commonly have associated injuries to the collateral ligaments. They may have associated fractures of the coronoid, capitellum, or proximal ulna as well.[76]

Assessment
A careful examination of an ROM is performed because the loss of forearm rotation is one of the primary indications for surgical intervention. In particular, the distal radioulnar joint and interosseous membrane should be palpated and assessed for both tenderness and instability.[7] Anteroposterior and lateral radiographs are typically sufficient to diagnose most displaced radial head fractures. Nondisplaced fractures may initially be challenging to diagnose, and they may only be suspected by the presence of an anterior and posterior fat pad sign. CT can be helpful to characterize the size, location, and displacement of radial head fractures. It is also useful to assess concomitant injuries of the coronoid, the capitellum, and the presence of associated osteochondral fragments.[7]

Classification
Several classification systems have been used to describe radial head fractures. The Mason classification and its subsequent modifications are commonly used. Mason's classification describes nondisplaced fractures (type I), partial fractures with displacement (type II), and comminuted and displaced fractures involving the entire radial head (type III) (Table 1).[71] Morrey modified the Mason classification and included the extent of articular fragment displacement (>2 mm) and fragment size (≥30% of the articular surface) (Fig. 16).[77] Johnston added a fourth

Table 1	
The Mason classification for radial head fractures	
Type 1	Fissure or marginal fractures without displacement
Type 2	Marginal sector fractures with displacement
Type 3	Comminuted fractures involving the whole head of the radius

type, which describes a radial head fracture with the dislocation of the elbow.[78]

Treatment

Nonoperative treatment

Nondisplaced or minimally displaced radial head fractures without a block to forearm rotation are treated nonsurgically.[79] The treatment includes immobilization for up to 2 or 3 days for comfort. Active motion is then encouraged with the use of a sling as needed between exercises. The natural course of Mason type I fractures is benign in general; however, persistent complaints have been reported in 20% of cases.[80]

Operative treatment

Operative treatment is indicated for most of these unstable radial head injuries and any isolated fractures with significant articular displacement, articular comminution, or mechanical block to motion.[81,82] Treatment options include radial head fragment excision, radial head excision, ORIF, and radial head arthroplasty. Fragment excision is indicated in patients with a block to forearm motion by a small (<25% of the articular diameter) non-reconstructible displaced articular fracture of the radial head

without instability.[83] Excision of any kind should never be performed in an instability pattern, and rarely, acutely. ORIF is indicated in patients with displaced, noncomminuted fractures of the radial head. In osteoporotic bone, even simple patterns can be fraught with impaction and relatively quick resorption. A radial head arthroplasty is the favored surgical treatment in patients with a comminuted (>3 parts) fracture, with poor bone quality, and with unstable elbow injuries or mechanical obstruction.[84] Radial head replacement had fewer complications than ORIF patients (13.9% vs 58.1%) and higher satisfaction rates (91.7% vs 51.6%) in Mason type III radial head fractures patients.[85]

ELBOW DISLOCATION/TERRIBLE TRIAD INJURY

Epidemiology

The elbow is the second most commonly dislocated joint in the adult population, with a reported rate of 5 to 6 per 100,000 person-years in the US population.[86,87] Elbow dislocation associated with radial head and coronoid fractures has been referred to as the "terrible triad injury"; it represents a pattern of complex elbow instability that has historically been associated with a poor prognosis.[88–90]

Mechanisms

Elbow dislocations are typically the result of a fall on an outstretched hand. The soft tissue injury begins on the lateral side of the elbow with the injury of the lateral collateral ligament (LCL) and then proceeds through the capsule to the medial side with the medial collateral ligament (MCL) being disrupted last.[91,92] A fall onto an outstretched arm with supination, valgus, and

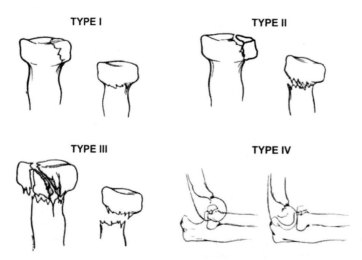

TYPE I   TYPE II

TYPE III   TYPE IV

Fig. 16. The Broberg-Morrey modification of the Mason classification.

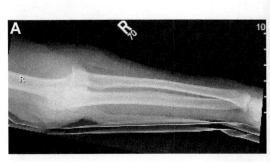
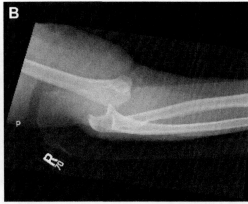

Fig. 17. Case 5: An 82-year-old woman who presented to clinic 10 days after a fall from standing height, sustaining a simple right elbow dislocation (see Fig. 15). The elbow was reduced, and a splint was applied (see Table 1). At 1 week follow-up, she was found to have a recurrent dislocation (see Fig. 16). She underwent closed reduction, and an external fixator was placed at 90° of flexion for 4 weeks (see Fig. 17; Fig. 18). Final ROM resulted in a flexion arc of 10° to 140°, pronation 90°, and supination 90°.

axial-directed force is a mechanism of terrible triad injury. It occurs by posterolateral rotatory displacement of the ulna, resulting in elbow subluxation or dislocation, a shear fracture of the coronoid with LCL injury, and radial head fracture.[7]

Treatment
Elbow dislocations
A relative consensus exists in favor of conservative treatment of simple elbow dislocations in the absence of any tendency to re-dislocate within the joint's functional arc.[93–95] Previous studies have reported good to excellent outcomes in most patients with a simple elbow dislocation.[93–95]

However, some research reported mild residual symptoms, including loss of motion, subjective stiffness, residual pain, and residual instability.[96–99] Prolonged immobilization after injury was associated with a worse result with increased flexion contracture and more severe

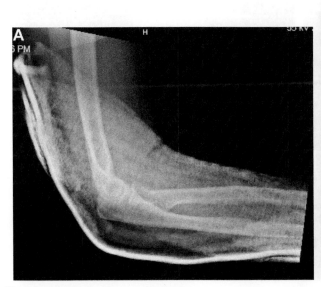
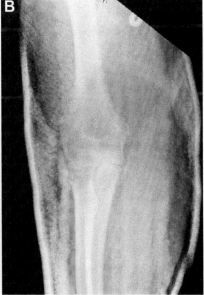

Fig. 18. Case 5: An 82-year-old woman.

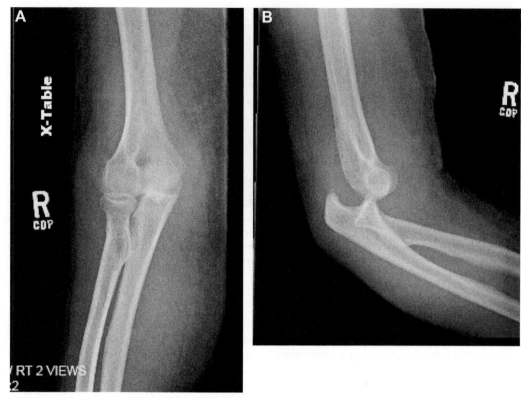

Fig. 19. Case 5: An 82-year-old woman.

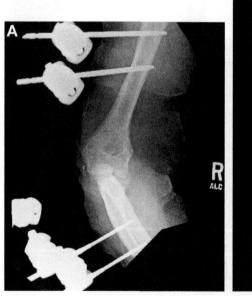
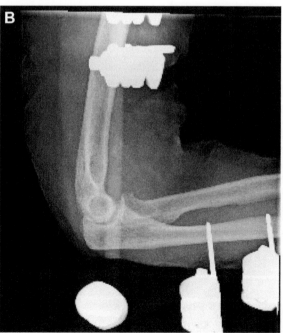

Fig. 20. Case 5: An 82-year-old woman.

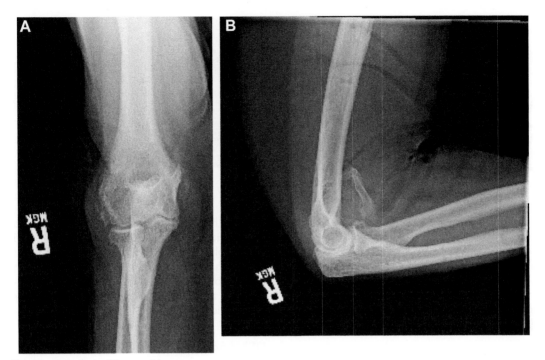

Fig. 21. Case 5: An 82-year-old woman.

residual pain.[99] The frailer patients are often quick to look past subtle functional losses but are vulnerable to loss of independence secondary to pain or instability.

The main indication for operative management is an inability to maintain a concentric elbow joint following closed reduction. Elbows that are so unstable that prolonged immobilization will be

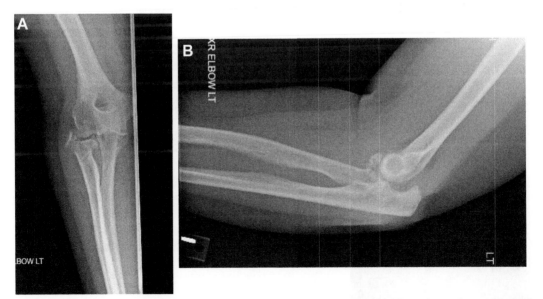

Fig. 22. Case 6: A 56-year-old right-handed woman sustained a ground level fall. Radiographs revealed left elbow dislocation with displaced radial head fracture, coronoid fracture, and olecranon fracture (see Figs. 19 and 20). She underwent ORIF of left coronoid, left olecranon, left radial head, and lateral ulnar collateral ligament repair (see Fig. 21). At 5-month follow-up, she achieved ROM of 10° to 138°, 70° supination, and 90° pronation with no pain.

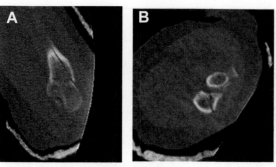
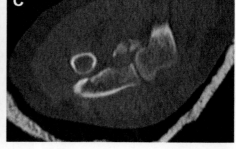

Fig. 23. Case 6: A 56-year-old woman.

required should also be considered for early surgical management to avoid stiffness. Because of soft tissue quality, simple elbow dislocation in the elderly may be more unstable, and careful follow-up is mandatory to recognize and promptly treat persistent instability with either closed reduction and external fixation or ligament repair (case 5, **Figs. 17–21**).

Terrible triad injury

Surgical treatment is preferred for most terrible triad injuries, as there are little contemporary data regarding the nonoperative treatment outcomes. A retrospective cohort study conducted by Chan and colleagues[100] reported nonoperative treatment of terrible triad injuries could be an option that can provide good function and restore stable elbow ROM for selected patients: (1) a concentric joint reduction, (2) a radial head

fracture that did not cause a mechanical block to the rotation, (3) a smaller coronoid fracture, and (4) a stable arc of motion to a minimum of 30° of extension. When doubt exists, early mobilization abiding by lateral ulnar collateral ligament precautions and repeat radiographs 1 week later can provide reassurance.

OPEN REDUCTION INTERNAL FIXATION

A systematic approach, including fixation or replacement of the radial head, fixation of the coronoid fragment, and repair of the LCL, is usually required (case 6, **Figs. 22–24**). The elbow is then evaluated intraoperatively for residual instability to determine if MCL repair is required. In many cases, the coronoid can be accessed and repaired from a lateral surgical exposure, particularly if a radial head replacement is

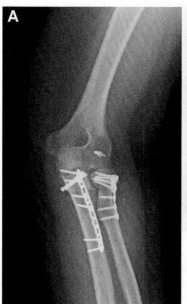
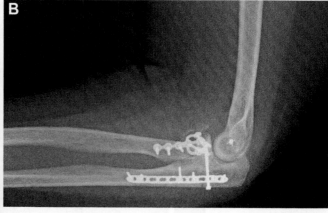

Fig. 24. Case 6: A 56-year-old woman.

required. Coronoid fractures too small or comminuted to be amenable to screw fixation can be repaired using sutures passed around the coronoid process and anterior capsule through transosseous tunnels on the dorsal ulna.

Some studies of triple triad injury reported satisfactory outcomes with few complications,[101,102] whereas other investigators have reported a high rate of symptomatic and asymptomatic complications.[103–112] Complications include stiffness (0%–22%), arthritis (0%–19.5%), ulnar nerve entrapment (0%–18%), and recurrent instability (4%–38%)[103–112] Gianicola and colleagues[113] reported that obesity, low compliance, delayed treatment, and extensive soft elbow tissue damage caused by a high-energy trauma represented negative prognostic factors that affect the surgical outcomes.

SPECIAL CONSIDERATION FOR GERIATRIC PATIENTS

Elderly patients should be evaluated and treated for the fall risk. Special attention should be directed toward identifying comorbidities and reversible illnesses that may impact the treatment recommendations and perioperative risk. In addition, a patient's preinjury functional abilities, demands, limitations related to the upper extremities, and hand dominance may affect the treatment decision making.

CLINICS CARE POINTS

- Approximately 4.1% of all fractures in the elderly involve the elbow.
- Elderly patients are at risk for elbow injuries following even low-energy falls.
- Approximately one-third of elbow injuries involves the distal humerus. Most of the distal humerus fractures in geriatric patients occur from low-energy injuries, such as falling from standing height.
- Fractures around the elbow in elderly patients are challenging because of poor bone quality, comminution, articular fragmentation, and preexisting conditions of the elbow.

DISCLOSURE

All the authors have declared no conflict of interest for this article.

REFERENCES

1. Court-Brown CM, Clement ND, Duckworth AD, et al. The spectrum of fractures in the elderly. Bone Joint J 2014;96-B(3):366–72.
2. Liman MNP, Avva U, Ashurst JV, et al. Elbow trauma. 2020 Aug 21. In: Morrey BF, editor. Stat-Pearls. Treasure Island (FL): StatPearls Publishing; 2021.
3. Palvanen M, Kannus P, Parkkari J, et al. The injury mechanisms of osteoporotic upper extremity fractures among older adults: a controlled study of 287 consecutive patients and their 108 controls. Osteoporos Int 2000;11(10):822–31.
4. Robinson CM, Hill RM, Jacobs N, et al. Adult distal humeral metaphyseal fractures: epidemiology and results of treatment. J Orthop Trauma 2003;17(1):38–47.
5. Court-Brown CM, Caesar B. Epidemiology of adult fractures: a review. Injury 2006;37(8):691–7.
6. Miller AN, Beingessner DM. Intra-articular distal humerus fractures. Orthop Clin North Am 2013; 44(1):35–45.
7. Rockwood and Green's Fractures in Adults. 9th edition. Tornetta P, Ricci W, Charles M. Court-Brown CM, McQueen M, McKee M. LWW.
8. McKee MD, Wilson TL, Winston L, et al. Functional outcome following surgical treatment of intra-articular distal humeral fractures through a posterior approach. J Bone Joint Surg Am 2000; 82(12):1701–7.
9. Min W, Ding BC, Tejwani NC. Comparative functional outcome of AO/OTA type C distal humerus fractures: open injuries do worse than closed fractures. J Trauma Acute Care Surg 2012;72(2): E27–32.
10. Gofton WT, Macdermid JC, Patterson SD, et al. Functional outcome of AO type C distal humeral fractures. J Hand Surg Am 2003;28(2):294–308.
11. Debus F, Karaman Y, Ruchholtz S, et al. The distal radius fracture: concomitant fractures and their relevancy. Technol Health Care 2014;22(6):877–84.
12. Brouwer KM, Lindenhovius AL, Dyer GS, et al. Diagnostic accuracy of 2- and 3-dimensional imaging and modeling of distal humerus fractures. J Shoulder Elbow Surg 2012;21(6):772–6.
13. Marsh JL, Slongo TF, Agel J, et al. Fracture and dislocation classification compendium - 2007: Orthopaedic Trauma Association classification, database and outcomes committee. J Orthop Trauma 2007;21(10 Suppl):S1–133.
14. Fracture and dislocation compendium. Orthopaedic Trauma Association Committee for Coding and Classification. J Orthop Trauma 1996; 10(Suppl 1):v-154.
15. Medvedev G, Wang C, Amdur R, et al. Operative distal humerus fractures in older patients:

predictors for early complications based on a national database. HSS J 2017;13(3):212–6.

16. Patino JM. Complex distal humerus fractures in elderly patients: open reduction and internal fixation versus arthroplasty. J Hand Surg Am 2012; 37(8):1699–701.

17. Brown RF, Morgan RG. Intercondylar T-shaped fractures of the humerus. Results in ten cases treated by early mobilisation. J Bone Joint Surg Br 1971;53(3):425–8.

18. Seth AK, Baratz ME. Fractures of the elbow. In: Trumble TE, Budoff JE, Hand CR, editors. Elbow & shoulder. Philadelphia: Mosby; 2006. p. 522–31.

19. Nauth A, McKee MD, Ristevski B, et al. Distal humeral fractures in adults. J Bone Joint Surg Am 2011;93(7):686–700.

20. Obert L, Ferrier M, Jacquot A, et al. Distal humerus fractures in patients over 65: complications. Orthop Traumatol Surg Res 2013;99(8):909–13.

21. Zagorski JB, Jennings JJ, Burkhalter WE, et al. Comminuted intraarticular fractures of the distal humeral condyles. Surgical vs. nonsurgical treatment. Clin Orthop Relat Res 1986;202:197–204.

22. John H, Rosso R, Neff U, et al. Operative treatment of distal humeral fractures in the elderly. J Bone Joint Surg Br 1994;76(5):793–6.

23. Hausman M, Panozzo A. Treatment of distal humerus fractures in the elderly. Clin Orthop Relat Res 2004;425:55–63.

24. Huang TL, Chiu FY, Chuang TY, et al. The results of open reduction and internal fixation in elderly patients with severe fractures of the distal humerus: a critical analysis of the results. J Trauma 2005;58(1):62–9.

25. Korner J, Lill H, Müller LP, et al. The LCP-concept in the operative treatment of distal humerus fractures–biological, biomechanical and surgical aspects. Injury 2003;34(Suppl 2):B20–30.

26. Srinivasan K, Agarwal M, Matthews SJ, et al. Fractures of the distal humerus in the elderly: is internal fixation the treatment of choice? Clin Orthop Relat Res 2005;434:222–30.

27. Githens M, Yao J, Sox AH, et al. Open reduction and internal fixation versus total elbow arthroplasty for the treatment of geriatric distal humerus fractures: a systematic review and meta-analysis. J Orthop Trauma 2014;28(8):481–8.

28. Kaiser T, Brunner A, Hohendorff B, et al. Treatment of supra- and intra-articular fractures of the distal humerus with the LCP distal humerus plate: a 2-year follow-up. J Shoulder Elbow Surg 2011; 20(2):206–12.

29. Leigey DF, Farrell DJ, Siska PA, et al. Bicolumnar 90-90 plating of low-energy distal humeral fractures in the elderly patient. Geriatr Orthop Surg Rehabil 2014;5(3):122–6.

30. Huang JI, Paczas M, Hoyen HA, et al. Functional outcome after open reduction internal fixation of intra-articular fractures of the distal humerus in the elderly. J Orthop Trauma 2011;25(5):259–65.

31. Moursy M, Wegmann K, Wichlas F, et al. Distal humerus fracture in patients over 70 years of age: results of open reduction and internal fixation [published online ahead of print, 2020 Nov 5]. Arch Orthop Trauma Surg 2020. https://doi.org/10.1007/s00402-020-03664-4.

32. Ducrot G, Bonnomet F, Adam P, et al. Treatment of distal humerus fractures with LCP DHP™ locking plates in patients older than 65 years. Orthop Traumatol Surg Res 2013;99(2):145–54.

33. Clavert P, Ducrot G, Sirveaux F, et al, SOFCOT. Outcomes of distal humerus fractures in patients above 65 years of age treated by plate fixation. Orthop Traumatol Surg Res 2013;99(7):771–7.

34. Athwal GS, Hoxie SC, Rispoli DM, et al. Precontoured parallel plate fixation of AO/OTA type C distal humerus fractures. J Orthop Trauma 2009; 23(8):575–80.

35. Theivendran K, Duggan PJ, Deshmukh SC. Surgical treatment of complex distal humeral fractures: functional outcome after internal fixation using precontoured anatomic plates. J Shoulder Elbow Surg 2010;19(4):524–32.

36. Rebuzzi E, Vascellari A, Schiavetti S. The use of parallel pre-contoured plates in the treatment of A and C fractures of the distal humerus. Musculoskelet Surg 2010;94(1):9–16.

37. Luegmair M, Timofiev E, Chirpaz-Cerbat JM. Surgical treatment of AO type C distal humeral fractures: internal fixation with a Y-shaped reconstruction (Lambda) plate. J Shoulder Elbow Surg 2008; 17(1):113–20.

38. Patel SS, Mir HR, Horowitz E, et al. ORIF of distal humerus fractures with modern pre-contoured implants is still associated with a high rate of complications. Indian J Orthop 2020;54(5):570–9.

39. Wilkinson JM, Stanley D. Posterior surgical approaches to the elbow: a comparative anatomic study. J Shoulder Elbow Surg 2001;10(4):380–2.

40. Meldrum A, Kwong C, Archibold K, et al. Olecranon osteotomy implant removal rates and associated complications [published online ahead of print, 2020 Oct 9]. J Orthop Trauma 2020. https://doi.org/10.1097/BOT.0000000000001979.

41. Coles CP, Barei DP, Nork SE, et al. The olecranon osteotomy: a six-year experience in the treatment of intraarticular fractures of the distal humerus. J Orthop Trauma 2006;20(3):164–71.

42. Kaiser PB, Newman ET, Haggerty C, et al. A limited fixation, olecranon sparing approach, for management of geriatric intra-articular distal humerus fractures. Geriatr Orthop Surg Rehabil 2020;11. 2151459320950063.

43. Ali A, Shahane S, Stanley D. Total elbow arthroplasty for distal humeral fractures: indications,

surgical approach, technical tips, and outcome. J Shoulder Elbow Surg 2010;19(2 Suppl):53–8.

44. Chalidis B, Dimitriou C, Papadopoulos P, et al. Total elbow arthroplasty for the treatment of insufficient distal humeral fractures. A retrospective clinical study and review of the literature. Injury 2009;40(6):582–90.

45. Cobb TK, Morrey BF. Total elbow arthroplasty as primary treatment for distal humeral fractures in elderly patients. J Bone Joint Surg Am 1997; 79(6):826–32.

46. Egol KA, Tsai P, Vazques O, et al. Comparison of functional outcomes of total elbow arthroplasty vs plate fixation for distal humerus fractures in osteoporotic elbows. Am J Orthop (Belle Mead Nj) 2011;40(2):67–71.

47. Gambirasio R, Riand N, Stern R, et al. Total elbow replacement for complex fractures of the distal humerus. An option for the elderly patient. J Bone Joint Surg Br 2001;83(7):974–8.

48. Garcia JA, Mykula R, Stanley D. Complex fractures of the distal humerus in the elderly. The role of total elbow replacement as primary treatment. J Bone Joint Surg Br 2002;84(6):812–6.

49. Gay DM, Lyman S, Do H, et al. Indications and reoperation rates for total elbow arthroplasty: an analysis of trends in New York State. J Bone Joint Surg Am 2012;94(2):110–7.

50. McKee MD, Veillette CJ, Hall JA, et al. A multicenter, prospective, randomized, controlled trial of open reduction–internal fixation versus total elbow arthroplasty for displaced intra-articular distal humeral fractures in elderly patients. J Shoulder Elbow Surg 2009;18(1):3–12.

51. Morrey BF. Total elbow arthroplasty did not differ from open reduction and internal fixation with regard to reoperation rates. J Bone Joint Surg Am 2009;91(8):2010.

52. Varecka TF, Myeroff C. Distal humerus fractures in the elderly population. J Am Acad Orthop Surg 2017;25(10):673–83.

53. Rommens PM, Küchle R, Schneider RU, et al. Olecranon fractures in adults: factors influencing outcome. Injury 2004;35(11):1149–57.

54. Duckworth AD, Clement ND, Aitken SA, et al. The epidemiology of fractures of the proximal ulna. Injury 2012;43(3):343–6.

55. Morrey BF. Current concepts in the treatment of fractures of the radial head, the olecranon, and the coronoid. Instr Course Lect 1995;44: 175–85.

56. Marot V, Bayle-Iniguez X, Cavaignac E, et al. Results of non-operative treatment of olecranon fracture in over 75-year-olds. Orthop Traumatol Surg Res 2018;104(1):79–82.

57. Duckworth AD, Bugler KE, Clement ND, et al. Nonoperative management of displaced olecranon fractures in low-demand elderly patients. J Bone Joint Surg Am 2014;96(1):67–72.

58. Gallucci GL, Piuzzi NS, Slullitel PA, et al. Non-surgical functional treatment for displaced olecranon fractures in the elderly. Bone Joint J 2014;96-B(4): 530–4.

59. Duckworth AD, Clement ND, McEachan JE, et al. Prospective randomised trial of non-operative versus operative management of olecranon fractures in the elderly. Bone Joint J 2017;99-B(7): 964–72.

60. Umer S, et al. Olecranon fractures in the elderly. Is tension band wiring the right treatment? Inj Extra 2011;42(9):122–3.

61. Duckworth AD, Clement ND, White TO, et al. Plate versus tension-band wire fixation for olecranon fractures: a prospective randomized trial. J Bone Joint Surg Am 2017;99(15):1261–73.

62. Ren YM, Qiao HY, Wei ZJ, et al. Efficacy and safety of tension band wiring versus plate fixation in olecranon fractures: a systematic review and meta-analysis. J Orthop Surg Res 2016; 11(1):137.

63. Hume MC, Wiss DA. Olecranon fractures. A clinical and radiographic comparison of tension band wiring and plate fixation. Clin Orthop Relat Res 1992;285:229–35.

64. Schliemann B, Raschke MJ, Groene P, et al. Comparison of tension band wiring and precontoured locking compression plate fixation in Mayo type IIA olecranon fractures. Acta Orthop Belg 2014; 80(1):106–11.

65. Hutchinson DT, Horwitz DS, Ha G, et al. Cyclic loading of olecranon fracture fixation constructs. J Bone Joint Surg Am 2003;85(5):831–7.

66. Niglis L, Bonnomet F, Schenck B, et al. Critical analysis of olecranon fracture management by pre-contoured locking plates. Orthop Traumatol Surg Res 2015;101(2):201–7.

67. Erturer RE, Sever C, Sonmez MM, et al. Results of open reduction and plate osteosynthesis in comminuted fracture of the olecranon. J Shoulder Elbow Surg 2011;20(3):449–54.

68. Wise KL, Peck S, Smith L, et al. Locked plating of geriatric olecranon fractures leads to low fixation failure and acceptable complication rates. JSES Int 2021;5(4):809–15.

69. Izzi J, Athwal GS. An off-loading triceps suture for augmentation of plate fixation in comminuted osteoporotic fractures of the olecranon. J Orthop Trauma 2012;26(1):59–61.

70. Siebenlist S, Buchholz A, Braun KF. Fractures of the proximal ulna: current concepts in surgical management. EFORT Open Rev 2019;4(1):1–9.

71. Mason ML. Some observations on fractures of the head of the radius with a review of one hundred cases. Br J Surg 1954;42(172):123–32.

72. Kodde IF, Kaas L, Flipsen M, et al. Current concepts in the management of radial head fractures. World J Orthop 2015;6(11):954–60.

73. Kaas L, van Riet RP, Vroemen JP, et al. The epidemiology of radial head fractures. J Shoulder Elbow Surg 2010;19(4):520–3.

74. Duckworth AD, Clement ND, Jenkins PJ, et al. The epidemiology of radial head and neck fractures. J Hand Surg Am 2012;37(1):112–9.

75. Morrey BF, An KN. Stability of the elbow: osseous constraints. J Shoulder Elbow Surg 2005;14(1 Suppl S):174S–8S.

76. van Riet RP, van den Bekerom M, Van Tongel A, et al. Radial head fractures. Shoulder Elbow 2020;12(3):212–23.

77. Morrey BF. Radial head fractures. In: BF M, editor. The elbow and its disorders. Philadelphia: WB Saunders; 1985. p. 355.

78. Johnston GW. A follow-up of one hundred cases of fracture of the head of the radius with a review of the literature. Ulster Med J 1962;31(1):51–6.

79. Mahmoud SS, Moideen AN, Kotwal R, et al. Management of Mason type 1 radial head fractures: a regional survey and a review of literature. Eur J Orthop Surg Traumatol 2014;24(7):1133–7.

80. Smits AJ, Giannakopoulos GF, Zuidema WP. Long-term results and treatment modalities of conservatively treated Broberg-Morrey type 1 radial head fractures. Injury 2014;45(10):1564–8.

81. Al-Burdeni S, Abuodeh Y, Ibrahim T, et al. Open reduction and internal fixation versus radial head arthroplasty in the treatment of adult closed comminuted radial head fractures (modified Mason type III and IV). Int Orthop 2015;39(8):1659–64.

82. Duckworth AD, Wickramasinghe NR, Clement ND, et al. Radial head replacement for acute complex fractures: what are the rate and risks factors for revision or removal? Clin Orthop Relat Res 2014;472(7):2136–43.

83. Solarino G, Vicenti G, Abate A, et al. Mason type II and III radial head fracture in patients older than 65: is there still a place for radial head resection? Aging Clin Exp Res 2015;27(Suppl 1):S77–83.

84. Lott A, Broder K, Goch A, et al. Results after radial head arthroplasty in unstable fractures. J Shoulder Elbow Surg 2018;27(2):270–5.

85. Li N, Chen S. Open reduction and internal-fixation versus radial head replacement in treatment of Mason type III radial head fractures. Eur J Orthop Surg Traumatol 2014;24(6):851–5.

86. Stoneback JW, Owens BD, Sykes J, et al. Incidence of elbow dislocations in the United States population. J Bone Joint Surg Am 2012;94(3):240–5.

87. Kuhn MA, Ross G. Acute elbow dislocations. Orthop Clin North Am 2008;39(2):155–v.

88. Broberg MA, Morrey BF. Results of treatment of fracture-dislocations of the elbow. Clin Orthop Relat Res 1987;216:109–19.

89. Regan W, Morrey B. Fractures of the coronoid process of the ulna. J Bone Joint Surg Am 1989;71(9):1348–54.

90. Terada N, Yamada H, Seki T, et al. The importance of reducing small fractures of the coronoid process in the treatment of unstable elbow dislocation. J Shoulder Elbow Surg 2000;9(4):344–6.

91. Schreiber JJ, Warren RF, Hotchkiss RN, et al. An online video investigation into the mechanism of elbow dislocation. J Hand Surg Am 2013;38(3):488–94.

92. O'Driscoll SW, Morrey BF, Korinek S, et al. Elbow subluxation and dislocation. A spectrum of instability. Clin Orthop Relat Res 1992;280:186–97.

93. de Haan J, Schep NW, Tuinebreijer WE, et al. Simple elbow dislocations: a systematic review of the literature. Arch Orthop Trauma Surg 2010;130(2):241–9.

94. Maripuri SN, Debnath UK, Rao P, et al. Simple elbow dislocation among adults: a comparative study of two different methods of treatment. Injury 2007;38(11):1254–8.

95. Taylor F, Sims M, Theis JC, et al. Interventions for treating acute elbow dislocations in adults. Cochrane Database Syst Rev 2012;2012(4):CD007908.

96. Kesmezacar H, Sarıkaya IA. The results of conservatively treated simple elbow dislocations. Acta Orthop Traumatol Turc 2010;44(3):199–205.

97. Mehlhoff TL, Noble PC, Bennett JB, et al. Simple dislocation of the elbow in the adult. Results after closed treatment. J Bone Joint Surg Am 1988;70(2):244–9.

98. Eygendaal D, Verdegaal SH, Obermann WR, et al. Posterolateral dislocation of the elbow joint. Relationship to medial instability. J Bone Joint Surg Am 2000;82(4):555–60.

99. Anakwe RE, Middleton SD, Jenkins PJ, et al. Patient-reported outcomes after simple dislocation of the elbow. J Bone Joint Surg Am 2011;93(13):1220–6.

100. Chan K, MacDermid JC, Faber KJ, et al. Can we treat select terrible triad injuries nonoperatively? Clin Orthop Relat Res 2014;472(7):2092–9.

101. Chemama B, Bonnevialle N, Peter O, et al. Terrible triad injury of the elbow: how to improve outcomes? Orthop Traumatol Surg Res 2010;96(2):147–54.

102. Jeong WK, Oh JK, Hwang JH, et al. Results of terrible triads in the elbow: the advantage of primary restoration of medial structure. J Orthop Sci 2010;15(5):612–9.

103. van Riet RP, Morrey BF, O'Driscoll SW. Use of osteochondral bone graft in coronoid fractures. J Shoulder Elbow Surg 2005;14(5):519–23.

104. Egol KA, Immerman I, Paksima N, et al. Fracture-dislocation of the elbow functional outcome

following treatment with a standardized protocol. Bull NYU Hosp Jt Dis 2007;65(4):263–70.

105. Forthman C, Henket M, Ring DC. Elbow dislocation with intra-articular fracture: the results of operative treatment without repair of the medial collateral ligament. J Hand Surg Am 2007;32(8):1200–9.

106. Lindenhovius AL, Jupiter JB, Ring D. Comparison of acute versus subacute treatment of terrible triad injuries of the elbow. J Hand Surg Am 2008;33(6):920–6.

107. Seijas R, Ares-Rodriguez O, Orellana A, et al. Terrible triad of the elbow. J Orthop Surg (Hong Kong) 2009;17(3):335–9.

108. Winter M, Chuinard C, Cikes A, et al. Surgical management of elbow dislocation associated with non-reparable fractures of the radial head. Chir Main 2009;28(3):158–67.

109. Wang YX, Huang LX, Ma SH. Surgical treatment of "terrible triad of the elbow": technique and outcome. Orthop Surg 2010;2(2):141–8.

110. Garrigues GE, Wray WH 3rd, Lindenhovius AL, et al. Fixation of the coronoid process in elbow fracture-dislocations. J Bone Joint Surg Am 2011;93(20):1873–81.

111. Zhang C, Zhong B, Luo CF. Treatment strategy of terrible triad of the elbow: experience in Shanghai 6th People's Hospital. Injury 2014;45(6):942–8.

112. Zeiders GJ, Patel MK. Management of unstable elbows following complex fracture-dislocations– the "terrible triad" injury. J Bone Joint Surg Am 2008;90(Suppl 4):75–84.

113. Giannicola G, Calella P, Piccioli A, et al. Terrible triad of the elbow: is it still a troublesome injury? Injury 2015;46(Suppl 8):S68–76.

Foot and Ankle

The Syndesmosis, Part I

Anatomy, Injury Mechanism, Classification, and Diagnosis

Lorena Bejarano-Pineda, MD[a,b],
Daniel Guss, MD, MBA[a,b], Gregory Waryasz, MD[a,b],
Christopher W. DiGiovanni, MD[a,b],
John Y. Kwon, MD[a,b],*

KEYWORDS

- Syndesmosis • Diagnosis • Syndesmotic injury • Classification • Advanced imaging
- Stress radiographs

KEY POINTS

- The syndesmosis has a complex osseoligamentous anatomy.
- Although the deltoid ligament is not formally part of the syndesmotic complex, concomitant injury is common and can significantly influence mortise instability.
- Diagnosis, in the absence of fracture or radiographic diastasis, can be difficult.
- Obtaining a history of injury mechanism, thorough physical examination and judicious use of adjunctive imaging modalities, aid in proper diagnosis.
- Conservative treatment modalities can be effective and should be trialed when gross instability or diastasis is not present.

INTRODUCTION

Ankle fractures are common injuries to the lower extremity, with approximately 20% sustaining a concomitant injury to the syndesmosis.[1–4] Suprasyndesmotic fibula fractures, when associated with a rotational injury mechanism, have an even higher incidence. In athletes, syndesmotic injuries account for up to 25% of ankle sprains with approximately 6500 syndesmotic injuries occurring yearly based on emergency room data.[5–8] Given the potential difficulties in diagnosis, the true incidence of syndesmotic injuries is likely higher than previously reported. Whether occurring with or without a concomitant fracture, syndesmotic injuries have prolonged recovery times[9,10] and increased potential for long-term sequela.[10]

If persistent diastasis or dynamic instability ensues, chronic pain and dysfunction are common and often require surgical intervention.[11] Malreduction has been demonstrated to result in poor outcomes.[11–14] Ray and colleagues[14] demonstrated the occurrence of symptomatic osteoarthritis within 7 years after injury in 11% of ankle fractures requiring syndesmotic fixation. Proper diagnosis and treatment is essential to allow for restoration of function and to avoid long-term complications.

ANATOMY

The syndesmosis is constituted by the distal tibia, distal fibula and 4 ligamentous structures: the anterior inferior tibiofibular ligament (AITFL), posterior inferior tibiofibular ligament (PITFL),

---

[a] Foot & Ankle Research and Innovation Laboratory - Harvard Medical School, Division of Foot and Ankle Surgery, Department of Orthopaedic Surgery, Massachusetts General Hospital - Newton-Wellesley Hospital, 40 2nd Avenue Building 52, Suite 1150, Waltham, MA 02451, USA; [b] Foot & Ankle Service, Department of Orthopaedic Surgery, Massachusetts General Hospital, 40 2nd Avenue Building 52, Suite 1150, Waltham, MA 02451, USA
* Corresponding author. Foot & Ankle Service, Department of Orthopaedic Surgery, Massachusetts General Hospital, 40 2nd Avenue Building 52, Suite 1150, Waltham, MA 02451.
E-mail address: johnkwonmd@gmail.com

Orthop Clin N Am 52 (2021) 403–415
https://doi.org/10.1016/j.ocl.2021.05.010
0030-5898/21/© 2021 Elsevier Inc. All rights reserved.

interosseous ligament (IOL), and interosseous membrane (IOM).[15] Although the deltoid ligament (DL) is not formally a part of the syndesmotic complex, it plays a key role in mortise stability and will be further discussed in this section.

Osseous Anatomy

The osseous anatomy consists of the incisura tibialis that articulates with the distal fibula. The proximal apex begins where the lateral tibial ridge bifurcates 6 to 8 cm proximal to the plafond forming the anterior and posterior margins that terminate distally as Chaput's and Volkmann's tubercles, respectively. Corresponding fibular anatomy matches the concave shape of the incisura tibialis. Chaput's tubercle is more prominent than Volkmann's tubercle and overlaps the anterior fibula.[15] The anterior fibular tubercle (Wagstaff–Le Fort tubercle) is more prominent than the posterior fibular tubercle.[15,16]

Although the tibiofibular contact area can be variable in size, it has been shown to consist of articulating cartilage facets in 100% of cadavers examined.[7,15,17] The presence of articular cartilage and the known dynamic nature of the syndesmosis illustrates its importance for normal ankle kinematics. Furthermore, these facets may provide visual landmarks for syndesmotic reduction when undergoing surgery.[15,17] The syndesmotic recess is a synovial joint contiguous with the ankle joint and bordered anteriorly by the AITFL and superiorly by the IOM.[7,17] Contrast leakage proximal to this synovial cavity, such as seen during arthrogram performed for suspected injury, may indicate significant syndesmotic disruption.[15] Similarly, proximal migration of joint fluid as seen on T2 sequencing on either coronal or MRI imaging can a give a similar appearance and may indicate syndesmotic disruption (Fig. 1).

Significant anatomic variation of the osseous articulation as described elsewhere in this article above and may influence predisposition to injury and risk of malreduction.[15,18] Additionally, significant anatomic variation of the incisura may make assessment of malalignment difficult even with axial advanced imaging.

Ligamentous Anatomy

The trapezoidal-shaped AITFL consists of 3 to 5 fascicles and runs distolaterally from the tibia to the fibula.[7,15] An anomalous distal band called Bassett ligament can exist and may cause symptomatic ankle impingement.[15] The AITFL

contributes approximately 35% of the tensile strength of the syndesmosis.[19]

The PITFL has superficial and deep components and contributes approximately 42% of syndesmotic strength.[19] The superficial portion is trapezoidal with multiple fascicles converging distally.[7] The deep portion (sometimes called the inferior transverse ligament) has more dense fibers and a thicker, rounder shape.[7,15] The PITFL has a broad attachment on Volkmann's tubercle. Given its tibial attachment, injury often results in an osseous avulsion rather than isolated rupture with rotational injuries.[15] Although posterior malleolus fracture morphology can vary,[20] the PITFL often remains largely intact according to MRI studies.[21] The PITFL's osseous attachments have important implications for posterior malleolar fixation affecting stability,[22] syndesmotic reduction,[21] and functional outcomes after ankle fractures.[23]

The IOL originates at the distal margin of the IOM. Biomechanical studies have demonstrated that the IOL contributes up to 22% of the strength of the syndesmosis.[19] The IOM lies between the lateral tibial ridge and the medial fibular ridge. Distally, it terminates as the IOL at the bifurcation of the tibial ridge of the incisura tibialis. Like the IOL, the IOM also seems to be loaded particularly during stance phase.[14] Although it contributes to syndesmotic stability, the IOM likely plays a lesser role compared with the other ligamentous components.[19]

Although not an anatomic component of the syndesmosis, the DL contributes directly to mortise stability and is often injured concomitant to the syndesmosis.[9,24] Approximately 50% of patients with DL disruption have an associated syndesmotic injury.[24] Massri-Pugin and colleagues[25] demonstrated that isolated DL disruption with or without sectioning of the AITFL did not render the syndesmosis unstable as assessed by Cotton testing. However, the syndesmosis became unstable if the DL was disrupted in combination with the AITFL and IOL. The same researchers demonstrated that isolated disruption of the AITFL and IOL was not enough to produce coronal instability.[26] Concomitant DL disruption may produce instability even in the presence of intact posterior structures.[25] Additionally, Goetz and colleagues,[27] using computed tomography (CT) imaging of loaded cadaveric specimens, demonstrated differences between instability patterns in the intact state, with isolated deep DL disruption, and with disruption of both the DL and syndesmotic ligaments. These and other investigations demonstrate the complex interplay between the DL in

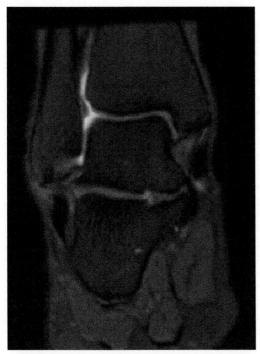

Fig. 1. A 31-year-old woman with history of chronic syndesmotic injury. T2 coronal imaging demonstrates extravasation of ankle joint fluid proximally consistent with syndesmotic disruption.

the setting of concomitant syndesmotic injury as it relates to subsequent instability.

MECHANISM OF INJURY

Syndesmotic injury typically results from supra-physiologic ankle external rotation.[9,28] Although a pronated foot position at time of injury has been postulated to lead to a higher incidence, syndesmotic injury can occur regardless of specific foot position.[29] Lauge-Hansen's mechanistic theory of ankle fractures postulated that a pronated foot puts the medial ankle ligamentous (DL) structures on tension, thus initially creating a medial-sided osseoligamentous disruption. As external rotation continues, the AITFL is disrupted followed by the posterior ligaments. Continued abnormal loading can result in disruption of the IOM and a suprasyndesmotic fibula fracture.[3,25] Syndesmotic injuries commonly occur during contact sports, which involve lateral movements and may be related to external foot constraint.[9,10,30]

CLASSIFICATION

There have been several classification systems to describe syndesmotic injury. A simple

grading system, based on symptoms and radiographic findings, has been used most commonly.[9,10,31–33] Grade I injuries demonstrate a stable syndesmosis, mild symptoms, and normal radiographs indicating ligamentous sprain. Conservative treatment as described elsewhere in this article is recommended. Grade II injuries have partial syndesmotic complex disruption with variable instability. Provocative examination tests may be positive, but radiographic findings are normal and generally conservative treatment is trialed. Given the interplay of the DL, some authors consider concomitant DL disruption, as visualized on MRI, as an indication for surgical stabilization in the setting of grade II injuries.[33] Some patients with grade II injuries, either after a trial of conservative treatment and/or with other mitigating factors, may be candidates for earlier surgical intervention. In grade III injuries, the entire anterior and posterior syndesmotic complex is disrupted with clear malalignment on plain radiographs requiring surgical stabilization.[9,33]

DIAGNOSIS

Subtle syndesmotic injuries can be difficult to diagnose, especially in the absence of fracture. This factor is compounded by a lack of consensus on criteria and variable reliability, sensitivity and specificity of diagnostic tests.[28] Although radiographic diastasis and gross instability on examination are obvious, careful history taking and physical examination may elucidate more subtle instability.

History

Although patients may recall a specific injury mechanism predisposing to syndesmotic injury,[28] many are often unable to recount a definitive mechanism, in contrast with patients sustaining simple inversion injuries. A history of trauma during impact or collision sports should increase the suspicion for occult syndesmotic injury. Signs and symptoms may include pain above the ankle joint, functional instability, and/or a history of protracted recovery.[33] Patients with chronic syndesmotic injury, although outside the focus of this work, may complain of a pain, a giving way sensation, difficulty ambulating on uneven ground, stiffness, and/or limited dorsiflexion.[34]

Physical Examination

In the acutely injured patient, either with or without a concomitant malleoli fracture, physical examination may be limited in assessing syndesmotic disruption. Patients with syndesmotic disruption classically have tenderness above the ankle joint at the level of the AITFL. They may also have tenderness with palpation of the posterior syndesmosis and associated swelling.[26,31] Tenderness along the entire lower leg is common with advanced disruption. Compartment syndrome should always be ruled out.

Several clinical tests have been described, mainly for patients without ankle fracture, albeit with variable sensitivity, specificity, and reliability.[28,33] Although they are described elsewhere in this article, these tests may be more applicable to patients without fracture. In the acutely traumatized patient, ensuring adequate neurovascular status and the absence of compartment syndrome takes priority. The external rotation stress test is performed by placing the ankle in a neutral position and externally rotating the foot with the knee flexed. Pain over the syndesmosis is considered a positive test. The dorsiflexion range of motion test involves passive ankle dorsiflexion with a positive test demonstrating reduced motion (as compared with the contralateral ankle) secondary to pain inhibition. The squeeze test is positive when proximal compression of the tibia and fibula causes pain distally at the syndesmosis. Despite these described maneuvers, Sman and colleagues[28] found low diagnostic accuracy of nearly all clinical tests. However, a positive squeeze test may be prognostic because it was associated with a longer time to return to sporting activities. The external rotation stress test and squeeze test both demonstrated high specificity but relatively low sensitivity for detecting injury when correlated with MRI findings. Furthermore, variable interobserver reliability has been demonstrated for most physical examination tests. As such, providers should not solely rely on physical examination to diagnose syndesmotic injury.

IMAGING
Plain Radiographs
Initial radiographic evaluation, especially in the acute trauma setting, should include non–weight-bearing anteroposterior (AP), mortise, and lateral views of the ankle. Weightbearing radiographs are preferred when a malleoli fracture is ruled out. AP and lateral tibia–fibula radiographs may be required to rule out a Maisonneuve injury. Given known anatomic variability, bilateral imaging is helpful especially in cases of subtle instability. Normal parameters include

(1) tibiofibular clear space (TFCS) of less than 5 mm or less than 44% of the fibular width on AP and mortise views; (2) medial clear space of no more than 4 mm or less than 2 mm than the contralateral side; and (3) tibiofibular overlap of more than 5 mm or more than 24% of the fibular width on AP and more than 1 mm on mortise view.[35] These parameters are measured 10 mm above the ankle joint line. Choi and colleagues[36] described preoperative findings associated to syndesmotic injuries in 191 patients with supination external rotation ankle fractures. The cutoff values for predicting unstable syndesmotic injuries were medial joint space of greater than 4.5 mm and fracture height of greater than 7 mm. Fracture height was defined as the vertical height between the distal tibial articular surface and the most inferior point of the fracture line of the lateral malleolus. Although some patients may not demonstrate more than 1 mm of tibiofibular overlap on the mortise view secondary to anatomic variation, any lack of overlap should be considered a syndesmotic injury unless proven otherwise (Fig. 2).

Standard techniques to assess syndesmotic instability under stress radiographs are (1) stress the fibula in external rotation, (2) lateral stress test (Cotton) by applying a laterally directed force over the fibula, and (3) sagittal stress test by applying an anterior/posterior directed force over the fibula.[37] An external rotation test and sagittal stress testing can be performed during clinical assessment, but the Cotton test is an intraoperative assessment. Studies have shown that the Cotton test may be superior to external rotation testing. Jiang and colleagues[38] demonstrated that the Cotton test produced significant

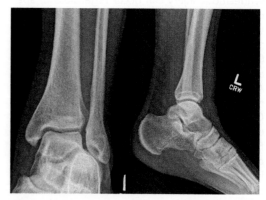

Fig. 2. An 18-year-old man status post-twisting injury while skiing. Mortise view of ankle radiographs demonstrates no tibiofibular overlap suspicious for syndesmotic injury. Stress fluoroscopy was subsequently performed, which demonstrated gross instability.

widening of the TFCS and medial clear space in the presence of IOM disruption. Likewise, Stoffel and colleagues[39] showed in a cadaveric study that the TFCS was more than 5 mm in 86% of specimens on the lateral stress test for Weber C injuries. Both studies demonstrated that the external rotation stress test is a poor indicator of syndesmotic disruption in the setting of associated DL injury. The use of radiostereometry for the external rotation test has shown fibular displacement after syndesmotic injury in the rotational plane,[40] which limits the usefulness of external rotation stress test with traditional radiographs. More recently, the role of sagittal stress testing has been studied. Lateral imaging seems to have greater sensitivity than mortise views in identifying syndesmotic injuries. LaMothe and colleagues[37] demonstrated that sagittal displacement of the fibula was twice as sensitive as compared with applied loads in coronal motion.

Although stress radiographs have proven helpful, there are several limitations described to their use. Coronal (and to a certain extent sagittal) stress maneuvers are difficult to perform in the clinical setting given the need to apply a mechanical force on the fibula directly. This factor limits its role in the diagnosis of subtle injuries. Additionally, the lack of consistency in position and interobserver reliability when defining stability may make the test less clinically useful. Lui and colleagues[41] compared intraoperative stress radiographs and ankle arthroscopy for the evaluation of syndesmotic injury in acute ankle fractures. They found that 30% of cases had positive stress radiographs as compared with 66% with positive arthroscopic findings for syndesmotic injury. Furthermore, Marmor and colleagues[42] showed in a cadaveric study that intraoperative fluoroscopy could not adequately detect rotational syndesmotic malreduction. Although plain radiographs should be part of the initial evaluation of the traumatized ankle, they may not be sensitive enough to detect subtle syndesmotic injuries as a sole diagnostic test.[43]

Computed Tomography Scans

Syndesmotic instability and malalignment is a multidimensional condition that affects the joint in the coronal, sagittal, and axial planes. CT scanning is a diagnostic tool that offers anatomic assessment in a multiplanar manner including 3-dimensional reformatting. A weight-bearing CT (WB-CT) scan adds the advantage of a more dynamic, physiologic evaluation allowing assessment in the standing position. Malhotra and

colleagues[44] compared supine and WB-CT images, demonstrating that the fibula translates laterally and posteriorly with external rotation in relation to the incisura in the standing position. This demonstrates potential enhanced benefit to WB-CT scans. Additional advantages include relatively low radiation exposure and reproducibility of measurements in less time by the use of automatic measurements that are generated by the device.[45]

There are several measurement methods described to assess the integrity of the syndesmosis on CT scan (Table 1). Lee and colleagues[46] evaluated the parameters to predict unstable syndesmotic injury in ankle fractures using a CT scan. They found that the syndesmotic area at 1 cm above the tibial plafond was the most reasonable parameter to predict syndesmotic injury (Fig. 3A). They described that a syndesmotic area 1.56 times larger than the contralateral side indicates a high possibility of injury. Abdelaziz and colleagues[47] also described that the syndesmotic area demonstrated the highest interobserver (0.96) and intraobserver agreement (>0.92) when assessing patients with unstable syndesmotic injuries. Similar results were found for fibular rotation with an interobserver and intraobserver reliability of 0.84 and more than 0.8, respectively. Volumetric measurements have recently been described. Bhimani and colleagues[48] reported WB-CT volumetric areas of the distal tibiofibular joint from the tibial plafond to 3 cm, 5 cm and 10 cm proximally. The authors found all volumetric measurements were significantly larger on the injured side as compared with the contralateral uninjured side (Fig. 3B). Volumetric analysis may be more accurate than previously used parameters.

Several authors have recommended obtaining bilateral ankle CT scans, especially in cases of subtle instability, given known significant anatomic variability of the syndesmosis.[49,50] Patel and colleagues[51] described reference values for the normal tibiofibular syndesmosis using WB-CT scans. In this retrospective review, the authors found that the upper limit of lateral translation in uninjured subjects was 5.27 mm, and the AP translation ranged between 1.48 mm and 3.44 mm anterior and posterior, respectively. There was no difference between the right and the left ankle, but men had significantly more lateral fibular translation. Likewise, Carrozzo and colleagues[52] showed that patients with a preoperative bilateral CT scan had better clinical outcomes and restoration of the tibiofibular joint anatomy as compared with those who

Table 1
Description of measurement methods in for syndesmotic injury

Method	Description	Definition of Injury
Anterior distance	Distance between the most anterior point of the fibula to the tibial border of the incisura in a line perpendicular to the fibular orientation line.[a]	
Posterior distance	Distance between the most posterior point of the fibula to the tibial border of the incisura in a line perpendicular to the fibular orientation line.[a]	
Middle distance	Distance between the most central point of the incisura and the nearest point of the fibula.	
Anterior tibiofibular tangential angle	The angle between the tangent to the anterior tibial surface at its most anterior point and the bisection of the vertical midline of the fibula.	
Tibiofibular line	A straight line placed along the anterolateral cortex of the fibula. The distance from the line to the anterior tubercle of the tibia determines syndesmotic instability.	Value ≥ 2 mm
Fibular sagittal translation	The distance between a line representing the direct anterior difference and the anterior border of tibial incisura.	Positive when the fibula is posterior to the anterior border of incisura
Syndesmotic area	The space between the lateral cortex of the tibial incisura, the medial cortex of the lateral malleolus, and 2 lines tangential to the anterior and posterior aspects of the tibia and fibula.	
Syndesmotic volume	Defined as the syndesmotic area spanning from the joint line to 5 cm proximally.	An absolute volume >14 cm^3 or $> 6 \pm 1.9$ cm^3 as compared with the contralateral ankle suggests syndesmotic instability
Fibular rotation	Angle between a line drawn between the anterior and posterior borders of the incisura and a line drawn in the fibula representing its orientation.	Positive when the fibula is internally rotated relative to the incisura

[a] Fibular orientation line, sagittal line connecting the most anterior point of the fibula with its most posterior point.

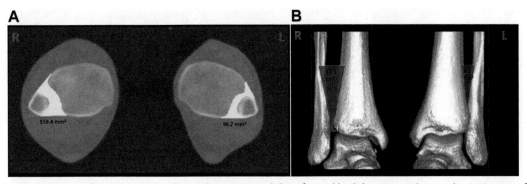

Fig. 3. A 33-year-old woman with right syndesmotic instability after ankle dislocation with a syndesmotic area of 159.4 mm^2 (*right*) versus 96.7 mm^2 (*left*) (*A*). Image demonstrating syndesmotic volume up to 5 cm from the tibial plafond of 13.1 cm^3 (*right*) versus 8.1 cm^3 (*left*) using WBCT (*B*). R, Right side; L, Left side.

had a CT scan of the injured ankle only. The lack of established measurements to determine syndesmosis instability or appropriate postoperative reduction accurately, underscores the importance and utility of contralateral imaging to detect syndesmotic injury. Furthermore, while beyond the scope of this work, increasing research is being performed examining the accuracy and validity of current measurement techniques to assess syndesmotic alignment on axial CT imaging. Recently, Wellman and colleagues used bilateral lower extremity CT imaging and demonstrated an apparent 35% rate of syndesmotic malalignment in patients with asymptomatic ankles questioning the validity of common measurement techniques as well as previously reported rates of syndesmotic malalignment.[53] Despite apparent limitations of specific measurement techniques, bilateral CT affords excellent comparative imaging and WB-CT may prove to be the best diagnostic test to determine syndesmotic malalignment.

MRI

Magnetic resonance imaging allows assessment with a high degree of sensitivity and specificity.[54,55] Findings vary based on acuity of injury. In the acute setting, high T2 signal in the location of the syndesmotic ligaments (associated with a wavy appearance or irregular contour) suggests complete ligament tear (Fig. 4A, B). Posterior malleolus bone edema is associated with PITFL injury and has been described in up to 93% of cases in acute injuries but only 54% of chronic conditions (Fig. 4C).[56] The presence of fluid signal within the distal tibiofibular joint space is considered suggestive of syndesmotic injury.[57] When signaling extends more than 12 mm proximal to the plafond, an IOL injury is likely present.[58–60]

The MRI slice orientation plays an important role in diagnosis. Ligament fiber obliqueness can lead to a false positive diagnosis of syndesmotic injury particularly when assessing the AITFL in the axial plane. Hermans and colleagues[59] demonstrated that, in the axial plane, the AITFL seemed to be partly discontinuous in 31% and completely discontinuous in 69% of healthy ankles. Instead, with a 45° oblique orientation the AITFL seemed to be continuous in 88% and partially discontinuous in only 12%. Another use of MRI in patients with presumed syndesmotic injury is to determine the presence of associated injuries (ie, tendon injury, lateral ligament disruption, osteochondral lesions) that may require surgical treatment and can be addressed concurrently.

Ultrasound Examination

Ultrasound examination is a readily available, low-cost test that offers dynamic evaluation of the distal tibiofibular joint. Ultrasound examination has the advantages of high-resolution imaging with no exposure to radiation. Particularly for the assessment of the ankle joint, it is recommended to use a high-frequency transducer of 15 to 18 MHz ($\geq$10 MHz) with a small footprint or transducer that allows for a more precise assessment.[60] During evaluation, the ankle ligaments should be slightly taut and are best evaluated in the long axis. The ankle is slightly inverted and the AITFL is identified in an oblique fashion from superomedial to inferolateral. Its normal thickness ranges from 2.6 to 4.0 mm and consists of multiple fascicles that can be confused with injury.[61] Fisher and colleagues[62] reported that TFCS widening of 6 mm or greater was diagnostic for syndesmotic injury in patients with supination–external rotation ankle injuries (Figs. 5 and 6). Although historically the greatest

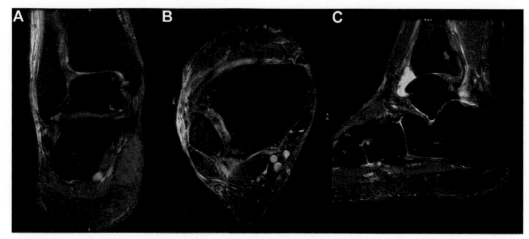

Fig. 4. A 40-year-old man with syndesmotic injury. Complete rupture of AITFL and IOL with irregular appearance (*A* & *B*, red arrow). Posterior malleolus bone marrow edema (*C*, red arrow).

limitation of ultrasound examination has been that it is operator dependent, Hagemeijer and colleagues[63] described excellent intraobserver and interobserver agreement (intraclass correlation coefficient of >0.8) in dynamic stress ultrasound examination when evaluating the syndesmosis. These findings highlight the ability of the test to diagnose syndesmotic injury, making it a viable alternative in patients with contraindications to other diagnostic tests as MRI or CT scan. Given its multiple advantages, increased familiarity and use among orthopedic surgeons may increase the use of ultrasound examination in diagnosing syndesmotic injury.

ARTHROSCOPIC AND INTRAOPERATIVE EVALUATION

Although a more comprehensive description of intraoperative evaluation is described in the article, we briefly include the use of arthroscopy and other modalities here given their diagnostic capabilities. Arthroscopy has hitherto been described as the gold standard in diagnosing subtle syndesmotic instability because it allows for the direct visualization of the distal tibiofibular articulation under an applied stress. Its invasive nature generally limits its use to scenarios in which there is a high index of clinical suspicion and/or if a

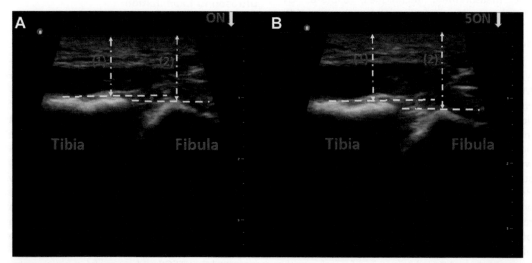

Fig. 5. Fibular translation measurements on ultrasound images under manually applied sagittal force from anterior to posterior direction in intact stage. (*A*) Under 0 N force. (*B*) Under 50 N of posteriorly directed force. (1) Distance from the ultrasound probe to the tibial osseous structure closest to the probe. (2) Distance from the ultrasound probe to the hyperechoic fibular osseous structure closest to the probe.

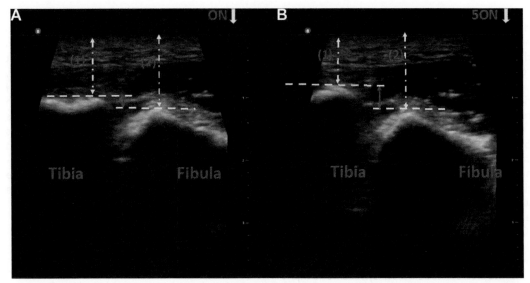

Fig. 6. Fibular translation measurements on ultrasound images under manually applied sagittal force from anterior to posterior direction after AITFL + OIL + PITFL transection. (*A*) Under 0 N force. (*B*) Under 50 N of posteriorly directed force. (1) Distance from the ultrasound probe to the hyperechoic tibial osseous structure closest to the probe. (2) Distance from the ultrasound probe to the hyperechoic fibular osseous structure closest to the probe.

patient is undergoing an operative procedure for concomitant pathology. Syndesmotic instability can readily be evaluated in the coronal and sagittal plane; rotational instability of the fibula can also occur, but is more challenging to visualize arthroscopically.

To assess coronal plane instability, the Cotton test is performed approximately 5 cm above the ankle joint with 100 N of force. This force value is based on cadaveric findings that forces greater than this amount do not result in an increased diastasis.[39] Other maneuvers such as external rotation tests may preferentially stress the DL.[38] Coronal plane measurements should be performed at the posterior one-third of the incisura rather than at the anterior one-third, where instability can be masked.[39] Although absolute values vary, a diastasis of more than 3 mm has been suggested as an appropriate threshold to detect subtle instability but avoid overdiagnosis.[39] The advantage of this threshold value is that it can be assessed using a probe size readily available in standard arthroscopy instrumentation sets.

Sagittal plane motion may be more sensitive than coronal plane diastasis in diagnosing syndesmotic instability.[64] To evaluate this factor, 100 N of force is applied 5 cm above the ankle joint in both an AP and posterior to anterior direction. Total fibular motion or more than 2 mm is not only suggestive of syndesmotic instability, but has demonstrated high sensitivity

and specificity (77.5% and 88.9%, respectively). Quantitative algorithms that incorporate both coronal and sagittal plane motion do exist and better reflect the 3-dimensional nature of syndesmotic instability, but are cumbersome to use in practice.[27]

Syndesmotic testing in the operating room can be performed by direct visualization or examination, radiography with or without stress evaluation, arthroscopic assessment, ultrasound examination, and/or intraoperative CT scan. Intraoperatively, it is important to continually assess instability and/or resultant stability after fixation.

CONSERVATIVE TREATMENT

Patients with syndesmotic injury with no evidence of instability nor diastasis can be treated nonoperatively. Some studies have suggested that isolated injury to the AITFL with an intact DL should be managed conservatively. Patients with syndesmotic injury with diastasis and/or concomitant fractures should generally be treated surgically. Conservative treatment consists of 3 stages: (1) a period of immobilization, limited weightbearing, rest, ice, elevation, compression, anti-inflammatories and therapeutic modalities, (2) functional and proprioceptive rehabilitation with associated brace wear, progression to full weightbearing and activity modification, and (3) progressive return to play.[65]

Electric stimulation and massage has been demonstrated to be efficacious.[33] Doughtie and colleagues[66] in a survey study reported that the most important modalities for reducing recovery time after syndesmotic sprains in National Football League athletes were immobilization followed by corticosteroid injection, ice, and rest.

Syndesmotic injury and injury severity have been associated with significant prolonged recovery times and delayed return to play. Knapik and colleagues[67] reported a return to competition in 2 to 6 weeks after stable syndemotic injuries in professional football players. Miller and colleagues[68] found that athletes with intact IOM had an average return to play of 12.6 days and those with an IOM injury had an average of 19.6 days. Likewise, the presence of heterotopic ossification after syndesmotic injury has been associated with higher rate of reinjuries, such as lateral ankle sprains and syndesmosis sprains.

Novel therapeutic modalities for conservative treatment of sport-related injuries have been described recently. However, the long-term impact is unknown and few comparative investigations exist. Dry needling is a relatively new procedure that involves using a needle to regulate trigger points.[67] Salom-Moreno and colleagues[69] described better functional outcomes after proprioceptive rehabilitation combined with dry needling compared with proprioceptive rehabilitation alone in patients with chronic lateral ankle instability. Blood flow restriction therapy is considered to assist in decreasing muscle atrophy and is increasingly being implemented for a variety of orthopedic conditions. In theory, this technique promotes protein synthesis through activation of the rapamycin complex (MTORC1) pathway via metabolic stress or muscle swelling.[70] Levels of growth hormone also have been seen to spike with blood flow restriction and low load training, which may facilitate collagen synthesis.[71]

There have been recent investigations into whether cortisone or platelet-rich plasma injections may improve symptoms. Periligamentous cortisone injections may in general be considered safe but only for short-term treatment and with limited application.[72] Local anesthetic injections have also been performed in high level athletes to assist with symptom relief with no significant known effects long-term. Platelet-rich plasma injections have limited data to date. Laver and colleagues[73] performed a randomized control trial using platelet-rich growth factors for high-level athletes with AITFL injury.

Athletes in the treatment group demonstrated a faster return to play from 41 days as compared with 60 days in the control group. Differences in residual pain also improved in the treatment group compared with the control. Similarly, Samra and colleagues[74] performed a level I investigation examining the role of platelet-rich plasma for syndesmotic sprains in rugby players and found that the return to play was 20 days sooner in the platelet-rich plasma group than in the control group. Further research in the usefulness of biologics as an adjuvant therapy in the conservative treatment of syndesmotic injury is warranted.

SUMMARY

The syndesmosis has a complex osseoligamentous anatomy and is commonly injured when associated with rotational ankle fractures. Even in the absence of concomitant fracture, syndesmotic injuries are common and likely underdiagnosed. Diagnosis, in the absence of radiographic diastasis, can be difficult. Obtaining a thorough history and physical examination as well as judicious use of adjunctive imaging modalities aid in diagnosis. Proper and timely diagnosis is critical in initiating appropriate treatment and optimizing outcomes. Conservative treatment modalities can be effective and should be trialed when surgery is not indicated.

CLINICS CARE POINTS

- The clinician cannot rely on a single test to diagnose syndesmotic injury. The clinical diagnosis should comprise clinical history with physical findings.
- Given the anatomic variability of the syndesmosis, imaging of the contralateral ankle provides very valuable information, especially in absence of fracture or frank diastasis.
- Stress radiographs can be difficult to perform in the clinical setting and they are not easily reproducible given the wide variation of the technique.
- Weight-bearing CT is a diagnostic tool that offers a dynamic and three-dimensional evaluation of the syndesmosis.
- Magnetic resonance imaging has a high sensitivity for acute syndesmotic injury and is useful to determine the presence of associated injuries.

REFERENCES

1. Shibuya N, Davis ML, Jupiter DC. Epidemiology of foot and ankle fractures in the United States: an analysis of the National Trauma Data Bank (2007 to 2011). J Foot Ankle Surg 2014;53(5):606–8.

2. Jennison T, Brinsden M. Fracture admission trends in England over a ten-year period. Ann R Coll Surg Engl 2019;101(3):208–14.

3. Dattani R, Patnaik S, Kantak A, et al. Injuries to the tibiofibular syndesmosis. J Bone Joint Surg Br 2008;90(4):405–10.

4. Ramsey DC, Friess DM. Cost-effectiveness analysis of syndesmotic screw versus suture button fixation in tibiofibular syndesmotic injuries. J Orthop Trauma 2018;32(6):e198–203.

5. Hootman JM, Dick R, Agel J. Epidemiology of collegiate injuries for 15 sports: summary and recommendations for injury prevention initiatives. J Athl Train 2007;42(2):311–9.

6. Fong DT, Hong Y, Chan LK, et al. A systematic review on ankle injury and ankle sprain in sports. Sports Med 2007;37(1):73–94.

7. Williams BT, Ahrberg AB, Goldsmith MT, et al. Ankle syndesmosis: a qualitative and quantitative anatomic analysis. Am J Sports Med 2015;43(1):88–97.

8. Vosseller JT, Karl JW, Greisberg JK. Incidence of syndesmotic injury. Orthopedics 2014;37(3):e226–9.

9. Hunt KJ, Phisitkul P, Pirolo J, et al. High ankle sprains and syndesmotic injuries in athletes. J Am Acad Orthop Surg 2015;23(11):661–73.

10. Gerber JP, Williams GN, Scoville CR, et al. Persistent disability associated with ankle sprains: a prospective examination of an athletic population. Foot Ankle Int 1998;19(10):653–60.

11. Weening B, Bhandari M. Predictors of functional outcome following transsyndesmotic screw fixation of ankle fractures. J Orthop Trauma 2005;19(2):102–8.

12. Kennedy JG, Soffe KE, Dalla Vedova P, et al. Evaluation of the syndesmotic screw in low Weber C ankle fractures. J Orthop Trauma 2000;14(5):359–66.

13. Sagi HC, Shah AR, Sanders RW. The functional consequence of syndesmotic joint malreduction at a minimum 2-year follow-up. J Orthop Trauma 2012;26(7):439–43.

14. Ray R, Koohnejad N, Clement ND, et al. Ankle fractures with syndesmotic stabilisation are associated with a high rate of secondary osteoarthritis. Foot Ankle Surg 2019;25(2):180–5.

15. Hermans JJ, Beumer A, de Jong TA, et al. Anatomy of the distal tibiofibular syndesmosis in adults: a pictorial essay with a multimodality approach. J Anat 2010;217(6):633–45.

16. Panchbhavi VK, Gurbani BN, Mason CB, et al. Radiographic assessment of fibular length variance: the case for "fibula minus. J Foot Ankle Surg 2018; 57(1):91–4.

17. Bartonicek J. Anatomy of the tibiofibular syndesmosis and its clinical relevance. Surg Radiol Anat 2003;25(5–6):379–86.

18. Boszczyk A, Kwapisz S, Krummel M, et al. Correlation of incisura anatomy with syndesmotic Malreduction. Foot Ankle Int 2018;39(3):369–75.

19. Ogilvie-Harris DJ, Reed SC. Disruption of the ankle syndesmosis: diagnosis and treatment by arthroscopic surgery. Arthroscopy 1994;10(5):561–8.

20. Haraguchi N, Haruyama H, Toga H, et al. Pathoanatomy of posterior malleolar fractures of the ankle. J Bone Joint Surg Am 2006;88(5):1085–92.

21. Fitzpatrick E, Goetz JE, Sittapairoj T, et al. Effect of posterior malleolus fracture on syndesmotic reduction: a cadaveric study. J Bone Joint Surg Am 2018; 100(3):243–8.

22. Miller AN, Carroll EA, Parker RJ, et al. Posterior malleolar stabilization of syndesmotic injuries is equivalent to screw fixation. Clin Orthop Relat Res 2010;468(4):1129–35.

23. Kang C, Hwang DS, Lee JK, et al. Screw fixation of the posterior malleolus fragment in ankle fracture. Foot Ankle Int 2019;40(11):1288–94.

24. Jeong MS, Choi YS, Kim YJ, et al. Deltoid ligament in acute ankle injury: MR imaging analysis. Skeletal Radiol 2014;43(5):655–63.

25. Massri-Pugin J, Lubberts B, Vopat BG, et al. Role of the deltoid ligament in syndesmotic instability. Foot Ankle Int 2018;39(5):598–603.

26. Massri-Pugin J, Lubberts B, Vopat BG, et al. Effect of sequential sectioning of ligaments on syndesmotic instability in the coronal plane evaluated arthroscopically. Foot Ankle Int 2017;38(12):1387–93.

27. Goetz JE, Vasseenon T, Tochigi Y, et al. 3D talar kinematics during external rotation stress testing in hindfoot varus and valgus using a model of syndesmotic and deep deltoid instability. Foot Ankle Int 2019;40(7):826–35.

28. Sman AD, Hiller CE, Refshauge KM. Diagnostic accuracy of clinical tests for diagnosis of ankle syndesmosis injury: a systematic review. Br J Sports Med 2013;47(10):620–8.

29. Ebraheim NA, Elgafy H, Padanilam T. Syndesmotic disruption in low fibular fractures associated with deltoid ligament injury. Clin Orthop Relat Res 2003;(409):260–7.

30. Mauntel TC, Wikstrom EA, Roos KG, et al. The epidemiology of high ankle sprains in National Collegiate Athletic Association Sports. Am J Sports Med 2017;45(9):2156–63.

31. Williams GN, Jones MH, Amendola A. Syndesmotic ankle sprains in athletes. Am J Sports Med 2007; 35(7):1197–207.

32. van Dijk CN, Longo UG, Loppini M, et al. Classification and diagnosis of acute isolated syndesmotic

injuries: ESSKA-AFAS consensus and guidelines. Knee Surg Sports Traumatol Arthrosc 2016;24(4): 1200–16.

33. Switaj PJ, Mendoza M, Kadakia AR. Acute and chronic injuries to the syndesmosis. Clin Sports Med 2015;34(4):643–77.

34. van den Bekerom MP, de Leeuw PA, van Dijk CN. Delayed operative treatment of syndesmotic instability. Current concepts review. Injury 2009;40(11): 1137–42.

35. Lin CF, Gross ML, Weinhold P. Ankle syndesmosis injuries: anatomy, biomechanics, mechanism of injury, and clinical guidelines for diagnosis and intervention. J Orthop Sports Phys Ther 2006;36(6): 372–84.

36. Choi Y, Kwon SS, Chung CY, et al. Preoperative radiographic and CT findings predicting syndesmotic injuries in supination-external rotation-type ankle fractures. J Bone Joint Surg Am 2014;96(14): 1161–7.

37. LaMothe JM, Baxter JR, Karnovsky SC, et al. Syndesmotic injury assessment with lateral imaging during stress testing in a cadaveric model. Foot Ankle Int 2018;39(4):479–84.

38. Jiang KN, Schulz BM, Tsui YL, et al. Comparison of radiographic stress tests for syndesmotic instability of supination-external rotation ankle fractures: a cadaveric study. J Orthop Trauma 2014;28(6):e123–7.

39. Stoffel K, Wysocki D, Baddour E, et al. Comparison of two intraoperative assessment methods for injuries to the ankle syndesmosis. A cadaveric study. J Bone Joint Surg Am 2009;91(11):2646–52.

40. Beumer A, Valstar ER, Garling EH, et al. External rotation stress imaging in syndesmotic injuries of the ankle: comparison of lateral radiography and radiostereometry in a cadaveric model. Acta Orthop Scand 2003;74(2):201–5.

41. Lui TH, Ip K, Chow HT. Comparison of radiologic and arthroscopic diagnoses of distal tibiofibular syndesmosis disruption in acute ankle fracture. Arthroscopy 2005;21(11):1370.

42. Marmor M, Hansen E, Han HK, et al. Limitations of standard fluoroscopy in detecting rotational malreduction of the syndesmosis in an ankle fracture model. Foot Ankle Int 2011;32(6):616–22.

43. Krahenbuhl N, Weinberg MW, Davidson NP, et al. Imaging in syndesmotic injury: a systematic literature review. Skeletal Radiol 2018;47(5):631–48.

44. Malhotra K, Welck M, Cullen N, et al. The effects of weight bearing on the distal tibiofibular syndesmosis: a study comparing weight bearing-CT with conventional CT. Foot Ankle Surg 2019;25(4):511–6.

45. Lintz F, de Cesar Netto C, Barg A, et al. Weight-bearing cone beam CT scans in the foot and ankle. EFORT Open Rev 2018;3(5):278–86.

46. Lee SW, Lee KJ, Park CH, et al. The valid diagnostic parameters in bilateral CT scan to predict unstable syndesmotic injury with ankle fracture. Diagnostics (Basel) 2020;10(10):812.

47. Abdelaziz ME, Hagemeijer N, Guss D, et al. Evaluation of syndesmosis reduction on CT Scan. Foot Ankle Int 2019;40(9):1087–93.

48. Bhimani R, Ashkani-Esfahani S, Lubberts B, et al. Utility of volumetric measurement via weight-bearing computed tomography scan to diagnose syndesmotic instability. Foot Ankle Int 2020;41(7): 859–65.

49. Hagemeijer NC, Chang SH, Abdelaziz ME, et al. Range of normal and abnormal syndesmotic measurements using Weightbearing CT. Foot Ankle Int 2019;40(12):1430–7.

50. Dikos GD, Heisler J, Choplin RH, et al. Normal tibiofibular relationships at the syndesmosis on axial CT imaging. J Orthop Trauma 2012;26(7): 433–8.

51. Patel S, Malhotra K, Cullen NP, et al. Defining reference values for the normal tibiofibular syndesmosis in adults using weight-bearing CT. Bone Joint J 2019;101-B(3):348–52.

52. Carrozzo M, Vicenti G, Pesce V, et al. Beyond the pillars of the ankle: a prospective randomized CT analysis of syndesmosis' injuries in Weber B and C type fractures. Injury 2018;49(Suppl 3):S54–60.

53. Kubik JF, Rollick NC, Bear J, et al. Assessment of malreduction standards for the syndesmosis in bilateral CT scans of uninjured ankles. Bone Joint J 2021;103-B(1):178–83.

54. Roemer FW, Jomaah N, Niu J, et al. Ligamentous injuries and the risk of associated tissue damage in acute ankle sprains in athletes: a cross-sectional MRI study. Am J Sports Med 2014;42(7):1549–57.

55. Brown KW, Morrison WB, Schweitzer ME, et al. MRI findings associated with distal tibiofibular syndesmosis injury. AJR Am J Roentgenol 2004;182(1): 131–6.

56. Randell M, Marsland D, Ballard E, et al. MRI for high ankle sprains with an unstable syndesmosis: posterior malleolus bone oedema is common and time to scan matters. Knee Surg Sports Traumatol Arthrosc 2019;27(9):2890–7.

57. Uys HD, Rijke AM. Clinical association of acute lateral ankle sprain with syndesmotic involvement: a stress radiography and magnetic resonance imaging study. Am J Sports Med 2002;30(6):816–22.

58. Perrich KD, Goodwin DW, Hecht PJ, et al. Ankle ligaments on MRI: appearance of normal and injured ligaments. AJR Am J Roentgenol 2009;193(3): 687–95.

59. Hermans JJ, Ginai AZ, Wentink N, et al. The additional value of an oblique image plane for MRI of the anterior and posterior distal tibiofibular syndesmosis. Skeletal Radiol 2011;40(1):75–83.

60. Alves T, Dong Q, Jacobson J, et al. Normal and injured ankle ligaments on ultrasonography

with magnetic resonance imaging correlation. J Ultrasound Med 2019;38(2):513–28.

61. Sconfienza LM, Orlandi D, Lacelli F, et al. Dynamic high-resolution US of ankle and midfoot ligaments: normal anatomic structure and imaging technique. Radiographics 2015;35(1):164–78.

62. Fisher CL, Rabbani T, Johnson K, et al. Diagnostic capability of dynamic ultrasound evaluation of supination-external rotation ankle injuries: a cadaveric study. BMC Musculoskelet Disord 2019;20(1):502.

63. Hagemeijer NC, Saengsin J, Chang SH, et al. Diagnosing syndesmotic instability with dynamic ultrasound - establishing the natural variations in normal motion. Injury 2020;51(11):2703–9.

64. Lubberts B, Massri-Pugin J, Guss D, et al. Arthroscopic assessment of syndesmotic instability in the sagittal plane in a cadaveric model. Foot Ankle Int 2020;41(2):237–43.

65. Vopat ML, Vopat BG, Lubberts B, et al. Current trends in the diagnosis and management of syndesmotic injury. Curr Rev Musculoskelet Med 2017;10(1):94–103.

66. Doughtie M. Syndesmotic ankle sprains in football: a survey of national football league athletic trainers. J Athl Train 1999;34(1):15–8.

67. Knapik DM, Trem A, Sheehan J, et al. Conservative management for stable high ankle injuries in professional football players. Sports Health 2018; 10(1):80–4.

68. Miller BS, Downie BK, Johnson PD, et al. Time to return to play after high ankle sprains in collegiate football players: a prediction model. Sports Health 2012;4(6):504–9.

69. Salom-Moreno J, Ayuso-Casado B, Tamaral-Costa B, et al. Trigger point dry needling and proprioceptive exercises for the management of chronic ankle instability: a randomized clinical trial. Evid Based Complement Alternat Med 2015;2015: 790209.

70. Gundermann DM, Walker DK, Reidy PT, et al. Activation of mTORC1 signaling and protein synthesis in human muscle following blood flow restriction exercise is inhibited by rapamycin. Am J Physiol Endocrinol Metab 2014;306(10):E1198–204.

71. Takarada Y, Takazawa H, Ishii N. Applications of vascular occlusion diminish disuse atrophy of knee extensor muscles. Med Sci Sports Exerc 2000; 32(12):2035–9.

72. Drakos M, Birmingham P, Delos D, et al. Corticosteroid and anesthetic injections for muscle strains and ligament sprains in the NFL. HSS J 2014;10(2): 136–42.

73. Laver L, Carmont MR, McConkey MO, et al. Plasma rich in growth factors (PRGF) as a treatment for high ankle sprain in elite athletes: a randomized control trial. Knee Surg Sports Traumatol Arthrosc 2015; 23(11):3383–92.

74. Samra DJ, Sman AD, Rae K, et al. Effectiveness of a single platelet-rich plasma injection to promote recovery in rugby players with ankle syndesmosis injury. BMJ Open Sport Exerc Med 2015;1(1): e000033.

The Syndesmosis, Part II
Surgical Treatment Strategies

Philip B. Kaiser, MD[a,b,*], Lorena Bejarano-Pineda, MD[a,b], John Y. Kwon, MD[a,b], Christopher W. DiGiovanni, MD[a,b], Daniel Guss, MD, MBA[a,b]

KEYWORDS

- Syndesmosis • Syndesmotic instability • Surgical repair • Flexible fixation • Rigid fixation
- Screw • Suture button

KEY POINTS

- The clinical consequences of undiagnosed syndesmotic instability far outweigh any incremental implications of its various fixation strategies.
- Effective treatment focuses on restoring fibular and periarticular anatomy, multiplanar fixation of the unstable syndesmosis, and ligamentoplasty or repair.
- Rigid screw and flexible suture button constructs can effectively treat syndesmotic instability.
- When destabilized, an overfixed syndesmosis works better than an underfixed or, worse, an unfixed one.
- Syndesmotic instability remains an incompletely understood continuum of disease severity, and is likely influenced by many other factors beyond injury to the syndesmotic ligaments themselves.

INTRODUCTION

Optimizing clinical outcomes after ankle fracture predicates restoring and maintaining the tibiotalar relationship. Even 1 mm of talar subluxation relative to the tibial plafond markedly alters contact areas.[1,2] Anatomic fixation of the affected malleoli and weight bearing surfaces is critical to this aim, but the ankle's mortise construct also requires that the fibula and tibia effectively bracket the talus. Very little stability is afforded by the tibial incisura itself, which is variable in morphology and can be concave or even convex.[3,4] Therefore, the stability of the distal tibiofibular articulation is instead enabled by a constellation of syndesmotic ligaments, including the anterior inferior tibiofibular ligament (AITFL), interosseous ligament (IOL), and posterior inferior tibiofibular ligament (PITFL).

Failure to diagnose and treat a destabilizing injury to the syndesmosis can result in significant and irreversible morbidity. The onus on the surgeon is, therefore, to first and foremost make the diagnosis given that the clinical implications of undiagnosed (and therefore untreated) syndesmotic instability arguably supersedes that of a slightly malreduced distal tibiofibular articulation.[5] In contrast, reduction and fixation strategies remain critical because patients with syndesmotic malreduction have been shown in some studies to have poorer clinical outcomes.[6] Effectively treating syndesmotic instability therefore requires an understanding of relevant anatomy, diagnostic strategies, reduction techniques, fixation options, as well as the implications of hardware choices and chronicity of injury.

[a] Department of Orthopaedic Surgery, Foot and Ankle Service, Harvard Medical School, Massachusetts General Hospital and Newton-Wellesley Hospital, Boston, MA, USA; [b] Foot & Ankle Research and Innovation Laboratory - Harvard Medical School, Division of Foot and Ankle Surgery, Department of Orthopaedic Surgery, Massachusetts General Hospital - Newton-Wellesley Hospital, Boston, MA, USA
* Corresponding author. MGH-NWH Foot & Ankle Center, Building 52, Suite 1150, 40 2nd Avenue, Waltham, MA 02451.
E-mail address: pkaiser@mgh.harvard.edu

Orthop Clin N Am 52 (2021) 417–432
https://doi.org/10.1016/j.ocl.2021.05.011
0030-5898/21/© 2021 Elsevier Inc. All rights reserved.

DIAGNOSIS

There is no sine qua non test to diagnose syndesmotic instability, and therefore a high index of suspicion is necessary. Physical examination remains critical, with findings including tenderness over the anterior syndesmosis or a positive squeeze test at the mid fibula.[6] Imaging modalities almost invariably supplement physical examination, and include radiographs, MRI, computed tomography (CT) scans, and ultrasound examination. These modalities vary along 3 primary characteristics, namely, their ability to (1) visualize the ankle joint under stress, (2) afford a contralateral comparison, and (3) evaluate the distal tibiofibular joint in 3 dimensions (3D). Although radiographs allow the application of weight-bearing or external rotation stress, as well as a contralateral comparison, their inherent 2-dimensional nature limits their sensitivity.[7] Although MRI can demonstrate injury, ligamentous disruption may not correlate with instability, and does not afford a contralateral comparison. A CT scan, especially when performed under weight bearing conditions, allows evaluation of the syndesmotic relationship under physiologic load in 3D, and allows bilateral assessment (Fig. 1). The latter is critical because the variability in morphology of the distal tibiofibular articulation between individual patients necessitates use of the contralateral, uninjured ankle as an internal control (Fig. 2).[8] weight bearing CT scan also allows 3D volumetric measurements that have a heightened sensitivity as compared with traditional 1-dimensional distance or even 2-dimensional area measurements.[9] Ultrasound examination may represent the future gold standard for diagnosing instability, especially as compared with invasive arthroscopy, because of its ability to evaluate bilateral tibiofibular articulations under stress and at the point of care, with minimal cost and no ionizing radiation exposure.

ANATOMY

As alluded to elsewhere in this article, the distal tibiofibular articulation has very little inherent bony stability. The tibial incisura that cradles the fibula demonstrates enormous variability in morphology and can be quite shallow in upwards of one-third of patients, implying the critical role of ligamentous constraints in preventing abnormal motion.[10] The AITFL, IOL, and PITFL work in concert to prevent fibular translation in the coronal and sagittal planes, as well as constraining fibular rotation and pistoning (Fig. 3).

Notably, the collateral ligaments of the ankle also help to stabilize the distal tibiofibular joint, presumptively by anchoring the fibula to the tibia through the talus. Injury to structures such as the deltoid ligament can contribute to syndesmotic instability.[11]

Much like the shoulder joint, this lack of inherent bony constraint implies that the fibula can and does submit to moving in multiple directions when the syndesmosis is rendered unstable. Although coronal plane diastasis has traditionally been used during fluoroscopic stress examination, sagittal plane fibular motion may be more sensitive in diagnosing instability.[12] The advantage of this preoperatively is that a Cotton maneuver is inherently invasive, and accessible surrogates such as an external rotation test may primarily test deltoid competence rather than syndesmotic ligament integrity.[13,14] Preoperative sagittal plane motion can be assessed using a fibular shuck maneuver and even visualized with ultrasound.[15] Intraoperatively, sagittal plane fibular motion can readily be visualized as the fibula moves relative to the anterior lip of the incisura.

REDUCTION STRATEGIES

The paucity of bony restraints at the distal tibiofibular articulation complicates anatomic reduction because, unlike many other joints, the distal syndesmosis does not simply click into place. A few points, however, are worth noting when considering the published literature on reduction strategies. First, no attempt at avoiding malreduction of the syndesmosis can overcome malreduction of associated fractures, especially of the fibula. Failure of syndesmotic fixation is often representative of fibular shortening and the associated loss of lateral talar buttress, rather than an actual failure of syndesmotic reduction technique (Fig. 4). Second, an assessment of reduction quality inherently requires a comparison with the contralateral, uninjured side given enormous variations in tibiofibular morphology between individuals. Not all published studies incorporated bilateral assessments. Third, qualitative side to side comparisons of bilateral ankle weight bearing CT scan imaging has been shown to have a very poor interobserver interclass correlation coefficient when assessing whether the syndesmosis is malreduced (correlation coefficient, 0.26), whereas advanced, quantitative 2-dimensional techniques such as syndesmotic area demonstrate excellent correlation (correlation coefficient, 0.96).[9] This factor may explain why some

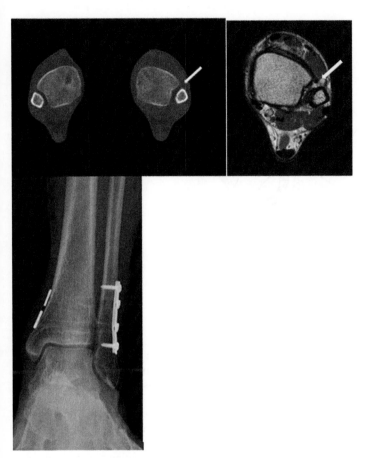

Fig. 1. Patient is a 21-year-old man who was injured while rock climbing and presented 9 months after injury with persistent ankle pain despite a period of immobilization and physical therapy alongside tenderness at the distal syndesmosis and positive fibular squeeze test. A weight bearing CT scan demonstrated subtle asymmetric widening at the distal tibiofibular articulation and MRI revealed chronic AITFL rupture (*white arrows*). Patient underwent surgical fixation of a chronically unstable syndesmosis with suture button fixation and direct AITFL imbrication. (*From* Ramsey P, Hamilton W. Changes in tibiotalar area of contact caused by lateral talar shift: The Journal of Bone & Joint Surgery. 1976;58(3):356-357. https://doi.org/10.2106/00004623-197658030-00010; with permission.)

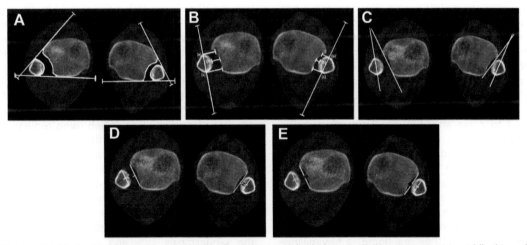

Fig. 2. Tibiofibular joint measurements. (*A*) Syndesmotic area (*shaded area*). (*B*) Direct anterior (a), middle (b), and direct posterior (c) differences. (*C*) Fibular rotation. (*D*) Sagittal translation (*dark line*). (*E*) Incisura depth (*dark line*). The patient had right-sided syndesmosis instability after an acute posterolateral ankle dislocation. (*From* Hagemeijer NC, Chang SH, Abdelaziz ME, et al. Range of Normal and Abnormal Syndesmotic Measurements Using Weightbearing CT. Foot Ankle Int. 2019;40(12):1430-1437. https://doi.org/10.1177/1071100719866831; with permission.)

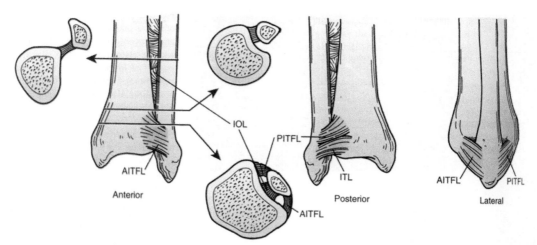

Fig. 3. Drawing of the ligamentous anatomy of the distal tibiofibular syndesmosis with anterior, posterior, lateral, and axial cut views. ITL, inferior transverse ligament. (*From* Davidovitch RI, Egol KA. Ankle fractures. In: Bucholz RW, Heckman JD, Court-Brown CM, Tornetta P, editors. Rockwood and Green's fractures in adults. 7th ed. Philadelphia: Lippincott Williams & Wilkins; 2010. Figure 57-12; with permission.)

studies have concluded that intraoperative use of a CT scan does not necessarily decrease the rate of malreduction.[16] Last, although it may seem intuitive that a malreduced syndesmosis may predicate poorer outcomes, there is a "chicken and the egg" component to such conclusions, wherein the severity of injury that made it more difficult to effectively decrease the syndesmosis may supersede the clinical implications of a malreduction, especially if subtle. It must also be pointed out when reviewing recent reports discussing this concept that gross syndesmotic malreduction is not the same as subtle syndesmotic malalignment. This concept is suggested implicitly by the fact that, although up to one-half of patients may demonstrate syndesmotic malreduction in some published studies, the majority of patients who undergo syndesmotic fixation nonetheless do well postoperatively—and syndesmotic malreduction is often defined as literally being off by a few degrees or 1 to 2 mm after fixation. Although these realignments are not ideal, applying reduction perfection standards to any other orthopedic procedure with 3-dimensional imaging would likely offer similar results, and in this case there are also data to suggest that when the hardware is removed, fails, loosens, or stretches out over time that many of these alignments may indeed end up finding "their real home" a few millimeters or a few degrees away if all other surrounding bony structures were fixed properly.[17] We still do not have the answer to the question "how close do we need to be?", let alone the question "how close can we actually ensure we

get?" What is clear, however, just like with routine fracture care, is that there is a big difference over the long term between minor malposition and gross residual malalignment or deformity. Therefore, making the diagnosis may arguably be more critical than the various fixation strategies themselves.

With these ideas in mind, some strategies do exist to minimize malreduction of the distal tibiofibular articulation. In 1 study, open visualization of the anterior fibula relative to the anterior incisura decreased the malreduction rates from 44% to 15% as compared with closed reduction without directly accessing the distal tibiofibular joint.[6] Some investigators have advocated for basing reduction based on a perfect fluoroscopic lateral of the contralateral talus before draping.[18] The distance between the posterior fibula and posterior tibia, as well as the converse anteriorly, is then used to assess the quality of reduction on the operative limb, resulting in a 6% rate of malreduction. When using reduction forceps, the placement of the medial tine is also critical toward achieving an anatomic reduction. Studies suggest that the medial tine should be placed in the anterior one-third of the medial tibia, resulting in 0% rates of malreduction in one study, while placing the tine in the middle or posterior third of the medial tibia will malreduce the syndesmosis 19% and 60% of instances, respectively.[19]

Broadly, effective reduction of the syndesmosis requires first and foremost anatomic reduction of associated fractures, with a special emphasis on avoiding fibular shortening. The

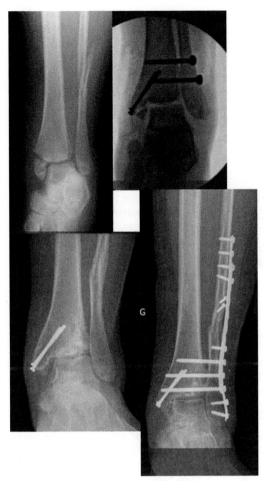

Fig. 4. Example of a 19-year-old patient who presented with an ankle fracture who underwent initial fixation with the fibula in a shortened position and without achieving articular congruency. One year later, she developed severe tibiotalar arthritis with valgus tilt and was referred for additional management. Attempted salvage entailed a fibular lengthening osteotomy and syndesmotic fixation. Initial repair of an unstable syndesmosis cannot overcome fibular or intra-articular malunion, and she will almost certainly need additional procedures in the future for severe posttraumatic arthritis.

diagnosis of instability is more readily based on a sagittal anterior–posterior and posterior–anterior stress than a Cotton maneuver, although both tactics may be pursued. An excess of 2 mm of total fibular motion in the sagittal plane is considered unstable.[12] The anterior lip of the incisura should always be visualized relative to the anterior fibula when performing a reduction, ensuring that a freer or other thin instrument cannot be readily inserted into this space. Especially when treating chronic instability, the distal tibiofibular joint should be formally debrided while protecting the articulation's cartilage; a laminar spreader can facilitate access with a pituitary rongeur. Preoperative, bilateral CT scans can be incredibly useful in more severe cases of distal tibiofibular diastasis, especially if the fibular fracture is proximal and will not be directly reduced, to facilitate an understanding of the reduction maneuver. The medial tine of a reduction clamp should be placed in the anterior one-third of the medial tibia but, if the fibula is significantly translated, a rotational motion of the clamp may also be necessary in addition to any simple, single vector compression.

RIGID FIXATION

Technical considerations inherent to screw fixation across the syndesmosis have included screw location, orientation, diameter, the number of screws used, and the number of cortices incorporated into the construct.[20,21] The most controversial topic, however, is the potential for syndesmotic malreduction using rigid fixation. Inextricable from this concern is the underlying reality that, if the syndesmosis is malreduced before the screw is placed, it will almost certainly stay malreduced after screw fixation.

Miller and colleagues examined the potential for syndesmotic malreduction with screws in a cadaveric study using a CT scan and found that the clamp must be placed from the posterolateral fibula to the anteromedial tibia angled at 15° relative to a direct lateral of the talus (as compared with 0° or 30°) to minimize malreduction (Fig. 5).[22] With the clamp in this position, they then went on to conclude that a syndesmotic screw placed from the lateral fibula should be angled 0° and a screw placed from the posterolateral fibula should be angled 30°. It should be noted that the absolute amount of malreduction averaged less than 1 mm in each instance. Therefore, a statistically significant malalignment may not translate into clinical significance. A separate study examining CT scans of uninjured syndesmoses among patients presenting with calcaneal fractures found that syndesmotic screws should be angled 18° relative to the coronal plane.[23] Given recent studies showing the usefulness of manual reduction, we preferentially use a lag screw technique rather than a clamp to reduce the syndesmosis when using rigid fixation unless displacement is severe, though one must avoid overtightening to prevent overcompression.[24]

Biomechanical and clinical studies have demonstrated no significant impact on the

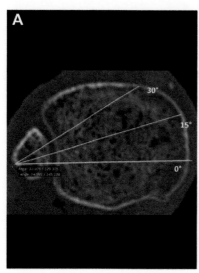
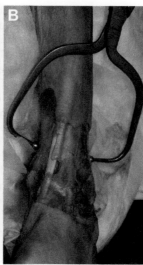

Fig. 5. Examples of angulation measurement for clamp and screw placement. (*A*) An axial CT scan measurement showing 0°, 15°, and 30° angulation from the posterolateral corner of the fibula. These are measured 2 cm proximal to the joint and compared with the Kirschner wires 4 cm proximal to the joint for clamp pilot hole placement. (*B*) A clinical example of a cadaver limb postdissection with clamp in place and ready for CT evaluation. (*From* Miller AN, Barei DP, Iaquinto JM, Ledoux WR, Beingessner DM. Iatrogenic syndesmosis malreduction via clamp and screw placement. J Orthop Trauma. 2013;27(2):100-106. https://doi.org/10.1097/BOT. 0b013e31825197cb; with permission.)

mechanical stability between tricortical versus quadricortical fixation. Likewise, although 4.5-mm screws afford greater resistance to breakage, this factor may not translate into better clinical outcomes when compared with 3.5-mm screws.[25] The composition of the screw has not shown differences in clinical or radiographic results.[26] However, bioabsorbable screws have been associated with increased foreign body reactions.[27]

Whether 1 or multiple screws are required to achieve adequate syndesmotic fixation is debatable. Multiple screws are usually considered in neuropathic, severely osteoporotic patients, or patients with Maisonneuve injuries to increase the stability of the construct. In grossly unstable syndesmotic injuries with severe fracture comminution or poor bone quality we lean toward screw fixation owing to the rigidity of the system, which also augments fixation of the fibula fracture. In the setting of rigid fixation, we recommend using two 3.5- or 4.0-mm screws starting at or slightly above the physeal scar. The screws may be placed in a slightly divergent direction to maximize fixation strength.

FLEXIBLE FIXATION

As discussed elsewhere in this article, the fixation principles designed to most closely restore natural syndesmotic ligament function for rigid fixation constructs apply equally well to implementation of any flexible construct. Flexible syndesmotic fixation has over the past 15 years become an increasingly popular method for

syndesmotic repair. Although there are multiple forms of flexible syndesmotic fixation, the suture button construct is the most commonly used. The purported advantage of flexible fixation, as implied by its name, is that it allows some degree of fibular motion relative to the tibia, more closely mimicking physiologic fibular motion. In theory, this factor also enables the fibula to reduce within the incisura without being entirely bound to its initial reduction position.[28–31] Suture button devices also potentially obviate the need for removal of hardware as is sometimes performed after rigid screw fixation.

Studies have indeed shown that flexible syndesmotic fixation can decrease malreduction rates at the distal tibiofibular joint. A cadaveric study by Westermann and colleagues[32] found that, even with deliberate malreduction using a clamp, suture button constructs can compensate for both anterior and posterior off-axis clamping (Fig. 6). With deliberate anterior off-axis clamping, sagittal malreduction was 2.7 ± 2.0 mm with screw fixation as compared with 1.0 ± 1.0 mm with suture button fixation (*P* = .02). With deliberate posterior off-axis clamping, sagittal malreduction was 7.2 ± 2.3 mm with screw fixation as compared with 0.5 ± 1.4 mm with suture button fixation (*P*<.01). The authors concluded that flexible syndesmotic fixation allowed for a self-reduction toward an anatomic distal tibia–fibula relationship.

By providing a tension vector across the distal tibiofibular articulation, a suture button construct attempts to mimic the constraint afforded by an intact ligament. In contrast,

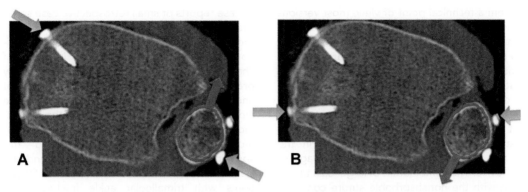

Fig. 6. Representative axial CT images 10 mm proximal to the tibiotalar joint illustrating the 2 malalignment conditions. To produce anterior displacement of the fibula (*orange arrow*) relative to the incisura fibularis (*A*), prongs of the tenaculum were placed engaging the posterior fibular screw head and the anterior tibial screw head (*blue arrows*). To produce posterior displacement of the fibula (*orange arrow*) relative to the incisura fibularis (*B*), prongs of the tenaculum were placed engaging the anterior fibular screw head and the posterior tibial screw head (*blue arrows*). (*From* Westermann RW, Rungprai C, Goetz JE, Femino J, Amendola A, Phisitkul P. The effect of suture-button fixation on simulated syndesmotic malreduction: a cadaveric study. J Bone Joint Surg Am. 2014;96(20):1732-1738. https://doi.org/10.2106/JBJS.N.00198; with permission.)

because the incisura itself offers very little bony constraint, a ligament that works under tension affords very little restraint to orthogonal forces. The AITFL, IOL, and PITFL overcome this by being divergent in orientation. Accordingly, Clanton and colleagues[33] compared 3 methods of syndesmotic fixation in a cadaver model: (1) one 3.5-mm syndesmotic screw, (2) 1 suture button construct, and (3) 2 divergent suture button constructs. They found similar resistance to internal and external rotation between all 3 constructs and the intact syndesmosis, but posterior sagittal plane translation was best constrained by screw fixation with only 2.5 mm of translation as compared with 4.6 mm with a single suture button construct and 2.9 mm with 2 suture buttons. Similarly, anterior sagittal translation was only 0.1 mm with screw fixation compared with 2.7 mm with a single suture button construct and 2.9 mm with 2 suture buttons. The authors concluded that a single suture button construct for syndesmotic repair was insufficient to control sagittal translation of the fibula.

A separate cadaveric study by Klitzman and colleagues[30] demonstrated that, after 100 cycles of loading, suture button fixation resulted in significantly increased sagittal plane motion (3.17 mm) as compared with the intact syndesmosis (2.77 mm, $P = .006$), but that screw fixation resulted in overconstraint (1.16 mm; $P \leq .001$). The relative advantage of overconstraint versus underconstraint during the initial healing period remains to be entirely elucidated.

The role of suture button constructs in obviating the need for hardware removal has been highlighted as a cost-saving benefit. Neary and colleagues[34] performed a cost-effectiveness analysis for the use of suture button versus syndesmotic screw fixation in supination–external rotation type IV ankle injuries. Through their comparative decision analysis model, assuming a 4% suture button hardware removal rate and 20% syndesmotic screw removal rate, the total cost for 2 syndesmotic screws was US$20,836 compared with $19,354 for syndesmotic repair using a suture button fixation. Therefore, it seemed that, when a return to the operating room for hardware removal was included in the cost of the implant, syndesmotic fixation using flexible options or screws are quite comparable in terms of overall costs. Their analysis modeled an estimated implant cost of 2 screws versus 1 suture button construct as $64.50 versus $880.00, respectively. The results of a cost analysis may change as surgeons start using multiple, divergent suture buttons to better approximately normal ligamentous orientation. In contrast, the indirect costs to the patient of a return to the operating room, such as lost wages, should also be taken into account.

One must note, however, that not all studies have replicated a low return to the operating room with suture button constructs. One early case series of 24 patients demonstrated suture button removal of rates of 25% and another case series of 19 patients demonstrated a removal rate of 26%, most frequently owing to skin irritation.[35,36] More recent studies have not necessarily replicated these high numbers, and it is possible that knotless constructs may obviate removal.

From a technical point of view, most versions of flexible syndesmotic fixation rely on fixation on the medial aspect of the distal tibia, which can put the saphenous neurovascular structures at risk.[37] Furthermore, tunnel placement on the relatively narrow fibula at an oblique angle can be challenging, especially because most forms of flexible syndesmotic fixation require drilling that is, larger than the comparable drill size for a standard syndesmotic screw, often in the 3.2 mm to 3.7 mm range to allow passage of the device. The combination of larger size tunnel along with the nonabsorbable suture construct and fibular motion can lead to tunnel widening and osteolysis.[35,38] Some of this may be mitigated by routinely using a fibular plate to act as a washer, even in Maisonneuve injuries when there is no distal fibular fracture. One should also have a low threshold for making small incisions medially, which not only protects the saphenous vein and nerve, but also has the secondary benefit of ensuring the medial hardware sits directly on bone rather than on soft tissue that can attenuate over time.

Allograft and Autograft Reconstruction

Allograft reconstruction of the syndesmosis is far less common than screw fixation or flexible syndesmotic fixation but some of its concepts of specific ligament repair such as the AITFL are being used readily with suture tape or allografts constructs. Recent biomechanical studies that have isolated the different ligamentous components of the ankle syndesmosis have demonstrated the importance of the AITFL and PITFL with regards to syndesmotic integrity. In a cadaveric study Clanton and colleagues,[33] under simulated physiologic conditions, tested the intact syndesmosis demonstrating 4.3° of fibular rotation and 3.3 mm of fibular sagittal translation. Sectioning of the AITFL resulted in the greatest reduction of resistance to external rotation—an average of 24% (Fig. 7). Similarly, Littlechild and colleagues[39] evaluated the effects of the individual syndesmotic components on preventing talar shift in ankle fractures. They found that division of the AIFTL resulted in a 3 times greater lateral talar shift when compared with the PITFL. Therefore, the authors concluded that repairing the PITFL—often through repair of a posterior malleolus fracture—may not be sufficient to prevent lateral talar shift and AITFL reconstruction should be considered as an augment to syndesmotic fixation.

Several studies have described different techniques for reconstruction of the syndesmosis using autograft or allograft tendon, but are limited to case reports or small retrospective case series without control or comparison groups. Nevertheless, they offer possible techniques for tendinous syndesmotic reconstruction in cases of chronic instability where prior screw holes may prevent or impair revision hardware placement and provide possible means to reconstruct the individual important components of the syndesmosis such as the AITFL in the acute syndesmotic injury as our understanding of this specific augmentation evolves. Nelson and colleagues[40] reported on a case series of 50 patients with trimalleolar ankle fractures who additionally underwent isolated AITFL repair using an extensor digitorum longus tendon autograft or suture that was anchored with screws and washers at the native AITFL footprints as the sole means of syndesmotic reconstruction. Forty-nine patients (98%) reportedly demonstrated stabilization of the ankle mortise intraoperatively after this procedure.[40] Yasui and colleagues[41] reported on 6 patients with chronic syndesmotic instability undergoing screw fixation alongside anatomic AITFL autograft reconstruction with bone tunnels. Patients demonstrated significant improvements in median AOFAS (AOFAS) scores from 53 preoperatively to 95 at the final follow-up.

Future studies are necessary, especially regarding the indications for ligament reconstructions and the relative usefulness to nonabsorbable suture tape constructs. Importantly, ligamentous procedures to supplement any additional fixation may become more critical in the chronic as compared with the acute state of syndesmotic instability.

CLINICAL OUTCOMES: RIGID VERSUS FLEXIBLE FIXATION

There have been multiple prospective, randomized clinical trials comparing suture button versus screw fixation. Anderson and colleagues[28] randomized 97 patients with acute syndesmotic injuries to stabilization with a suture button or with a single quadricortical 4.5 mm syndesmotic screw. Full weight bearing was initiated at 6 weeks postoperatively and the syndesmotic screw was removed 10 to 12 weeks after surgery. The median AOFAS score at 2 years postoperatively was higher in the suture button group at (96; interquartile range, 90–100) compared with the syndesmotic screw group (86; interquartile range, 80–96; $P = .001$), and similar differences were seen in other legacy scales such as the Olerud-Molander Ankle (OMA) Scale, a self-reported

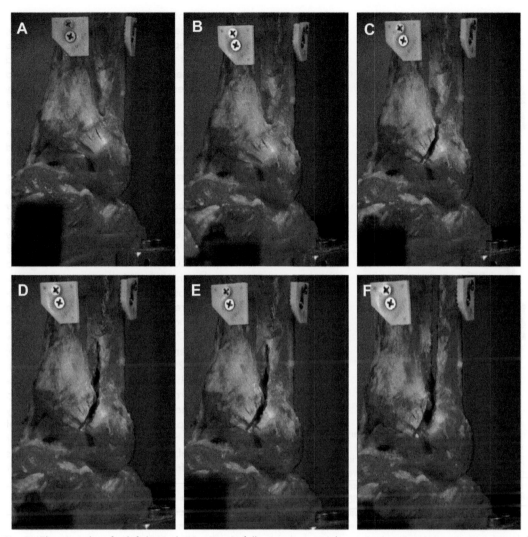

Fig. 7. Photographs of a left lower leg specimen following sequential anterior-to-posterior sectioning. Neutral rotation. (*A*) Intact syndesmosis with 15° external rotation. (*B*) Intact syndesmosis. (*C*) AITFL sectioned (state 1AP). (*D*) AITFL + ITFL sectioned (state 2AP). (*E*) AITFL, ITFL, deep PITFL, and superficial PITFL sectioned (state 4AP). (*F*) IOM sectioned (all cut). (*From* Clanton TO, Williams BT, Backus JD, et al. Biomechanical Analysis of the Individual Ligament Contributions to Syndesmotic Stability. Foot Ankle Int. 2017;38(1):66-75. https://doi.org/10.1177/1071100716666277; with permission). IOM, interosseous membrane.

functional scale. Additionally, they found that the suture button group reported less pain with walking (but not daily activity) at 2 years postoperatively, although pain scores were low in both groups with a median visual analog scale scores of 1 or less. They also attained bilateral, non-weightbearing CT scans at 2 weeks or less, 1 year, and 2 years with a threshold of 2 mm of asymmetry between the injured and uninjured side defining malalignment. Whereas no significant difference in alignment was seen at the initial CT scan at 2 weeks or less, 20 of 40 patients in the syndesmotic screw group had a difference in the tibiofibular distance 2 mm or greater compared with 8 of 40 patients in the suture button group (*P* = .009) (Fig. 8). There were no cases of symptomatic recurrent diastasis in the suture button group compared with 7 in the screw group. The authors concluded that the suture button group demonstrated better clinical outcomes and radiographic alignment then the screw fixation group. They additionally performed a subgroup multivariable analysis because, despite randomization, the screw fixation group included more patients who also sustained posterior malleolar

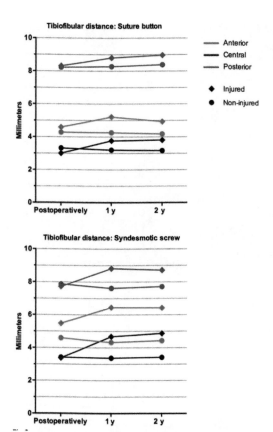

Fig. 8. Graphs comparing the mean anterior, central, and posterior tibiofibular distances between the injured and uninjured ankles over time in the 2 groups. At 1 and 2 years, the differences between the injured and uninjured ankles with respect to the anterior (P = .01) and central (P = .01) tibiofibular distances in the SS group were significantly greater than those in the SB group. The differences in the anterior, central, and posterior tibiofibular distances between the injured and uninjured ankles increased from the radiographs made within 2 weeks postoperatively to those made at 1 year in both the SS group (P = .003 for anterior, P < .001 for central, and P < .001 for posterior) and the SB group (P = .02 for anterior, P < .001 for central, and P = .03 for posterior). (*From* Andersen MR, Frihagen F, Hellund JC, Madsen JE, Figved W. Randomized Trial Comparing Suture Button with Single Syndesmotic Screw for Syndesmosis Injury. J Bone Joint Surg Am. 2018;100(1):2-12. https://doi.org/10.2106/JBJS.16.01011; with permission.)

fractures (73% vs 52%) and combined posterior/medial malleolar fractures (43% vs 25%). They still found that the method of fixation was the single determining aspect.

Notably, contemporaneous commentary about the study cautioned against the use of legacy scales (such as the AOFAS hindfoot score) that are nonvalidated and hampered by the fact that data becomes skewed when the

subelements of the score (in this case "categories of measurement, surgeon evaluation, and patient report" that make up the AOFAS score) interact with each other. It also noted that in this specific study the data was skewed when examined for normality, and that the magnitude of differences in pain were quite small.

Laflamme and colleagues[42] conducted a prospective, multicenter randomized double-blind controlled trial to compare the clinical and radiographic outcomes of acute syndesmotic injuries stabilized with a suture button (n = 33) versus 1 quadricortical 3.5-mm syndesmotic screw (n = 32). Better OMA scores were seen at 3 months (68.8 vs 60.2; P = .067), 6 months (84.2 vs 76.8; P = .082), and 12 months (93.3 vs 87.6; P = .046) in the suture button group compared with the syndesmotic screw group. However, although the AOFAS scores were better in the suture button group as compared with the screw fixation group at 3 months postoperatively (78.6 vs 70.6; P = .016), there was no significant difference at 6 months (87.1 vs 83.8; P = .26) or 12 months (93.1 vs 89.9; P = .26). They reported loss of reduction in the syndesmotic screw group in 4 cases (11.1%) compared with none in the suture button group, defined by plain radiographs. They also noted that in 3 of those 4 cases the loss of reduction was after screw removal, and that if these 3 patients were omitted from the analysis, radiographic differences were no longer present. Additionally, there was a higher implant failure rate, described as screw breakage, in the screw group compared with the suture button group (36.1% vs 0%; P<.05), although none of these breakages were associated with the loss of radiographic reduction. There were no significant differences in return to sporting activities. The authors concluded that suture button fixation was a reliable method of repair and seemed to have slightly better clinical and radiographic outcomes compared with screws with a lower failure and reoperation rate.

The explicit clinical consequences of syndesmotic malreduction, and therefore the benefit of suture buttons, can be difficult to tease out given the myriad of factors that may interplay in predicating malreduction. One study by Sagi and colleagues[6] identified 68 patients who were at least 2 years status post surgical treatment of an ankle fracture with syndesmotic fixation and invited them for clinical, radiographic, and bilateral CT evaluation. They found a malreduction rate of 39.7% overall, although this rate decreased to 15% among patients who had open rather than closed reduction of the distal tibiofibular articulation, and statistically poorer outcomes on the Selective Functional Movement Assessment general health questionnaire and OMA scale in malreduced patients. Malreduction was subjectively defined by 1 reviewer, and it was unclear whether injury severity predicated the malreduction and therefore confounded clinical outcomes. A study by Andersen and colleagues[28] examined 87 patients who had undergone syndesmotic screw fixation and found that a diastasis of more than 2 mm on a CT scan measured at the anterior incisura (but not the posterior incisura) seemed to correlate with poorer outcomes on OMA and AOFAS scores. In contrast, a study by Warner and colleagues[43] failed to find significant differences in Foot and Ankle Outcome Scores among patients who had undergone screw fixation and had residual malreduction on a CT scan as defined by a series of quantitative measurements. They had set out to redefine the 2-mm threshold that traditionally described clinically impactful malreduction, and were unable to do so. They concluded that adequacy of fracture and articular reduction may play a much more significant role.

It should be noted that many of these studies found that malreduction rates increase over time. In the study by Anderson and colleagues there was no significant difference in measured tibiofibular distance on CT between screws and suture buttons at the 2-week scan, but such differences manifested at 1 year when only screws had been routinely removed. The study by Laflamme and colleagues[42] used radiographic measurements and similarly found no significant differences immediately postoperatively nor at 3 months, but did note differences starting at 6 months. This finding may suggest that the length of time during which stabilizing hardware is necessary across the syndesmosis may be longer than traditionally thought.

From these authors' point of view, although it has been reported that less rigid fixation better enables the body to finds its natural position after fixation, it does not state that using flexible fixation enables better anatomic reduction. In both cases, we are still falling short in achieving perfect reduction, and rather than aspiring to such, perhaps more focus and debate in the years ahead should focus on the manner in which we insert fixation and restore bony and ligamentous balance instead of the kind of fixation we use. Said differently, these authors feel that our most effective treatment strategy would focus on (1) restoring fibular and periarticular fracture anatomy, (2) providing multiplanar syndesmotic fixation to confer sufficient stability after reduction in a manner that is most consistent with the uninjured state, and (3) restoring normal resting length and orientation to the distal syndesmotic ligament complex through either direct reapposition, repair, or ligamentoplasty when necessary (depending on whether this is done in the acute or chronic setting). If these 3 tenets are followed during any syndesmotic fixation procedure, then on a relative scale of import, it is probably a matter of personal preference what "kind" of hardware one ultimately chooses to insert.

REMOVAL OF HARDWARE

Generally speaking, arguments supporting removal of syndesmotic screws are based on concerns that rigid trans-syndesmotic fixation may contribute to abnormal ankle kinematics.[44–46] Functionally, screw fixation immobilizes the distal tibia–fibula articulation allowing for ligamentous healing. Rigid fixation, however, inhibits physiologic fibular translation and rotation and may also limit dorsiflexion.[44,45] Hardware removal after successful healing may serve to restore physiologic motion of the syndesmosis and ankle joint. As such, some investigators continue to support removal before weight-bearing at 6 to 8 weeks.[47] Unfortunately, formal recommendations, as well as the timing of removal if indicated, have not been well-established in the literature and clinical practice remains highly variable.

The removal of syndesmotic fixation has been examined extensively with a range of levels of evidence present in the current literature. The majority of such studies are level IV evidence and have focused on removal of metal screws. To the best of our knowledge, no study has examined outcomes after removal of suture button devices. Although an exhaustive review is beyond the scope of this article, the literature supports the fact that there is little clinical, radiographic, or functional benefit to screw removal for the majority of patients. However, the more recent literature seems to support the notion that syndesmotic screw removal should be considered in symptomatic patients with intraosseous screw breakage (where pain can be directly attributable to the screw), well-fixed screws limiting motion, and/or in cases of syndesmotic malreduction. Furthermore, newer studies have revisited the effects of screw removal on ankle dorsiflexion.

Boyle and colleagues[48] performed a level I investigation examining syndesmotic screw removal. The authors randomized 51 patients to either screw retention or removal at approximately 3 months postoperatively. Clinical, radiographic, and patient-reported outcome measures such as the OMA score, American Orthopedic Foot and Ankle Society ankle–hindfoot score, American Academy of Orthopedic Surgeons foot and visual analog score were used. Trans-syndesmotic screw removal yielded no significant functional, clinical, or radiologic benefit in adult patients at the 1-year follow-up.

Several systematic reviews have similarly echoed these findings. Schepers[49] challenged the practice of routine screw removal in their 2011 review drawing evidence from 7 studies published from January 2000 to October 2010. Six of those studies found no difference in outcomes in patients when comparing screw retention versus removal.[50–54] Only 1 study showed favorable outcomes with screw removal, demonstrating that an intact screw was associated with worse functional outcome as compared with loose, broken, or removed screws.[55] These authors provided evidence that screw removal is unlikely to benefit patients with loose or fractured screws, but may be indicated in patients with intact screws and that removal should be pursued if still intact after 6 months. The mean time of removal for all 7 studies was approximately 3 months. Walley and colleagues[56] examined the literature from 2010 to 2016. A total of 9 studies were included. Overall, there was no difference in the functional, clinical, or radiographic outcomes in patients who had screw removal. The authors reported a higher likelihood of recurrent syndesmotic diastasis when screws were removed between 6 and 8 weeks and higher rates of postoperative infections when screws were removed without administering preoperative antibiotics.

Ankle range of motion after screw removal, in particular dorsiflexion, continues to be examined in the literature. Although improving ankle motion is a commonly considered clinical indication for screw removal, the current literature is conflicting. Miller and colleagues[45] examined range of motion after removal of a locking plate/screw construct for syndesmotic stabilization in 2010. Although the authors noted significant improvements in range of motion, Foot and Ankle Outcome, and OMA scores at the immediate postoperative visit in 25 patients, methodologic issues existed. A less commonly used locking screw construct was used in their study. Furthermore, range of motion was assessed by

an unblinded researcher using goniometric measurements and unmeasured applied ankle dorsiflexion force, which has been demonstrated to be of relatively poor reliability. In 2019, Briceno and colleagues[57] examined ankle dorsiflexion before and after nonlocked screw removal using a standardized dorsiflexion force with range of motion assessed radiographically. A standardized torque force was applied to the ankle and a perfect lateral radiograph was obtained immediately before removal, immediately after removal, and at 3 months after removal (**Fig. 9**). The authors demonstrated no statistically significant difference in ankle dorsiflexion at all 3 time points. Most recently, Kohring and colleagues[58] published results of a 2020 investigation compared 58 patients with ankle fractures who underwent syndesmotic screw removal with 71 patients who did not undergo removal. The authors demonstrated significant improvements in Patient-Reported Outcomes Measurement Information System physical function outcomes and mean improvement of total arc ankle range of motion by 17°.

Syndesmotic screw breakage may be more problematic than previously reported. Ibrahim

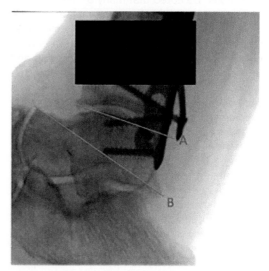

Fig. 9. Example of lateral ankle radiograph edited to blind syndesmotic screw presence (*black box*) with reference lines for angle measurement. The tibial reference line connects the 2 most distal points on the anterior and posterior tibial plafond (A). The talus reference line connects the points between the posterior process (lateral tubercle) of the talus and the anterodorsal aspect of the talus head (B). (*From* Briceno J, Wusu T, Kaiser P, et al. Effect of Syndesmotic Implant Removal on Dorsiflexion. Foot Ankle Int. 2019;40(5):499-505. https://doi.org/10.1177/1071100718818572; with permission.)

and colleagues[59] examined 43 patients (with 58 screws) experiencing postoperative screw breakage. Intraosseous screw breakage, as defined by breakage within either the fibula or tibia, occurred in 32 patients (74.4%). Screw breakage occurred exclusively in the tibiofibular clear space in the remaining 11 instances (25.6%). Intraosseous breakage was associated with significantly higher rates of implant removal secondary to pain.

Patients with retained syndesmotic screws with known syndesmotic malreduction should be considered for screw removal. Although limited by a small patient cohort, Song and colleagues[60] demonstrated that screw removal may lead to auto-reduction of the malaligned syndesmosis. Nine patients demonstrated evidence of tibiofibular malreduction on initial postoperative CT scans. After removal, 8 of 9 showed adequate reduction of the tibiofibular syndesmosis on CT scans. Although promising, further investigations are required to assess effects of implant removal on alignment in a larger patient cohort.

SUMMARY

As one examines the literature exploring syndesmotic instability, including studies comparing rigid versus flexible syndesmotic fixation, a few critical points must be considered. Poor outcomes after a destabilizing syndesmotic injury are much more likely to result from failure to diagnose (and therefore treat) syndesmotic instability, technical malreduction of a concomitant fibular fracture (eg, failure to attain length), or failure to attain articular congruency, than it is to arise from a malreduction of the syndesmosis itself. Malreduction of the distal tibiofibular articulation has been correlated with poorer outcomes in some but not all studies, and its independent contribution is more difficult to elucidate. Importantly, the distinction between gross malreduction and more subtle malreductions are often confounded in the literature but likely entail very different clinical consequences. Ultimately, both rigid and flexible fixation of syndesmotic instability are excellent approaches to treat the unstable syndesmosis. Less discussed is the role of repair or reconstruction of the syndesmotic ligaments themselves, which may play an increasingly important role in the setting of chronic instability. Furthermore, both the lateral ankle ligaments and the deltoid ligamentous complex contribute toward stabilizing the syndesmosis, and yet they are rarely discussed in treatment algorithms.

Suture button constructs are less likely to result in syndesmotic malreduction and this may partly stem from their ability to compensate for an error in surgical technique during clamping or manual reduction maneuvers. In contrast, especially if using only 1 suture button construct, they afford less stability than screws, especially in the sagittal plane, and multiple suture buttons with divergent orientation should be considered.

Flexible constructs also have significantly lower rates of removal of hardware. Many of the well-designed, prospective studies that describe loss of reduction with screw fixation compare a screw cohort in which hardware is electively removed, often before 3 months, with a suture button cohort in which it is not. Additional studies may be necessary to understand the timing of screw removal as well as its necessity, especially given that many studies show increased tibiofibular diastasis over time after screw removal. Furthermore, the description of screw breakage because a hardware failure may overshadow a natural phenomenon that enables normal fibular motion rather than representing an actual complication.

The cost savings inherent to avoiding an elective removal of hardware are overshadowed by the higher cost of flexible implants, especially if multiple suture buttons are used. In contrast, such analyses should also take into account the indirect patient costs, not just the direct healthcare costs, of a return to the operating room for the removal of hardware.

Ultimately, both rigid and flexible fixation seem to have excellent clinical outcomes, with the majority of patients enjoying significant long term pain relief. Both have an integral role, wherein more complex fractures and patients with neuropathy or osteoporosis may benefit from the rigidity of screw constructs and their contribution toward maintaining fibular length, whereas other patients may benefit from the ability of flexible constructs to better replicate normal fibular motion and distal tibiofibular alignment.

CLINICS CARE POINTS

- Diagnosis of syndesmotic instability associated with ankle injuries is critically important to maximize patient outcome and minimize morbidity.
- Weight bearing x-rays and CT complement the role of the physical exam in diagnosing subtle syndesmotic injuries.

- The benefits of flexible over screw fixation remains an ongoing area of debate and study at this time.

DISCLOSURE

The authors have nothing to disclose.

REFERENCES

1. Lloyd J, Elsayed S, Hariharan K, Tanaka H. Revisiting the concept of talar shift in ankle fractures. Foot Ankle Int 2006;27(10):793–6.
2. Ramsey P, Hamilton W. Changes in tibiotalar area of contact caused by lateral talar shift. J Bone Joint Surg Am 1976;58(3):356–7.
3. Hermans JJ, Beumer A, de Jong TAW, Kleinrensink G-J. Anatomy of the distal tibiofibular syndesmosis in adults: a pictorial essay with a multimodality approach. J Anat 2010;217(6):633–45.
4. Sora M-C, Strobl B, Staykov D, Förster-Streffleur S. Evaluation of the ankle syndesmosis: a plastination slices study. Clin Anat 2004;17(6):513–7.
5. Olson KM, Dairyko GH, Toolan BC. Salvage of chronic instability of the syndesmosis with distal tibiofibular arthrodesis: functional and radiographic results. J Bone Joint Surg Am 2011;93(1):66–72.
6. Sagi HC, Shah AR, Sanders RW. The functional consequence of syndesmotic joint malreduction at a minimum 2-year follow-up. J Orthop Trauma 2012;26(7):439–43.
7. Lui TH, Ip K, Chow HT. Comparison of radiologic and arthroscopic diagnoses of distal tibiofibular syndesmosis disruption in acute ankle fracture. Arthroscopy 2005;21(11):1370.
8. Hagemeijer NC, Chang SH, Abdelaziz ME, et al. Range of normal and abnormal syndesmotic measurements using weightbearing CT. Foot Ankle Int 2019;40(12):1430–7.
9. Abdelaziz ME, Hagemeijer N, Guss D, El-Hawary A, El-Mowafi H, DiGiovanni CW. Evaluation of syndesmosis reduction on CT scan. Foot Ankle Int 2019;40(9):1087–93.
10. Elgafy H, Semaan HB, Blessinger B, Wassef A, Ebraheim NA. Computed tomography of normal distal tibiofibular syndesmosis. Skeletal Radiol 2010;39(6):559–64.
11. Massri-Pugin J, Lubberts B, Vopat BG, Wolf JC, DiGiovanni CW, Guss D. Role of the deltoid ligament in syndesmotic instability. Foot Ankle Int 2018;39(5):598–603.
12. Lubberts B, Massri-Pugin J, Guss D, et al. Arthroscopic assessment of syndesmotic instability in the sagittal plane in a cadaveric model. Foot Ankle Int 2020;41(2):237–43.
13. Goetz JE, Vasseenon T, Tochigi Y, Amendola A, Femino JE. 3D talar kinematics during external rotation stress testing in hindfoot varus and valgus using a model of syndesmotic and deep deltoid instability. Foot Ankle Int 2019;40(7):826–35.
14. Jiang KN, Schulz BM, Tsui YL, Gardner TR, Greisberg JK. Comparison of radiographic stress tests for syndesmotic instability of supination-external rotation ankle fractures: a cadaveric study. J Orthop Trauma 2014;28(6):e123–7.
15. Hagemeijer NC, Saengsin J, Chang SH, et al. Diagnosing syndesmotic instability with dynamic ultrasound - establishing the natural variations in normal motion. Injury 2020;51(11):2703–9.
16. Davidovitch RI, Weil Y, Karia R, et al. Intraoperative syndesmotic reduction: three-dimensional versus standard fluoroscopic imaging. J Bone Joint Surg Am 2013;95(20):1838–43.
17. Gardner MJ, Demetrakopoulos D, Briggs SM, Helfet DL, Lorich DG. Malreduction of the tibiofibular syndesmosis in ankle fractures. Foot Ankle Int 2006;27(10):788–92.
18. Summers HD, Sinclair MK, Stover MD. A reliable method for intraoperative evaluation of syndesmotic reduction. J Orthop Trauma 2013;27(4):196–200.
19. Cosgrove CT, Putnam SM, Cherney SM, et al. Medial clamp tine positioning affects ankle syndesmosis malreduction. J Orthop Trauma 2017;31(8):440–6.
20. Hansen M, Le L, Wertheimer S, Meyer E, Haut R. Syndesmosis fixation: analysis of shear stress via axial load on 3.5-mm and 4.5-mm quadricortical syndesmotic screws. J Foot Ankle Surg 2006;45(2):65–9.
21. Thompson MC, Gesink DS. Biomechanical comparison of syndesmosis fixation with 3.5- and 4.5-millimeter stainless steel screws. Foot Ankle Int 2000;21(9):736–41.
22. Miller AN, Barei DP, Iaquinto JM, Ledoux WR, Beingessner DM. Iatrogenic syndesmosis malreduction via clamp and screw placement. J Orthop Trauma 2013;27(2):100–6.
23. Park YH, Choi WS, Choi GW, Kim HJ. Ideal angle of syndesmotic screw fixation: a CT-based cross-sectional image analysis study. Injury 2017;48(11):2602–5.
24. Park YH, Ahn JH, Choi GW, Kim HJ. Comparison of clamp reduction and manual reduction of syndesmosis in rotational ankle fractures: a prospective randomized trial. J Foot Ankle Surg 2018;57(1):19–22.
25. Stuart K, Panchbhavi VK. The fate of syndesmotic screws. Foot Ankle Int 2011;32(5):S519–25.
26. Litrenta J, Saper D, Tornetta P, et al. Does syndesmotic injury have a negative effect on functional outcome? A multicenter prospective evaluation.

J Orthop Trauma 2015;29(9):410–3. https://doi.org/10.1097/BOT.0000000000000295.

27. Jones CR, Nunley JAI. Deltoid ligament repair versus syndesmotic fixation in bimalleolar equivalent ankle fractures. J Orthop Trauma 2015;29(5):245.

28. Andersen MR, Frihagen F, Hellund JC, Madsen JE, Figved W. Randomized trial comparing suture button with single syndesmotic screw for syndesmosis injury. J Bone Joint Surg Am 2018;100(1):2–12.

29. Kaiser PB, Cronin P, Stenquist DS, Miller CP, Velasco BT, Kwon JY. Getting the starting point right: prevention of skiving and fibular cortical breach during suture button placement for syndesmotic ankle injuries. Foot Ankle Spec 2020;13(4):351–5.

30. Klitzman R, Zhao H, Zhang L-Q, Strohmeyer G, Vora A. Suture-button versus screw fixation of the syndesmosis: a biomechanical analysis. Foot Ankle Int 2010;31(1):69–75.

31. Teramoto A, Suzuki D, Kamiya T, Chikenji T, Watanabe K, Yamashita T. Comparison of different fixation methods of the suture-button implant for tibiofibular syndesmosis injuries. Am J Sports Med 2011;39(10):2226–32.

32. Westermann RW, Rungprai C, Goetz JE, Femino J, Amendola A, Phisitkul P. The effect of suture-button fixation on simulated syndesmotic malreduction: a cadaveric study. J Bone Joint Surg Am 2014;96(20):1732–8.

33. Clanton TO, Williams BT, Backus JD, et al. Biomechanical analysis of the individual ligament contributions to syndesmotic stability. Foot Ankle Int 2017;38(1):66–75.

34. Neary KC, Mormino MA, Wang H. Suture button fixation versus syndesmotic screws in supination-external rotation type 4 injuries: a cost-effectiveness analysis. Am J Sports Med 2017;45(1):210–7.

35. Degroot H, Al-Omari AA, El Ghazaly SA. Outcomes of suture button repair of the distal tibiofibular syndesmosis. Foot Ankle Int 2011;32(3):250–6.

36. Förschner PF, Beitzel K, Imhoff AB, et al. Five-year outcomes after treatment for acute instability of the tibiofibular syndesmosis using a suture-button fixation system. Orthop J Sports Med 2017;5(4). 2325967117702854.

37. Kaiser PB, Riedel MD, Qudsi R, et al. Consideration of medial anatomical structures at risk when placing quadricortical syndesmotic fixation: a cadaveric study. Injury 2020;51(2):527–31.

38. Storey P, Gadd RJ, Blundell C, Davies MB. Complications of suture button ankle syndesmosis stabilization with modifications of surgical technique. Foot Ankle Int 2012;33(9):717–21.

39. Littlechild J, Mayne A, Harrold F, Chami G. A cadaveric study investigating the role of the anterior inferior tibio-fibular ligament and the posterior inferior tibio-fibular ligament in ankle fracture syndesmosis stability. Foot Ankle Surg 2020;26(5):547–50.

40. Nelson OA. Examination and repair of the AITFL in transmalleolar fractures. J Orthop Trauma 2006;20(9):637–43.

41. Yasui Y, Takao M, Miyamoto W, Innami K, Matsushita T. Anatomical reconstruction of the anterior inferior tibiofibular ligament for chronic disruption of the distal tibiofibular syndesmosis. Knee Surg Sports Traumatol Arthrosc 2011;19(4):691–5.

42. Laflamme M, Belzile EL, Bédard L, van den Bekerom MPJ, Glazebrook M, Pelet S. A prospective randomized multicenter trial comparing clinical outcomes of patients treated surgically with a static or dynamic implant for acute ankle syndesmosis rupture. J Orthop Trauma 2015;29(5):216–23.

43. Warner SJ, Fabricant PD, Garner MR, et al. The Measurement and Clinical Importance of Syndesmotic Reduction After Operative Fixation of Rotational Ankle Fractures. J Bone Joint Surg Am 2015;97(23):1935–44.

44. Hooper J. Movement of the ankle joint after driving a screw across the inferior tibiofibular joint. Injury 1983;14(6):493–506.

45. Miller AN, Paul O, Boraiah S, Parker RJ, Helfet DL, Lorich DG. Functional outcomes after syndesmotic screw fixation and removal. J Orthop Trauma 2010;24(1):12–6.

46. Needleman RL, Skrade DA, Stiehl JB. Effect of the syndesmotic screw on ankle motion. Foot Ankle 1989;10(1):17–24.

47. Tile M. Fractures of the ankle. In: Schatzker J, Tile M, editors. The rationale of operative fracture care. Berlin: Springer; 2005. p. 551–90. https://doi.org/10.1007/3-540-27708-0_22.

48. Boyle MJ, Gao R, Frampton CMA, Coleman B. Removal of the syndesmotic screw after the surgical treatment of a fracture of the ankle in adult patients does not affect one-year outcomes: a randomised controlled trial. Bone Joint J 2014;96-B(12):1699–705.

49. Schepers T. To retain or remove the syndesmotic screw: a review of literature. Arch Orthop Trauma Surg 2011;131(7):879–83.

50. Bell DP, Wong MK. Syndesmotic screw fixation in Weber C ankle injuries–should the screw be removed before weight bearing? Injury 2006;37(9):891–8.

51. Hamid N, Loeffler BJ, Braddy W, Kellam JF, Cohen BE, Bosse MJ. Outcome after fixation of ankle fractures with an injury to the syndesmosis: the effect of the syndesmosis screw. J Bone Joint Surg Br 2009;91(8):1069–73.

52. Høiness P, Strømsøe K. Tricortical versus quadricortical syndesmosis fixation in ankle fractures: a

prospective, randomized study comparing two methods of syndesmosis fixation. J Orthop Trauma 2004;18(6):331–7.

53. Moore JA, Shank JR, Morgan SJ, Smith WR. Syndesmosis fixation: a comparison of three and four cortices of screw fixation without hardware removal. Foot Ankle Int 2006;27(8):567–72.

54. Weening B, Bhandari M. Predictors of functional outcome following transsyndesmotic screw fixation of ankle fractures. J Orthop Trauma 2005;19(2):102–8.

55. Manjoo A, Sanders DW, Tieszer C, MacLeod MD. Functional and radiographic results of patients with syndesmotic screw fixation: implications for screw removal. J Orthop Trauma 2010;24(1):2–6.

56. Walley KC, Hofmann KJ, Velasco BT, Kwon JY. Removal of hardware after syndesmotic screw fixation: a systematic literature review. Foot Ankle Spec 2017;10(3):252–7.

57. Briceno J, Wusu T, Kaiser P, et al. Effect of syndesmotic implant removal on dorsiflexion. Foot Ankle Int 2019;40(5):499–505.

58. Kohring JM, Greenstein A, Gorczyca JT, Judd KT, Soles G, Ketz JP. Immediate improvement in physical function after symptomatic syndesmotic screw removal. J Orthop Trauma 2020; 34(6):327–31.

59. Ibrahim IO, Velasco BT, Ye MY, Miller CP, Kwon JY. Syndesmotic screw breakage may be more problematic than previously reported: increased rates of hardware removal secondary to pain with intraosseous screw breakage. Foot Ankle Spec 2020. https://doi.org/10.1177/1938640020932049. 1938640020932049.

60. Song DJ, Lanzi JT, Groth AT, et al. The effect of syndesmosis screw removal on the reduction of the distal tibiofibular joint: a prospective radiographic study. Foot Ankle Int 2014;35(6):543–8.

Calcaneal Fractures—Which Approach for Which Fracture?

Stefan Rammelt, MD, PhD[a],*, Michael P. Swords, DO[b]

KEYWORDS

- Displaced calcaneus fracture • Subtalar joint • Less invasive fixation • Percutaneous fixation
- Control of reduction

KEY POINTS

- The management of calcaneal fractures is demanding, and the best treatment is still subject to debate. It has become apparent that there is no single method that is suitable for all calcaneal fracture variants. Treatment must be tailored to the individual fracture pathoanatomy, accompanying soft tissue damage, associated injuries, functional demand, and comorbidities of the patient.
- If operative treatment is chosen, anatomic reconstruction of the overall shape and joint surfaces of the calcaneus are of utmost importance to obtain a good functional result. For severely comminuted fractures with multiple joint fragmentation, an extensile lateral approach offers excellent exposure and allows for lateral buttressing with a plate but requires meticulous soft tissue handling.
- For most of the displaced, intraarticular fractures, less invasive reduction and fixation via a direct approach over the sinus tarsi has successfully lowered soft tissue complications while ensuring exact anatomic reduction. This approach may be extended to the calcaneocuboid joint and over the tip of the fibula along the "lateral utility" line, if warranted for calcaneocuboid joint involvement or calcaneal fracture-dislocations, respectively.
- Purely percutaneous reduction and fixation is the treatment of choice for displaced extraarticular fractures and simple intraarticular fractures with adequate control of joint reduction.
- Specific approaches for rare calcaneal fracture variants include a direct medial approach for isolated sustentacular fractures, a posterolateral approach for superior tuberosity avulsion ("beak") fractures, and a posteromedial approach for displaced medial plantar tuberosity avulsions.

BACKGROUND

The management of displaced calcaneal fractures is a challenging task, and operative treatment is fraught with a considerable learning curve. Reasons include the irregular shape of the calcaneus and its joint surfaces, the delicate but unique soft tissue cover, and the great variety of fracture patterns.[1,2] Despite all controversy, there is consensus that there is no single treatment that is suitable for all types of calcaneal fractures[3-5]; this may be one of the reasons why studies comparing a uniform operative treatment, mostly open reduction and plate fixation via an extensile lateral approach, with nonoperative treatment including randomized trials and meta-analyses are for a great part inconclusive.[6-8] Consequently, recent meta-analyses failed to produce

---

[a] University Center of Orthopaedics, Trauma and Plastic Surgery, University Hospital Carl Gustav Carus at TU Dresden, Fetscherstrasse 74, Dresden 01307, Germany; [b] Michigan Orthopedic Center, Sparrow Hospital, 2815 S. Pennsylvania Avenue, Suite 204 Lansing, MI 48910, USA
* Corresponding author.
E-mail address: strammelt@hotmail.com

Orthop Clin N Am 52 (2021) 433–450
https://doi.org/10.1016/j.ocl.2021.05.012
0030-5898/21/© 2021 Elsevier Inc. All rights reserved.

a clear recommendation in the treatment of these injuries; however, operative treatment was favored if anatomic reduction could be achieved.[9,10] Several clinical studies have shown that only anatomic reconstruction of the calcaneal shape and joint congruity will lead to acceptable functional results and thus merit the effort of operative treatment with its possible complications.[11–20] In particular, restoration of the subtalar joint congruity is essential for postoperative foot function.[21,22]

To achieve favorable results, treatment has to be tailored individually not only to the fracture pattern and soft tissue conditions but also to patient demands, expectations, comorbidities, and compliance with the postoperative protocol. The worst results are to be expected, if operative treatment with extensive soft tissue dissection and protruding implants fails to reconstruct the anatomic shape of the calcaneus and its joints.[8,23–25]

PATIENT EVALUATION OVERVIEW
Clinical Examination
In patients with acute calcaneal fractures, the soft tissue status must be documented and monitored meticulously. Typically, there is marked swelling and hematoma around the heel and malleoli. Blisters may develop within a few hours and indicate pressure from the inside by hematoma or grossly displaced fragments (Fig. 1). In particular, marked upward displacement of the posterior tuberosity fragment as seen in tongue type and beak fractures may rapidly progress into a full-thickness skin necrosis over the insertion of the Achilles tendon.[26,27]

Progressive soft tissue swelling with loss of skin wrinkling and pain out of proportion despite

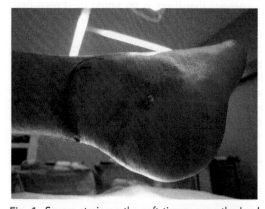

Fig. 1. Severe strain on the soft tissues over the heel with a small open wound (sutured in the referring hospital) from a grossly displaced tuberosity avulsion fracture of the calcaneus.

adequate rest, elevation, and local cooling highly indicate a foot compartment syndrome.[28] The diagnosis of a compartment syndrome is established clinically. Multistick invasive measurements of compartment pressures are only needed in unconscious patients. Repeat clinical examinations are suggested to not overlook calcaneal fractures and other foot injuries in multiple injured or polytraumatized patients.

Imaging
Clinical suspicion of a calcaneal fracture is confirmed with standard lateral and axial radiographs. Anteroposterior radiographs of the ankle show broadening of the heel and the amount of fibulocalcaneal abutment and talar tilt in case of fracture-dislocations.[29] Brodén views of the subtalar joint are useful for intraoperative fluoroscopic assessment of joint reconstruction.[30] The foot is placed in neutral flexion and internal rotation of 45°, whereas the x-ray tube is angled 10° to 40°, the former showing the posterior and the latter the anterior portion of the subtalar joint.

With suspected or confirmed diagnosis of a calcaneal fracture, computed tomography (CT) imaging is indispensable for a precise analysis of the fracture morphology and treatment planning (Fig. 2).[12,13]

INDICATIONS AND CONTRAINDICATIONS TO SURGERY
Indications
Although there is no general consensus on the choice of treatment, given the available evidence, most agree that, in the absence of local or systemic contraindications, intraarticular calcaneal fractures should be reduced anatomically and fixed if there is a step-off in the subtalar joint of 2 mm or greater in order to avoid restricted hindfoot motion and posttraumatic arthritis of the subtalar joint, provided that an anatomic reduction can be obtained.[10–24,30] There is no clear cutoff for the displacement of Böhler or Gissane angles but marked deformities regularly go along with joint displacement.

Severely displaced extraarticular fractures lead to hindfoot deformities with functional limitations, painful callosities, shoewear conflict, and soft tissue impingement.[8,31,32] Extraarticular fractures should therefore be reduced with substantial varus or valgus (>10°) and broadening or shortening of the heel (more than 20%), preferably via small or percutaneous approaches.[3,8,26]

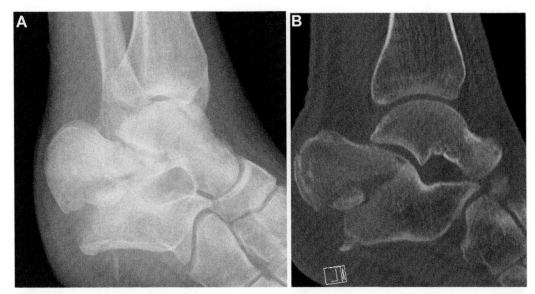

Fig. 2. (*A*) Lateral radiograph of a tuberosity avulsion fracture of the calcaneus. (*B*) CT imaging reveals no subtalar joint displacement but a large intercalary fragment from the medial plantar tuberosity warranting open reduction (same patient as in **Fig. 1**).

Contraindications

Systemic contraindications to open reduction and internal fixation include severe peripheral vascular disease, poorly controlled insulin-dependent diabetes mellitus, in particular with complications such as neuropathy and nephropathy, poor patient compliance (eg, substance abuse), and severe systemic disorders with immunodeficiency and/or a poor overall prognosis.[1,3] Heavy smokers should be counseled that they have a higher risk of soft tissue–related complications.[33,34]

If open reduction and internal fixation of severely displaced calcaneal fractures is impossible because of critical soft tissue conditions or an overall critical condition of the patient—for example, with polytrauma—gross reduction and temporary fixation by percutaneous methods reduces soft tissue strain and prevents severe contractures. In these cases, a staged open reduction and internal fixation is feasible after stabilization of the overall conditions of the patient and/or local soft tissue conditions.[35]

Nonoperative treatment is a good choice in nondisplaced or minimally displaced fractures where the calcaneus is centered beneath the talus and there is only mild flattening of Böhler angle and step-off in the subtalar joint of less than 2 mm.[3,4,8,36,37]

EMERGENCY PROCEDURES
Tuberosity Avulsion Fractures
Emergency treatment of calcaneal fractures is directed at avoiding severe soft tissue

complications. It is indicated either with open fractures or with closed fractures with severe soft tissue compromise through pressure from severely displaced fragments.[2,35,38] The latter is frequently seen with avulsion fractures of the tuberosity. Because of the characteristic appearance of the displaced fragment in the lateral radiograph, they are also called "beak" fractures. The superior portion of the tuberosity is pulled upward by the Achilles tendon, thus exerting a massive strain on the vulnerable skin over the posterior heel. In a recent study of 41 calcaneal avulsion fractures, almost 50% had either an open fracture or a severe soft tissue compromise necessitating urgent surgery.[38] These fractures are a result of either a high-velocity injury in younger patients or a low-velocity injury in elderly patients with reduced bone quality as in osteoporosis and neuropathic conditions. Both conditions can lead to a full-thickness necrosis over the Achilles tendon insertion with catastrophic outcomes if the soft tissue strain is not released urgently through reduction of the fragment.[3,26,27]

These mostly extraarticular fractures are typically approached through a vertical posterolateral incision lateral to the Achilles tendon (**Fig. 3**). Purely percutaneous lag screw fixation may lead to catastrophic failure of fixation, particularly with osteoporotic bone quality in elderly patients.[38] In these cases, supplementary tension band wiring or lateral interlocking plates are preferred.[2,38,39] Intercalary fragments may also prevent percutaneous treatment and even

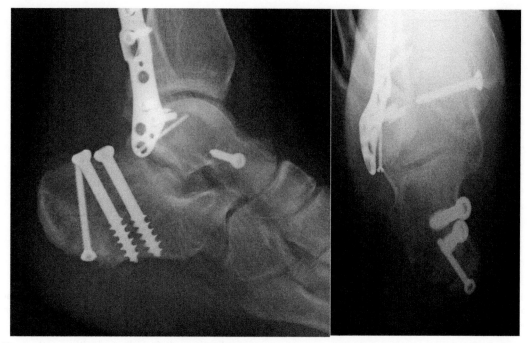

Fig. 3. Fixation of the superior tuberosity avulsion in a young patient with adequate bone stock can be achieved with 2 large (6.5 mm) cancellous lag screws. The medial plantar tuberosity avulsion was fixed with a bicortical 3.5 mm screw. Additional fractures of the fibula and the talar body were treated in the same session (same patient as in **Figs. 1** and **2**).

require an additional small medial approach as detailed later.[3]

Open Calcaneal Fractures

The surgical approach in open calcaneal fractures is dictated by the site of the open wound. Most of these have a medial wound inflicted by sharp fragments of the thick medial wall.[26,40] Treatment consists of debridement of contaminated and devitalized tissue, copious lavage, gross reduction by percutaneous leverage or direct manipulation, and temporary fixation with Kirschner wires (K-wires) or screws supplemented by tibio(calcaneo)metatarsal external fixation.[35,41] In selected cases, definite minimally invasive fixation can be achieved. Depending on the size of the wound, vacuum-assisted closure is applied until definite wound closure or soft tissue coverage, if needed.[40,42] With staged treatment protocols, complication rates could be substantially reduced in recent studies.[43,44]

Foot Compartment Syndrome

Between 1% and 10% of all calcaneal fractures are reportedly complicated by acute foot compartment syndrome.[45,46] The deep posterior (calcaneal) compartment containing the quadratus plantae muscle will always be involved in calcaneal fractures.[47] Treatment consists of emergent decompression via a medial incision

(Henry approach), which allows release of the medial, central, and lateral compartments.[28] The surgeon then critically assesses the dorsal aspect of the foot for the necessity of an additional dorsal compartment release. It should further be borne in mind that there is a direct communication between the deep posterior compartments of the foot and the lower leg via the flexor tendons that may result in a combined compartment syndrome of the foot and ankle.[48]

TIMING OF SURGERY

In the absence of an emergency, internal fixation of closed calcaneal fractures is traditionally performed within 2 weeks after the injury when hematoma and swelling have markedly decreased and skin blisters healed. With further delay, anatomic reduction will become more difficult due to early fibrous union, soft tissue contracture, and calf muscle tightness, which, in turn, may increase the risk of wound-healing problems.[49,50] With the advent of less invasive approaches, the time to surgery has decreased, and a substantial number of calcaneal fractures can be considered for early surgical fixation.[2] If purely percutaneous fixation is considered, surgery should generally be performed within 7 days after the injury.[35,51]

CHOICE OF APPROACH AND FIXATION
Open Reduction and Lateral Plate Fixation via an Extensile Lateral Approach

The extensile lateral approach[11] allows excellent exposure of the lateral aspect of the calcaneus, subtalar, and calcaneocuboid joints in complex fractures with severe displacement of the lateral wall and multiple articular fragments (Fig. 4).[12,13,52] It is less useful for the treatment of fracture-dislocations and isolated fractures of the sustentaculum tali.[5,29,53] The major drawback of this approach lies in the potential for early soft tissue–related complications such as wound edge necrosis, deep soft tissue, and bone infection as well as late complications including arthrofibrosis and stiffness of the subtalar joint because of the extensile soft tissue dissection despite a meticulous surgical technique.[19,54,55]

The patient is placed in a lateral decubitus position on the uninjured side. The incision for the vertical limb begins approximately 2 cm proximal to the tip of the lateral malleolus, just lateral to the Achilles tendon and thus posterior to the sural nerve and the lateral calcaneal artery. The horizontal limb is drawn along the junction of the hairy skin of the lateral foot and glabrous skin of the heel pad. The demarcation between the 2 can be easily identified by compressing the heel. The incision is gently curved where these 2 limbs combine in an obtuse angle to avoid apical necrosis of the resulting flap

(Fig. 5A). A full-thickness, subperiosteal flap is raised to the sinus tarsi, subtalar, and calcaneocuboid joints. The use of sharp retractors and any separation of the skin from the underlying subcutaneous tissue should be avoided. The calcaneofibular ligament and inferior peroneal retinaculum are sharply released from the lateral calcaneal wall. The peroneal tendons are exposed and released at the peroneal tubercle, from where they are mobilized within their sheath.[56] For gentle and continuous retraction of the flap, K-wires are placed into the fibular tip, the talar neck, and the cuboid. The lateral wall fragment is gently separated from the adjacent affected superolateral articular fragment, reflected inferiorly and secured with a suture.

In many cases, direct manipulation of the tuberosity fragment with 4.5 mm cancellous Schanz screw with T-handle introduced via a stab incision into the posterior tuberosity from either posterior[13] or lateral[11] is most helpful. Levering of the handle loosens the affected intraarticular fragments. The affected superolateral articular fragment is carefully elevated from the body of the calcaneus with either a posterior Schanz screw or a periosteal elevator placed beneath the entire fragment for gentle disimpaction. The fragments are cleared from hematoma and debris.

Reduction step 1
In a crucial first step, the main tuberosity fragment is brought downward and medially

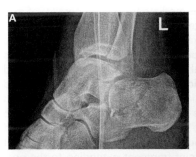
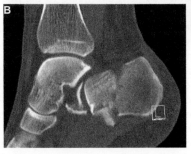
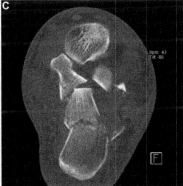
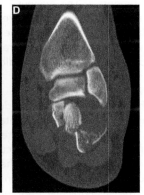

Fig. 4. (*A*) Lateral radiograph, (*B*) sagittal, (*C*) semicoronal, and (*D*) coronal CT section of a displaced, intraarticular calcaneal fracture with multiple joint fragments and severe blowout of both the medial and lateral calcaneal wall.

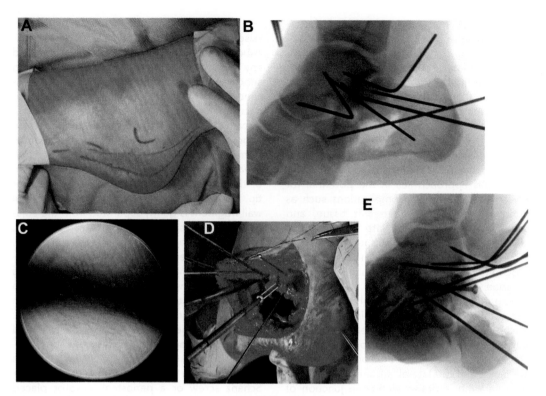

Fig. 5. (A) The extensile lateral approach is marked on the skin with the patient in lateral decubitus position. (B) Temporary fixation is achieved with K-wires after step-wise reduction of the subtalar joint and calcaneal body. (C) Dry arthroscopy can be used to precisely control subtalar joint reconstruction, particularly with a fracture line running far medially. (D, E) A first, independent screw is introduced parallel to the posterior facet and aimed at the sustentaculum tali in order to stabilize the joint (same patient as in **Fig. 4**).

beneath the sustentacular fragment with an elevator introduced as a lever between these 2 fragments.[1,3] This maneuver restores the medial wall and enables anatomic reduction of the articular fragments. The fragments are fixed along the medial wall with K-wires, and reduction is controlled with an axial radiograph.

Reduction step 2
The subtalar joint is then reduced stepwise starting medially with the sustentacular fragment that is either angulated, translated medially, or fractured in 42% of intraarticular calcaneal fractures.[57] Reduction of the medial wall as outlined earlier will result in correct positioning of the sustentacular fragment in most cases. If still tilted or shifted, reduction must be repeated until the sustentaculum is congruent to the medial facet of the talus. In rare cases, comminuted fractures of the sustentaculum require an additional direct medial approach in order to anatomically reduce the medial facet.[13]

The intermediate joint fragments in Sanders type III and IV fractures are then reduced to the sustentacular fragment and fixed with one or two K-wires that are drilled through the medial cortex and the skin until they are flush with the intermediate fragment laterally.[56] Small intermediate fragments that are not amenable to screw fixation but display an intact cartilage cover may be definitely fixed with "lost" K-wires or absorbable pins.[58] Finally, the depressed lateral portion of the posterior facet is reduced to the medial and intermediate fragments, and the K-wires are drilled back from medial to lateral (see **Fig. 5B**). In severely displaced tongue type fractures, anatomic reduction of the lateral joint fragment extending to the posterior tuberosity at the joint level may be impossible because of soft-tissue restraints, particularly with delayed surgery. In these cases, an osteotomy through that fragment posterior to the joint facet facilitates exact reduction of the posterior facet.[59] Rotational reduction of the posterior component of the tongue fragment is essential to prevent long-term irritation with shoe wear.

Anatomic reduction of the subtalar joint is controlled visually by tilting the reconstructed joint block into varus and with intraoperative

Brodén projections.[12] With medial extension or multiple fragmentation of the subtalar joint the quality of reduction may be checked more reliably by open subtalar arthroscopy.[60] For this, a small diameter arthroscope (2.7 mm, 30°) is introduced into the exposed subtalar joint from the angle of Gissane or from the posterior joint (see **Fig. 5**C). If a residual intraarticular step-off is found at this stage, the K-wires are removed and joint reduction repeated. This may be warranted in about 20% of cases even though joint reduction had been judged as being anatomic with fluoroscopy.[60] After exact reduction is confirmed, 1 or 2 independent screws are inserted parallel to the joint from the lateral wall into the sustentaculum to stabilize the articular portion of the calcaneus (see **Fig. 5**D, E).

Reduction step 3
The tuberosity fragment is then aligned to the reconstructed subtalar joint block. At this stage, any residual loss of height, varus or valgus of the tuberosity is corrected by using the inserted Schanz screw as a lever. The tuberosity is fixed temporarily to the joint block with K-wires.

Reduction step 4
The calcaneocuboid joint, if displaced, is reconstructed from medial to lateral using the cuboid as a template. The fragments are held temporarily with K-wires that are introduced into the subchondral bone so that they are not interfering with later plate positioning.

Reduction step 5
Finally, the reconstructed anterior process is aligned with the reduced posterior part and the calcaneus is fixed with axial K-wires. This realigns the strong cortical bone at the angle of Gissane. The small bone fragments that have been cleared initially from the fracture are now brought back into the calcaneal body. There is no general need of additional bone grafting or the use of bone substitutes for subcortical defect filling.[12,61,62] When the bulged lateral wall fragments are folded back, the fragments should fit anatomically along the fracture lines.

Fixation is completed with a calcaneal plate that fits the lateral wall and mimics the anatomic shape of the calcaneus without protruding laterally.[12,52,56,63–65] The plate is fixed with screws to the subthalamic portion, the tuberosity, and the anterior process, providing a 3-point stabilization (**Fig. 6**). Most current plate designs are interlocking and allow variable angle screw placement.[5,66]

Less Invasive Fixation via a Sinus Tarsi Approach
Over the last decade, a small oblique lateral approach over the sinus tarsi has gained

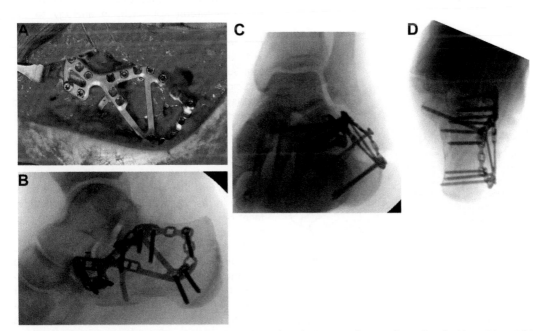

Fig. 6. (A) A lateral plate is used for final fixation. Most plate designs used currently are interlocking with variable angle screw placement. Restoration of the anatomic shape of the calcaneus is confirmed fluoroscopically with a (B) lateral, (C) Brodén, and (D) axial view (same patient as in **Figs. 4** and **5**).

increasing popularity for less invasive reduction and fixation of calcaneal fractures.[1,2,65-67] It allows a direct vision on the subtalar joint and manipulation of the articular fragments from the sinus tarsi. It may also be used for direct access to the joint if an attempted percutaneous reduction proves impossible.[35] The sinus tarsi approach may be applied for all Sanders type II and most of the Sanders type III fractures. For Sanders type IV fractures, an individual decision has to be made between internal fixation via an extensile lateral or sinus tarsi approach and primary subtalar fusion.[8,52,68]

Patient placement is exactly the same as described earlier for the extensile lateral approach. The incision starts at the tip of the fibula above the peroneal tendons and extends 2 to 3 cm distally toward the anterior process. It follows along the superior aspect of the calcaneus to allow placement of a small plate at the end of the procedure. The sural nerve and lateral calcaneal artery are situated below the incision, and the lateral branches of the superficial peroneal nerve are well dorsal. The incision has to be directed toward the fourth metatarsal (Fig. 7). If required, the approach can be extended distally along the "lateral utility" line between the tip of the fibula and the fourth metatarsal base allowing reduction of the calcaneocuboid joint under direct vision.[69] With an incision running toward the fifth metatarsal base, more wound complications and sural

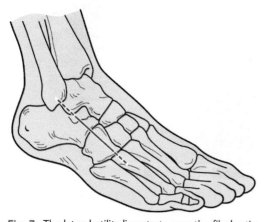

Fig. 7. The lateral utility line starts over the fibular tip and continues to the sinus tarsi (*dotted line*), the calcaneocuboid joint and cuboid (*solid line*), and the fourth tarsometatarsal joint (*dotted line*), if needed. (*From* Rammelt S, Zwipp H, Hansen ST. Posttraumatic reconstruction of the foot and ankle. In: Browner BD, Jupiter JB, Krettek C, Anderson PA (eds.): Skeletal Trauma, 6th Edition, Philadelphia, Elsevier Saunders, 2019, pp 2641-2690, with permission).

nerve lesions are reported.[70] The peroneal tendons are gently elevated off the lateral wall of the calcaneus and released from their sheath only at the peroneal tubercle on the lateral aspect of the calcaneus. They are then retracted distally within their sheath. The fat pad in the sinus tarsi is removed to allow adequate visualization. The lateral capsule of the subtalar joint, if still intact, is incised. Joint visualization can be improved by exerting a varus stress on the heel or placing a colinear distractor via stab incisions into the distal fibula and calcaneal tuberosity.

It is imperative that the same sequence of reduction (steps 1–5) is observed as with an extensile approach. The same instruments may be used—that is, an elevator or osteotome inserted into the fracture line just below the posterior facet and through the primary fracture line between the joint fragments exiting out the medial wall, a Schanz screw with T-handle placed from lateral (or posterior) into the calcaneal tuberosity, K-wires for temporary fragment fixation (Fig. 8). K-wires are typically advanced up to the fracture line and then across the fracture after reduction has been achieved. In analogy to the extensile lateral approach, 1 or 2 independent screws are placed through the existing incision or through an additional stab incision toward the sustentaculum tali to fix the reconstructed subtalar joint. Visual control of joint reduction is at least as efficient as with an extensile lateral approach. In analogy to the latter, an even more precise control of reduction can be achieved with dry arthroscopy.[8,71]

Definite fixation is achieved with either percutaneous screws,[8,66] an intramedullary nail with locking screws,[72–74] or a small plate (Fig. 9) that is slid in through the approach and tunneled beneath the peroneal tendons.[5,65,67]

Purely Percutaneous Fixation

Percutaneous reduction and screw fixation is the treatment of choice for displaced extraarticular fractures and Sanders type IIC fractures, that is, simple intraarticular fractures with the posterior facet being displaced as a whole.[35,75] With precise control of joint reduction with the use of subtalar arthroscopy, this technique can also be applied to simple (Sanders types IIA and IIB) intraarticular fractures with just one displaced fracture line across the subtalar joint.[51,60,76,77] Most studies, including one systematic review, report wound complication rates that are close to zero.[78]

Percutaneous techniques also have a role in patients with critical soft tissue conditions.

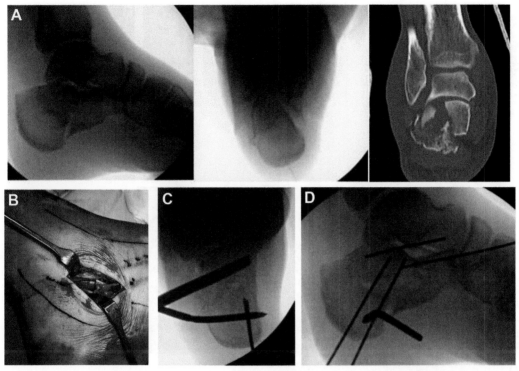

Fig. 8. (A) Preoperative lateral, axial, and axial CT view demonstrating a displaced closed displaced Sanders II joint depression fracture. (B) A sinus tarsi approach provides access to the displaced subtalar joint. (C) The medial wall height is restored using a Schanz pin and elevator. (D) Reduction is complete, and provisional fixation is achieved with K wires.

Performing percutaneous reduction and fixation irrespective of the type of calcaneal fracture and without adequate control of reduction carries the risk of inadequate reduction and loss of fixation.[35,79,80]

Dislocation Approach

Calcaneal fracture-dislocations result in a direct compression of the fibular tip by the calcaneal body fragment carrying the tuberosity and most of the subtalar joint and subsequent dislocation of the peroneal tendons.[5,29] In these cases, a posterior extension of the sinus tarsi approach along the lateral utility line (dislocation approach) allows access to the displaced tuberosity and lateral joint fragment from above.[1,56] The incision starts over the lateral malleolus. Because fracture-dislocations are frequently

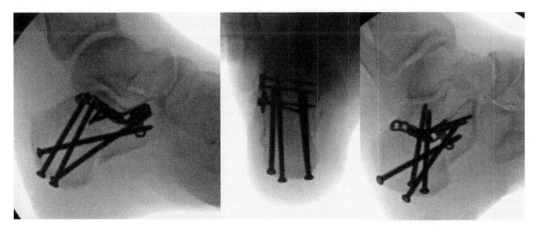

Fig. 9. Final fixation is obtained with a 2.7 mm variable angle calcaneal plate and independent 4.0 mm screws with restoration of normal anatomy in lateral, axial, and Brodén view (same patient as in Fig. 8).

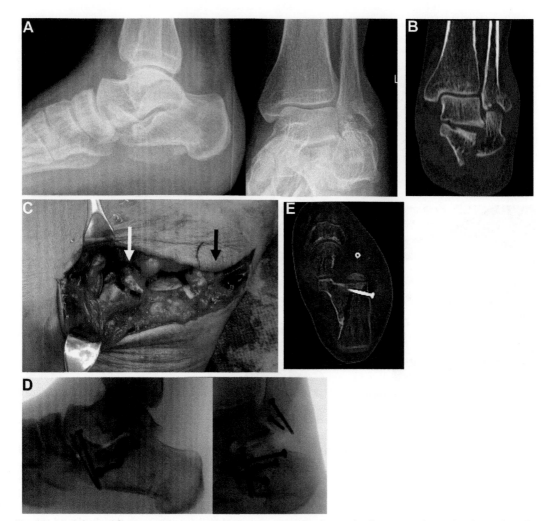

Fig. 10. (*A*) Calcaneal fracture-dislocation displaying the typical radiographic features such as talocalcaneal overlap (double density sign) in the lateral view and lateral dislocation of the calcaneal body abutting the distal fibula producing a direct fibular fracture in the anteroposterior ankle radiograph. (*B*) Coronal CT scan showing the dislocated calcaneal body fragment with the sustentacular fragment being still in place. (*C*) The dislocated fragments of the calcaneus and distal fibula (*black arrow*) are visualized via a dislocation approach that is extended anteriorly to expose the displaced calcaneocuboid joint (*white arrow*). (*D*) Fixation is achieved with 3.5 mm screws across the main body and sustentacular fragments and 2.7 mm screws in the distal fibula and anterior process. A "lost" K-wire stabilizes the small fragments along the cuboidal joint facet. (*E*) Postoperative axial (semicoronal) CT scan showing anatomic reduction of the calcaneal body and subtalar joint.

accompanied by direct compression fractures of the distal fibula with avulsions of the peroneal retinacula and fractures of the anterior process running into the calcaneocuboid joint, the approach can be extended posteriorly and/or anteriorly along the lateral utility line (see **Fig. 7**) to address these additional fractures (**Fig. 10**).

The fragments are best reduced early.[2] After cleaning the main fragments, a pointed reduction clamp placed between the sustentaculum tali and the lateral calcaneal body is most useful to close the fracture gap.[1] Fixation of the main fragments is achieved with compression screws inserted from lateral to medial, with at least one screw being placed into the sustentaculum tali.[29] Accompanying anterior process and fibular fractures are then fixed with screws or small plates. The peroneal tendons are rerouted behind the fibula, and the peroneal retinaculum is reattached after fracture reduction. When performed early, fixation of calcaneal fracture-dislocations is straightforward and favorable results can be expected.[29]

Sustentacular Approach

Isolated, displaced fractures of the sustentaculum tali cannot be reasonably addressed from lateral. In these cases, a small medial approach directly over the palpable sustentaculum is used.[26,53] The incision of about 3 cm is placed horizontally over the sustentaculum. (Fig. 11) The nearby posterior tibial and flexor digitorum longus tendons are held away with vessel loops. The posterior tibial neurovascular bundle lies plantar and usually is not exposed. The medial joint facet is reduced under direct vision using the medial talar facet as a template. A pointed reduction clamp is applied.[5,53] After visual and fluoroscopic control of reduction, the sustentaculum is generally fixed with compression screws if the fracture pattern is relatively simple or with a small plate if comminution is present.[26,53,81]

Medial Plantar Tuberosity Fractures

These fractures may result from direct plantar impaction or represent an avulsion of the plantar fascia. Surgery is indicated for displaced fractures (see Fig. 2) that will result in plantar pressure sores, conflict with shoewear, or even tarsal tunnel syndrome if left unreduced.[3,82,83]

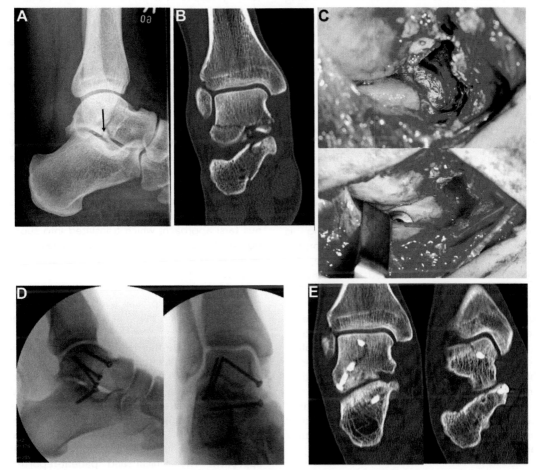

Fig. 11. (*A*) Lateral view of a sustentacular fracture combined with a talar body fracture. Note the irregular contour of the sustentaculum (*arrow*) that does not overlap with the contour of the lateral facet due to the impression. (*B*) Coronal CT scans show impression of both the sustentaculum tali and the medial facet of the talus. Failure to reconstruct the original height on the medial side will inevitably result in varus malalignment at the hindfoot. (*C*) Intraoperative aspect of the sustentacular approach showing impression of the medial facet of both the talus and calcaneus resulting in gaping of the joint space. (*C*) After lifting up the sustentaculum and buttressing the medial facet of the talus, congruity of the medial aspect of the subtalar joint is restored. (*D*) Internal fixation of the talus and sustentaculum is achieved with screws. Note that the contour of the sustentaculum now overlaps with the lateral facet of the subtalar joint. (*E*) Postoperative CT scan showing restoration of the height of both the sustentaculum and talus with congruent subtalar joint. (*From* Rammelt S, Pitakveerakul A. Hindfoot injuries: How to avoid post-traumatic varus deformity? Foot Ankle Clin 2019;24: 325-345, with permission).

The medial process of the calcaneal tuberosity is accessed by a small medial approach of 3 cm parallel to the sole at the transition to the glabrous skin.[5] A plantar incision should be avoided, because it may result in a painful scar and hyperkeratosis. Care is taken to avoid the terminal branches of the lateral plantar nerve that are running obliquely down the medial calcaneal wall. The superior margin of the fracture is visualized, and the plantar fragments are reduced anatomically to the main tuberosity fragment, starting with the fragment that is situated more laterally, if there is more than one. The forefoot is held in maximal plantar flexion during reduction to ease reduction by relaxing the pull of the plantar aponeurosis. The fragments are fixed with 2.7 mm (or 3.5 mm) small fragment screws placed from medial.[3,5] The screw heads must be flush with the plantar-medial aspect of the fragments (see **Fig. 3**).

Postoperative Care, Rehabilitation, and Implant Removal

Postoperative treatment aims at early mobilization of the patient, with active and passive range of motion exercises in the ankle, subtalar, and midtarsal joints beginning with the second postoperative day. Continuous passive motion of the subtalar joint is initiated. A lower leg cast or splint is applied for soft tissue protection until the swelling subsides. Weight-bearing is restricted for 6 to 12 weeks, depending on the fracture pattern and bone quality. Active, reliable patients can be mobilized on crutches in their own shoes, particularly following less invasive approaches. Otherwise, a removable boot or walker is applied. If patients are unable to restrict weight-bearing to about 20 kg, offloading is preferred until bone healing. Implant removal at 1 year is advocated only in cases of hardware irritation or restricted range of motion, mostly after plate fixation via extensile approaches. In these cases, implant removal is combined with extraarticular and intraarticular arthrolysis and debridement using subtalar arthroscopy.[1,60]

EVALUATION OF OUTCOME

The literature is abundant with clinical studies reporting the short-term to midterm results after various kinds of calcaneal fractures treatment. Several series with more than 100 patients followed-up for more than 1 year showed good to excellent results with open reduction and plate fixation via an extensile lateral approach (**Fig. 12**) in 60% to 85% of cases using different outcome measurements.[12,13,50,84] These results seem to prevail on the long term with an average follow-up of 8 to 15 years.[18,19,52,85]

Several studies have identified surgeon experience as an important prognostic factor for both functional outcome and the occurrence of complications.[12,34,86,87] Negative prognostic factors that have been identified in different clinical studies include a severe fracture pattern (as Sanders type 4), open and bilateral fractures, eligibility for workers' compensation, high workload, failure to reconstruct Böhler angle, and residual step-offs in the subtalar joint of 2 mm or more.[10–24,88–90] Axial impaction at the time of surgery results in a primary cartilage damage that may lead to posttraumatic arthritis irrespective of the kind of treatment.[52,91] Higher patient age by itself does not negatively affect outcome after operative treatment of calcaneal fractures.[19,92,93] However, care has to be taken not to misjudge low-velocity injuries in the elderly population with avulsion or beak fractures associated with osteoporosis or diabetes that are challenging to treat and prone to complications.[94,95] Lower bone mineral density negatively affected functional outcome in a retrospective study.[96]

A multitude of studies including several meta-analyses has demonstrated significantly less wound complications and infections with the sinus tarsi approach, which translated into superior outcome in most of these studies,[97–102] whereas some others did not find significant differences between the 2 approaches.[103] The favorable outcomes with less invasive approaches seem to prevail over time as shown by the results of the first long-term clinical studies.[104–106]

It is imperative that less invasive techniques are not traded off with less-than-ideal reduction in order to obtain favorable outcomes. Park and colleagues,[107] in a recent randomized controlled trial, found no differences in the restoration Böhler angle but significantly better restoration of calcaneal width with an extensile lateral approach compared with the sinus tarsi approach. The clinical and patient-reported scores as well as subtalar range of motion in this study were significantly better in patients treated via sinus tarsi approach compared with extensile lateral approach. Busel and colleagues,[108] in a retrospective study, found significantly better reduction of Böhler angle in Sanders type III fractures but not type II fractures with the extensile lateral approach compared with the sinus tarsi approach. Schepers and colleagues[98] found a similar quality of reduction

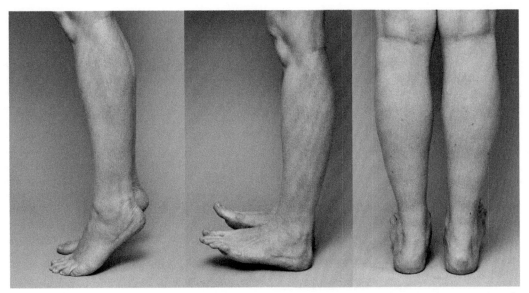

Fig. 12. Functional result 1 year after bilateral open reduction and internal fixation of displaced intraarticular calcaneal fractures with lateral interlocking plating. With meticulous soft tissue handling, anatomic reduction of the calcaneal shape, and joint facets, good clinical results can be expected (same patient as in **Figs. 4–6**).

when using either the sinus tarsi approach or extensile lateral approach. Without anatomic reduction, results after percutaneous procedures may be even worse than outcomes after using an extensile lateral approach for obtaining anatomic reduction.[109]

SUMMARY

Fractures of the calcaneus require an individualized treatment approach and precise preoperative planning. Nondisplaced and mildly displaced extraarticular fractures, intraarticular fractures with step-offs of less than 2 mm, and patients with general contraindications to surgery are best treated nonoperatively. Open fractures and closed fractures with compartment syndrome or severe soft tissue incarceration resulting from internal fragment pressure are treated as emergencies. Severely displaced extraarticular and less severe intraarticular fractures may be treated with percutaneous reduction and fixation. The latter is also a useful temporary measure in more severe fracture patterns with severe soft tissue damage or a critical overall condition of the patient. In the absence of contraindications, most of the displaced, intraarticular fractures are best treated by open reduction and internal fixation. Selected, less invasive approaches and novel fixation techniques have the potential to minimize soft-tissue complications while ensuring anatomic

reduction and stable fixation. For best outcomes the procedure should be performed by an experienced surgeon. Nonoperative treatment of severely displaced fractures or failure to achieve anatomic reduction with surgical treatment regularly results in painful malunions with rapidly evolving subtalar arthritis.

CLINICS CARE POINTS

- The management of calcaneal fractures is challenging, and the best treatment is still subject to debate. There is no single method that is suitable for all calcaneal fracture variants.

- If operative treatment is chosen, anatomic reconstruction of the overall shape and joint surfaces of the calcaneus is imperative to obtain a good functional result. For severely comminuted fractures with multiple joint fragmentation, an extensile lateral approach offers excellent exposure and allows for lateral buttressing with a plate but requires meticulous soft tissue handling.

- For most of the displaced, intraarticular fractures, less invasive reduction and fixation via a direct approach over the sinus tarsi has the potential to significantly lower the rate of soft tissue complications while ensuring exact anatomic reduction. This approach may be extended to the calcaneocuboid joint and over the tip of the fibula along the "lateral utility" line, if warranted for calcaneocuboid joint involvement or calcaneal fracture-dislocations, respectively.

- Purely percutaneous reduction and fixation is the treatment of choice for displaced extraarticular fractures and simple intraarticular fractures with adequate control of joint reduction, for example, by using subtalar arthroscopy.

- Specific approaches are used for rare calcaneal fracture variants. These include a direct medial ("sustentacular") approach for isolated fractures of the sustentaculum tali, a posterolateral approach for superior tuberosity avulsion ("beak") fractures, and a small medial approach for displaced medial plantar tuberosity avulsions.

REFERENCES

1. Rammelt S, Zwipp H. Fractures of the calcaneus: current treatment strategies. Acta Chir Orthop Traumatol Cech 2014;81(3):177–96.
2. Swords MP, Penny P. Early Fixation of Calcaneus Fractures. Foot Ankle Clin 2017;22(1):93–104.
3. Sanders R, Rammelt S. Fractures of the Calcaneus. In: Coughlin MJ, Saltzman CR, Anderson JB, editors. Mann's surgery of the foot & ankle. 9th edition. St Louis (MO): Elsevier; 2013. p. 2041–100.
4. Sharr PJ, Mangupli MM, Winson IG, et al. Current management options for displaced intra-articular calcaneal fractures: Non-operative, ORIF, minimally invasive reduction and fixation or primary ORIF and subtalar arthrodesis. A contemporary review. Foot Ankle Surg 2016;22(1):1–8.
5. Rammelt S, Swords M, Dhillon M, et al, editors. AO manual of fracture management: foot & ankle. Stuttgart – New York: Thieme; 2020.
6. Griffin D, Parsons N, Shaw E, et al. UK Heel Fracture Trial Investigators. Operative versus non-operative treatment for closed, displaced, intra-articular fractures of the calcaneus: randomised controlled trial. BMJ 2014;349:g4483.
7. Pearce CJ, Wong KL, Calder JD. Calcaneal fractures: selection bias is key. Bone Joint J 2015;97-B(7):880–2.
8. Rammelt S, Sangeorzan BJ, Swords MP. Calcaneal Fractures - Should We or Should We not Operate? Indian J Orthop 2018;52(3):220–30.
9. Jiang N, Lin QR, Diao XC, et al. Surgical versus nonsurgical treatment of displaced intra-articular calcaneal fracture: a meta-analysis of current evidence base. Int Orthop 2012;36(8):1615–22.
10. Zhang W, Lin F, Chen E, et al. Operative Versus Nonoperative Treatment of Displaced Intra-Articular Calcaneal Fractures: A Meta-Analysis of Randomized Controlled Trials. J Orthop Trauma 2016;30(3):e75–81.
11. Benirschke SK, Sangeorzan BJ. Extensive intraarticular fractures of the foot. Surgical management of calcaneal fractures. Clin Orthop 1993;292(292):128–34.
12. Sanders R, Fortin P, DiPasquale T, et al. Operative treatment in 120 displaced intraarticular calcaneal fractures. Results using a prognostic computed tomography scan classification. Clin Orthop Relat Res 1993;290:87–95.
13. Zwipp H, Tscherne H, Thermann H, et al. Osteosynthesis of displaced intraarticular fractures of the calcaneus. Results in 123 cases. Clin Orthop Relat Res 1993;290:76–86.
14. Song KS, Kang CH, Min BW, et al. Preoperative and postoperative evaluation of intra-articular fractures of the calcaneus based on computed tomography scanning. Clin Orthop Relat Res 1997;11(6):435–40.
15. Thordarson DB, Krieger LE. Operative vs. nonoperative treatment of intra-articular fractures of the calcaneus: a prospective randomized trial. Foot Ankle Int 1996;17(1):2–9.
16. Kurozumi T, Jinno Y, Sato T, et al. Open reduction for intra-articular calcaneal fractures: evaluation using computed tomography. Foot Ankle Int 2003;24(12):942–8.
17. Jardé O, Havet E, Alovor G, et al. Intra-articular calcaneal fractures: clinical and radiological results of 54 cases with a minimum follow-up of 7 years. Med Chir Pied 2005;21:107–17.
18. Makki D, Alnajjar HM, Walkay S, et al. Osteosynthesis of displaced intra-articular fractures of the calcaneum: a long-term review of 47 cases. J Bone Joint Surg Br 2010;92(5):693–700.
19. Rammelt S, Zwipp H, Schneiders W, et al. Severity of injury predicts subsequent function in surgically treated displaced intraarticular calcaneal fractures. Clin Orthop Relat Res 2013;471(9):2885–98.
20. Agren PH, Mukka S, Tullberg T, et al. Factors Affecting Long-Term Treatment Results of Displaced Intra-Articular Calcaneal Fractures A Post-hoc Analysis of a Prospective, Randomized, Controlled Multicenter Trial. J Orthop Trauma 2014;28:564–8.
21. van Hoeve S, de Vos J, Verbruggen JP, et al. Gait Analysis and Functional Outcome After Calcaneal Fracture. J Bone Joint Surg Am 2015;97(22):1879–88.
22. Dürr C, Apinun J, Mittlmeier T, et al. Foot Function After Surgically Treated Intraarticular Calcaneal Fractures: Correlation of Clinical and

Pedobarographic Results of 65 Patients Followed for 8 Years. J Orthop Trauma 2018;32(12):593–600.

23. Paul M, Peter R, Hoffmeyer P. Fractures of the calcaneum. A review of 70 patients. J Bone Joint Surg Br 2004;86(8):1142–5.

24. Agren PH, Wretenberg P, Sayed-Noor AS. Operative versus nonoperative treatment of displaced intra-articular calcaneal fractures: a prospective, randomized, controlled multicenter trial. J Bone Joint Surg Am 2013;95(15):1351–7.

25. Rammelt S, Marx C. Managing Severely Malunited Calcaneal Fractures and Fracture-Dislocations. Foot Ankle Clin 2020;25(2):239–56.

26. Rammelt S, Zwipp H. Calcaneus fractures: facts, controversies and recent developments. Injury 2004;35(5):443–61.

27. Gardner MJ, Nork SE, Barei DP, et al. Secondary soft tissue compromise in tongue-type calcaneus fractures. J Orthop Trauma 2008;22(7):439–45.

28. Sands AK, Rammelt S, Manoli A. Foot compartment syndrome – a clinical review. Fuss Sprungg 2015;13(1):11–21.

29. Rammelt S, Marx C, Swords G, et al. Calcaneal fracture dislocation: Recognition, treatment and outcome. Foot Ankle Int 2021;42(6):706–13.

30. Sanders R. Intra-articular fractures of the calcaneus: present state of the art. J Orthop Trauma 1992;6(2):252–65.

31. Squires B, Allen PE, Livingstone J, et al. Fractures of the tuberosity of the calcaneus. J Bone Joint Surg Br 2001;83(1):55–61.

32. Ketz J, Clare M, Sanders R. Corrective Osteotomies for Malunited Extra-Articular Calcaneal Fractures. Foot Ankle Clin 2016;21(1):135–45.

33. Folk JW, Starr AJ, Early JS. Early wound complications of operative treatment of calcaneus fractures: analysis of 190 fractures. J Orthop Trauma 1999;13(5):369–72.

34. Fischer S, Meinert M, Neun O, et al. Surgical experience as a decisive factor for the outcome of calcaneal fractures using locking compression plate: results of 3 years. Arch Orthop Trauma Surg 2020. https://doi.org/10.1007/s00402-020-03649-3.

35. Rammelt S, Amlang M, Barthel S, et al. Minimally-invasive treatment of calcaneal fractures. Injury 2004;35(Suppl 2):SB55–63.

36. Buckley R, Tough S, McCormack R, et al. Operative compared with nonoperative treatment of displaced intra- articular calcaneal fractures: a prospective, randomized, controlled multicenter trial. J Bone Joint Surg Am 2002;84-A(10):1733–44.

37. Crosby LA, Fitzgibbons T. Intraarticular calcaneal fractures. Results of closed treatment. Clin Orthop Relat Res 1993;290:47–54.

38. Mitchell PM, O'Neill DE, Branch E, et al. Calcaneal Avulsion Fractures: A Multicenter Analysis of Soft-Tissue Compromise and Early Fixation Failure. J Orthop Trauma 2019;33(11):e422–6.

39. Giordano V, Godoy-Santos AL, de Souza FS, et al. Combined Lag Screw and Cerclage Wire Fixation for Calcaneal Tube rosity Avulsion Fractures. Case Rep Orthop 2018;2018:6207024.

40. Spierings KE, Min M, Nooijen LE, et al. Managing the open calcaneal fracture: A systematic review. Foot Ankle Surg 2019;25(6):707–13.

41. Heier KA, Infante AF, Walling AK, et al. Open fractures of the calcaneus: soft-tissue injury determines outcome. J Bone Joint Surg Am 2003;85-A(12):2276–82.

42. Brenner P, Rammelt S, Gavlik JM, et al. Early soft tissue coverage after complex foot trauma. World J Surg 2001;25(5):603–9.

43. Mehta S, Mirza AJ, Dunbar RP, et al. A staged treatment plan for the management of Type II and Type IIIA open calcaneus fractures. J Orthop Trauma 2010;24(3):142–7.

44. Beltran MJ, Collinge CA. Outcomes of high-grade open calcaneus fractures managed with open reduction via the medial wound and percutaneous screw fixation. J Orthop Trauma 2012;26(11):662–70.

45. Mittlmeier T, Mächler G, Lob G, et al. Compartment syndrome of the foot after intraarticular calcaneal fracture. Clin Orthop Relat Res 1991;(269):241–8.

46. Park YH, Lee JW, Hong JY, et al. Predictors of compartment syndrome of the foot after fracture of the calcaneus. Bone Joint J 2018;100-B(3):303–8.

47. Manoli A 2nd, Weber TG. Fasciotomy of the foot: an anatomical study with special reference to release of the calcaneal compartment. Foot Ankle 1990;10(5):267–75.

48. Manoli A 2nd, Fakhouri AJ, Weber TG. Concurrent compartment syndromes of the foot and leg. Foot Ankle 1993;14(6):339.

49. Tennent T, Calder P, Salisbury R, et al. The operative management of displaced intra-articular fractures of the calcaneum: a two-centre study using a defined protocol. Injury 2001;32(6):491–6.

50. Rammelt S, Barthel S, Biewener A, et al. Calcaneus fractures. Open reduction and internal fixation. Zbl Chir 2003;128:517–28.

51. Rammelt S, Amlang M, Barthel S, et al. Percutaneous treatment of less severe intraarticular calcaneal fractures. Clin Orthop Relat Res 2010;468(4):983–90.

52. Sanders R, Vaupel Z, Erdogan M, et al. The Operative Treatment of Displaced Intra-articular Calcaneal Fractures (DIACFs): Long Term (10-20 years) Results in 108 Fractures using a Prognostic CT Classification. J Orthop Trauma 2014;28:551–63.

53. Dürr C, Zwipp H, Rammelt S. Fractures of the sustentaculum tali. Operat Orthop Traumatol 2013; 25(6):569–78.

54. Abidi NA, Dhawan S, Gruen GS, et al. Wound-healing risk factors after open reduction and internal fixation of calcaneal fractures. Foot Ankle Int 1998;19(12):856–61.

55. Harvey EJ, Grujic L, Early JS, et al. Morbidity associated with ORIF of intra-articular calcaneus fractures using a lateral approach. Foot Ankle Int 2001;22(11):868–73.

56. Zwipp H, Rammelt S, Barthel S. Calcaneal fractures–open reduction and internal fixation (ORIF). Injury 2004;35(Suppl 2):SB46–54.

57. Berberian W, Sood A, Karanfilian B, et al. Displacement of the sustentacular fragment in intra-articular calcaneal fractures. J Bone Joint Surg Am 2013;95(11):995–1000.

58. Min W, Munro M, Sanders R. Stabilization of displaced articular fragments in calcaneal fractures using bioabsorbable pin fixation: a technique guide. J Orthop Trauma 2010;24(12):770–4.

59. Sanders R. Turning tongues into joint depressions: a new calcaneal osteotomy. J Orthop Trauma 2012;26(3):193–6.

60. Rammelt S, Gavlik JM, Barthel S, et al. The value of subtalar arthroscopy in the management of intra-articular calcaneus fractures. Foot Ankle Int 2002;23(10):906–16.

61. Longino D, Buckley RE. Bone graft in the operative treatment of displaced intraarticular calcaneal fractures: is it helpful? J Orthop Trauma 2001; 15(4):280–6.

62. Thordarson DB, Latteier M. Open reduction and internal fixation of calcaneal fractures with a low profile titanium calcaneal perimeter plate. Foot Ankle Int 2003;24(3):217–21.

63. Rammelt S, Bartoníček J, Park KH. Traumatic injury to the subtalar joint. Foot Ankle Clin 2018; 23:353–74.

64. Richter M, Droste P, Goesling T, et al. Polyaxially-locked plate screws increase stability of fracture fixation in an experimental model of calcaneal fracture. J Bone Joint Surg Br 2006;88(9):1257–63.

65. Nosewicz T, Knupp M, Barg A, et al. Mini-open sinus tarsi approach with percutaneous screw fixation of displaced calcaneal fractures: a prospective computed tomography-based study. Foot Ankle Int 2012;33(11):925–33.

66. Weber M, Lehmann O, Sagesser D, et al. Limited open reduction and internal fixation of displaced intra-articular fractures of the calcaneum. J Bone Joint Surg Br 2008;90(12):1608–16.

67. Swords MP, Rammelt S, Sands AK. Nonextensile techniques for treatment of calcaneus fractures. In: Pfeffer GB, Easley ME, Hintermann B, et al,

editors. Operative techniques: foot and ankle surgery. Philadelphia: Elsevier; 2017. p. 319–26.

68. Buckley R, Leighton R, Sanders D, et al. Open reduction and internal fixation compared with ORIF and primary subtalar arthrodesis for treatment of Sanders type IV calcaneal fractures: a randomized multicenter trial. J Orthop Trauma 2014; 28(10):577–83.

69. Rammelt S, Zwipp H, Hansen ST. Posttraumatic reconstruction of the foot and ankle. In: Browner BD, Jupiter JB, Krettek C, et al, editors. Skeletal Trauma. 6th edition. Philadelphia: Elsevier Saunders; 2019. p. 2641–90.

70. Li S. Wound and Sural Nerve Complications of the Sinus Tarsi Approach for Calcaneus Fractures. Foot Ankle Int 2018;39(9):1106–11.

71. Park CH, Yoon DH. Role of Subtalar Arthroscopy in Operative Treatment of Sanders Type 2 Calcaneal Fractures Using a Sinus Tarsi Approach. Foot Ankle Int 2018;39(4):443–9.

72. Goldzak M, Mittlmeier T, Simon P. Locked nailing for the treatment of displaced articular fractures of the calcaneus: description of a new procedure with calcanail((R)). Europ J Orthop Surg Traumatol 2012;22(4):345–9.

73. Zwipp H, Paša L, Žilka L, et al. Introduction of a New Locking Nail for Treatment of Intraarticular Calcaneal Fractures. J Orthop Trauma 2016; 30(3):e88–92.

74. Veliceasa B, Filip A, Pinzaru R, et al. Treatment of Displaced Intra-articular Calcaneal Fractures With an Interlocking Nail (C-Nail). J Orthop Trauma 2020;34(11):e414–9.

75. Tornetta P 3rd. Percutaneous treatment of calcaneal fractures. Clin Orthop Relat Res 2000;375: 91–6.

76. Woon CY, Chong KW, Yeo W, et al. Subtalar arthroscopy and flurosocopy in percutaneous fixation of intra-articular calcaneal fractures: the best of both worlds. J Trauma 2011;71(4): 917–25.

77. Yeap EJ, Rao J, Pan CH, et al. Is arthroscopic assisted percutaneous screw fixation as good as open reduction and internal fixation for the treatment of displaced intra-articular calcaneal fractures? Foot Ankle Surg 2016;22(3):164–9.

78. Marouby S, Cellier N, Mares O, et al. Percutaneous arthroscopic calcaneal osteosynthesis for displaced intra-articular calcaneal fractures: Systematic review and surgical technique. Foot Ankle Surg 2020;26(5):503–8.

79. Buch J. Bohrdrathosteosynthese des Fersenbeinbruches. Akt Chir 1980;15:285–96.

80. Magnan B, Bortolazzi R, Marangon A, et al. External fixation for displaced intra-articular fractures of the calcaneum. J Bone Joint Surg Br 2006;88(11):1474–9.

81. Della Rocca GJ, Nork SE, Barei DP, et al. Fractures of the sustentaculum tali: injury characteristics and surgical technique for reduction. Foot Ankle Int 2009;30(11):1037–41.

82. Adams MR, Koury KL, Mistry JB, et al. Plantar Medial Avulsion Fragment Associated With Tongue-Type Calcaneus Fractures. Foot Ankle Int 2019;40(6):634–40.

83. Walley KC, Johns WL, Jackson JB, et al. Plantar Medial Avulsion Fracture of the Calcaneus With Acute Tarsal Tunnel: Case Report and Technique Tip. Foot Ankle Int 2020;41(8):1002–6.

84. Brattebo J, Molster AO, Wirsching J. Fractures of the calcaneus: A retrospective study of 115 fractures. Orthop Int 1995;3:117–26.

85. Potter MQ, Nunley JA. Long-term functional outcomes after operative treatment for intra-articular fractures of the calcaneus. J Bone Joint Surg Am 2009;91(8):1854–60.

86. Poeze M, Verbruggen JP, Brink PR. The relationship between the outcome of operatively treated calcaneal fractures and institutional fracture load. A systematic review of the literature. J Bone Joint Surg Am 2008;90(5):1013–21.

87. Ahn J, Kim TY, Kim TW, et al. Learning Curve for Open Reduction and Internal Fixation of Displaced Intra-articular Calcaneal Fracture by Extensile Lateral Approach Using the Cumulative Summation Control Chart. Foot Ankle Int 2019; 40(9):1052–9.

88. Janzen DL, Connell DG, Munk PL, et al. Intraarticular fractures of the calcaneus: value of CT findings in determining prognosis. AJR Am J Roentgenol 1992;158(6):1271–4.

89. Ojeda-Jiménez J, Rendón-Díaz D, Martín-Vélez P, et al. Surgically treated calcaneal joint fractures: what does postoperative computed tomography give us? Rev Esp Cir Ortop Traumatol 2020;64(6): 393–400.

90. Schindler C, Schirm A, Zdravkovic V, et al. Outcomes of intra-articular calcaneal fractures: surgical treatment of 114 consecutive cases at a maximum care trauma center. BMC Musculoskelet Disord 2021;22(1):234.

91. Borrelli JJ, Torzilli PA, Grigiene R, et al. Effect of impact load on articular cartilage: development of an intra-articular fracture model. J Orthop Trauma 1997;11:319–26.

92. Herscovici DJ, Widmaier J, Scaduto JM, et al. Operative treatment of calcaneal fractures in elderly patients. J Bone Joint Surg Am 2005;87(6):1260–4.

93. Gaskill T, Schweitzer K, Nunley J. Comparison of surgical outcomes of intra-articular calcaneal fractures by age. J Bone Joint Surg Am 2012;92(18):2884–9.

94. Hedlund LJ, Maki DD, Griffiths HJ. Calcaneal fractures in diabetic patients. J Diabetes Complic 1998;12(2):81–7.

95. Rammelt S. Management of acute hindfoot fractures in diabetics. In: Herscovici D Jr, editor. The surgical management of the diabetic foot and ankle. Switzerland: Springer International Publishing; 2016. p. 85–102.

96. Lee SM, Seo JS, Kwak SH, et al. Bone density of the calcaneus correlates with radiologic and clinical outcomes after calcaneal fracture fixation. Injury 2020;51(8):1910–8.

97. Kline AJ, Anderson RB, Davis WH, et al. Minimally invasive technique versus an extensile lateral approach for intra-articular calcaneal fractures. Foot Ankle Int 2013;34(6):773–80.

98. Schepers T, Backes M, Dingemans SA, et al. Similar Anatomical Reduction and Lower Complication Rates With the Sinus Tarsi Approach Compared With the Extended Lateral Approach in Displaced Intra-Articular Calcaneal Fractures. J Orthop Trauma 2017;31(6):293–8.

99. Nosewicz TL, Dingemans SA, Backes M, et al. A systematic review and meta-analysis of the sinus tarsi and extended lateral approach in the operative treatment of displaced intra-articular calcaneal fractures. Foot Ankle Surg 2019;25(5):580–8.

100. Yu T, Xiong Y, Kang A, et al. Comparison of sinus tarsi approach and extensile lateral approach for calcaneal fractures: A systematic review of overlapping meta-analyses. J Orthop Surg (Hong Kong) 2020;28(2). 2309499020915282.

101. Seat A, Seat C. Lateral extensile approach versus minimal incision approach for open reduction and internal fixation of displaced intra-articular calcaneal fractures: a meta-analysis. J Foot Ankle Surg 2020;59(2):356–66.

102. Steinhausen E, Martin W, Lefering R, et al. C-Nail versus plate osteosynthesis in displaced intra-articular calcaneal fractures-a comparative retrospective study. J Orthop Surg Res 2021;16(1):203.

103. Lv Y, Zhou YF, Li L, et al. Sinus tarsi approach versus the extended lateral approach for displaced intra-articular calcaneal fractures: a systematic review and meta-analysis. Arch Orthop Trauma Surg 2020. https://doi.org/10.1007/s00402-020-03554-9.

104. Richter I, Krähenbühl N, Ruiz R, et al. Mid- to long-term outcome in patients treated with a mini-open sinus-tarsi approach for calcaneal fractures. Arch Orthop Trauma Surg 2021;141(4):611–7.

105. Bremer AK, Kraler L, Frauchiger L, et al. Limited Open Reduction and Internal Fixation of Calcaneal Fractures. Foot Ankle Int 2020;41(1):57–62.

106. Weng QH, Dai GL, Tu QM, et al. Comparison between Percutaneous Screw Fixation and Plate Fixation via Sinus Tarsi Approach for Calcaneal Fractures: An 8-10-Year Follow-up Study. Orthop Surg 2020;12(1):124–32.

107. Park CH, Yan H, Park J. Randomized comparative study between extensile lateral and sinus tarsi approaches for the treatment of Sanders type 2 calcaneal fracture. Bone Joint J 2021;103-B(2):286–93.

108. Busel G, Mir HR, Merimee S, et al. Quality of Reduction of Displaced Intra-Articular Calcaneal Fractures Using a Sinus Tarsi versus Extensile Lateral Approach. J Orthop Trauma 2021;35(6):285–8.

109. Biz C, Barison E, Ruggieri P, et al. Radiographic and functional outcomes after displaced intra-articular calcaneal fractures: a comparative cohort study among the traditional open technique (ORIF) and percutaneous surgical procedures (PS). J Orthop Surg Res 2016;11(1):92.

Spine Section

Upper Cervical Trauma

Catherine Olinger, MD[a],*, Richard Bransford, MD[b,c,d]

KEYWORDS

- Craniocervical junction • Craniocervical dissociation • Odontoid fractures • Hangman fractures
- Atlas fractures • Atlantoaxial dislocation

KEY POINTS

- Trauma to the craniocervical junction is defined as an injury involving the occiput to the axis, involving both intricate bony and ligamentous connections.
- Careful evaluation of patients sustaining high energy mechanisms including helical CT and MRI of the CCJ allow for identification and classification of these injuries.
- Treatment of traumatic injuries to the craniocervical junction rely on the ability to withstand physiologic loads while reducing the potential for neurologic deficits or progressive deformity.
- Goals of surgical fixation include internal fixation only of the involved unstable segments that do not require access to the vertebral canal or intracranial space with simultaneous decompression, while performing fixation and providing sufficient mechanical stability with no additional need for external fixation.

ANATOMY INTRODUCTION

The craniocervical junction (CCJ) is the uppermost articulation of the cervical spine, involving the occipital bone, the occipitoatlantal articulation, the atlas, the axis, and the ligaments that span from the occiput to the axis.[1] Trauma to the CCJ can be defined as any injury involving the region from the skull base to the axis.[2] Spinal stability generally infers the spine's ability to withstand physiologic loads without the potential for neurologic deficits, progressive deformity, or long-term dysfunction from pain and disability.[3] Goals of intervention can be formulated into four specific entities: 1. decompression of the spinal cord or nerve roots, 2. realignment or maintenance of physiologic alignment of injured vertebral segments, 3. stabilization of disrupted discoligamentous segments, and 4. enable rapid return to functional recovery.[4]

Upper CCJ injuries account for 10% to 30% of cervical spine trauma. There are an increasing number of patients surviving these devastating injuries due to advancements in automobile technology, resuscitation techniques, and diagnostic modalities.[4,5] Cervical spine trauma is estimated to account for 25,000 new fractures per year in the United States and occurs in 2% to 3% of all patients with blunt trauma. Ultimately, this accounts for an estimated incidence of 10 to 50 fractures per 1 million persons. The leading injury mechanisms are motor vehicle crashes, falls from height, and sports-related events.[6]

Current treatment with urgent rigid posterior fixation of the occiput to the cervical spine has resulted in a substantial reduction in management delays, which has resulted in much more expedited treatment of CCJ injuries. Severely neurologically impaired patients are surviving in greater numbers due to these advances, however, long-term neurologic outcomes are more dependent on the severity of the presenting neurologic injury. Logic would dictate that survivors have less displaced or spontaneously

[a] Harborview Medical Center, University of Washington Department of Orthopaedics and Sports Medicine, 908 Jefferson Street, Fifth Floor, Seattle, WA, USA; [b] Department of Orthopaedics and Sports Medicine, University of Washington, Seattle, WA, USA; [c] Department of Neurological Surgery, University of Washington, Seattle, WA, USA; [d] Spine Fellowship Program, University of Washington Department of Orthopaedics and Sports Medicine, 908 Jefferson Street, Fifth Floor, Seattle, WA, USA
* Corresponding author.
E-mail address: colinger@uw.edu

Orthop Clin N Am 52 (2021) 451–479
https://doi.org/10.1016/j.ocl.2021.05.013
0030-5898/21/© 2021 Elsevier Inc. All rights reserved.

reduced injuries and neurologic deficits in survivors are less likely to be as severe.[7]

Within CCJ injuries is a spectrum of instability, ranging from isolated nondisplaced occipital condyle fractures treated nonoperatively to highly unstable injuries with severely distracted craniocervical dissociation. Despite the evolution of understanding and improvement in management of cases regarding catastrophic failure to diagnose, subsequent neurologic deterioration still occurs even in experienced trauma centers.[8]

The purpose of this article is to review the injuries that occur at the CCJ with the accompanying anatomy, presentation, imaging, classification, management, and outcomes.

The CCJ protects the brain stem, cranial nerves, and cranial blood supply, while allowing complicated motion between the five unconstrained joints including the paired occipitoatlantal joints, atlantoodontoid joint, and the paired atlantoaxial joints.[1,7,9] A larger lever arm induced by the mass and immobility of the cranium, combined with the relative freedom of movement more caudal, relies on ligamentous structures rather than bony stability for the maintenance of CCJ alignment[7] (Fig. 1). The vertebral artery may progressively erode the medial body support of the lateral mass of the axis, hollowing out the inferior lateral mass below its articular surface, which could significantly impact the selection types of screw fixation into the axis putting the vertebral artery at risk. The left vertebral artery is more likely to become dominant at adult age.[3]

OCCIPUT

The occiput is the most cranial aspect of the CCJ. The occipital condyles are anterolateral to the foramen magnum, and project caudally to form convex bony surfaces that articulate with the matched concave superior articular facet of the atlas, which allows the condyles to move like a rocking chair on the lateral masses.[1,7] Lateral and ventral to the occipital condyles are the hypoglossal foramen through which cranial nerve XII exits and is prone to injury with fractures of the occipital condyle, atlantooccipital dissociations (AODs), and with occiput-C1 transarticular screw fixation. The ventral aspect of the occipital condyle is bound by the basion, which is the caudal extent of the clival plate. The dorsal boundary of the foramen magnum is the opisthion.[7]

ATLAS

The atlas, which consists of a fragile bony ring structure, assumes a washer-like function and serves as a modulator between the occipital condyles and axis.[4] From the coronal view the lateral masses are narrow medially and project out laterally similar to a bowtie shape from the anterior view. Within the ring, the transverse atlantal ligament (TAL) bridges the lateral masses of the atlas while passing posteriorly to the dens. Lateral to the lateral mass is the transverse foramen, in which the vertebral arteries pass rostrally from the axis to posteriorly over the ring of the atlas and enter the foramen magnum to form the basilar arteries.[1,7]

Anatomic variants can exist and surgeons are advised to be mindful when treating injuries of the CCJ. The ponticulus posticus, an anatomic variant of the posterolateral arch of the atlas, forms an arcuate posterior foramen of the vertebral artery and can be mistaken for a portion of the posterior ring.[3] Case reports advise that there may be patients with assimilation of the atlas to the skull. These variants are exposed to an increased risk of injury and delay in diagnosis due to the abnormal anatomy. Congenital assimilation of the atlas is caused by failure of segmentation between the last occipital and first cervical sclerotome, more commonly found in males with a reported incidence of 0.75% to 3%. Anatomic variation, such as occipitalization of the atlas, can be associated with other abnormalities such as the location of the vertebral arteries. In one such case, the vertebral arteries were identified coursing bilaterally below the C1 ring, with the posterior ring of C1 completely coalesced to the occiput. The case report of this presentation of these anatomic findings was associated with the right atlantooccipital fracture dislocation, and the C1 lateral mass screws were not placed.[10]

AXIS

The axis is unique anatomically compared to other cervical levels. The dens extends behind the anterior arch of the atlas and is kept in position by the TAL, which primarily serves as a flexion-extension stabilizer.[1] The axis is an essential component of the cranial cervical articulation. The vertebral arteries extend along the inferior lateral border of the axis body and exit laterally through the transverse foramen.[7] The axis is the linchpin of the CCJ because all of the major restraining ligaments attach between the axis and the occiput.[8]

LIGAMENTOUS ANATOMY

The ligamentous anatomy of the CCJ can be divided into internal, within the canal, and

A

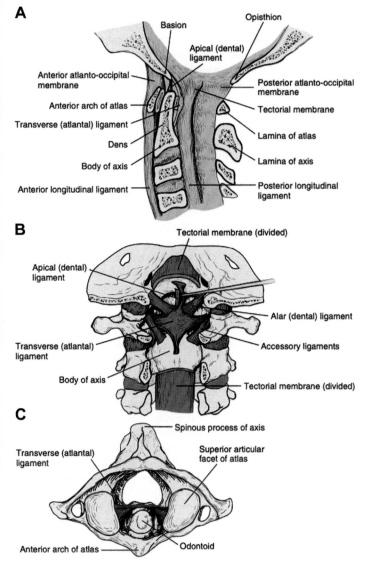

Basion
Opisthion
Apical (dental) ligament
Anterior atlanto-occipital membrane
Posterior atlanto-occipital membrane
Anterior arch of atlas
Tectorial membrane
Transverse (atlantal) ligament
Lamina of atlas
Dens
Lamina of axis
Body of axis
Anterior longitudinal ligament
Posterior longitudinal ligament

B

Tectorial membrane (divided)
Apical (dental) ligament
Alar (dental) ligament
Transverse (atlantal) ligament
Accessory ligaments
Body of axis
Tectorial membrane (divided)

C

Spinous process of axis
Transverse (atlantal) ligament
Superior articular facet of atlas
Anterior arch of atlas
Odontoid

Fig. 1. (*A*): Sagittal anatomy of CCJ; (*B*) coronal anatomy of CCJ; (*C*) axial anatomy of CCJ. (*From* Cheng CW, Bellabarba C, Bransford RJ. Cranio-cervical Injuries: Atlas Fractures, Atlanto-Occipital Injuries, and Atlan-toaxial Injuries. SKELETAL TRAUMA: Basic science, management, and reconstruction, 2 vol. set. ELSEVIER; 2019; with permission.)

external ligaments outside the canal. The external ligaments include ligamentum nuchae, the anterior and dorsal occipitoatlantal membrane, and the occipitoatlantal and atlantoaxial facet joint capsules. The facet capsules are thin and redundant to facilitate wide-range motion, yet are key stabilizers in the stability of the CCJ.[1,7]

The internal ligaments are the key stabilizers. The alar ligaments are oblique fibers which connect the dens to occipital condyles. The cruciate ligament, which connects the posterior dens to anterior atlas arch, is composed of the TAL and vertical fibers connecting the posterior atlas to the foramen magnum. The tectorial membrane is the cranial insertion of the

posterior longitudinal ligament, which inserts from the posterior axis to the ventral foramen magnum.[1,11]

The alar (butterfly) ligaments are thick, paired, cordlike structures that project laterally and ventrally from the tip of the dens to the ventral medial aspect of the occipital condyles and act as the primary rotational restraints of the CCJ. In vitro, load to failure of the alar ligament is 210 N, however the ligaments tolerate less than 50% of the load to failure compared with the cruciate ligament of the knee. The tectorial membrane, which constitutes the rostral extension of the posterior longitudinal ligament, effectively limits axial distraction and atlantooccipital flexion.[1,7]

The TAL is more robust than the alar ligaments, crosses the odontoid waist, and allows rotation while limiting atlantoaxial flexion, translation, and distraction. Although the joint capsules have long been considered secondary stabilizers of the CCJ, recent biomechanical cadaveric study indicated that they share equal importance with the tectorial membrane and alar ligaments in stabilizing the craniocervical junction.[7] The atlantoaxial joint capsule plays a role in maintaining stability of the atlantoaxial joint.[12,13]

In an attempt to characterize tectoral membrane injury, a retrospective radiographic review was performed to determine the level of injury between adult and pediatric patients. Adult patients sustained complete disruptions inferior to the clivus, with 22% of tears at the level of the basion and 78% of the level of the odontoid tip. In contrast, 83% of the pediatric patients suffered a "stripping" injury of the tectorial membrane posterior to the clivus. Stretch injuries of the tectorial membrane were identified in 10% of the adults and 17% of the pediatric patients. Classification of tectorial membrane injury was identified as type I retroclival (more common in pediatric patients), type IIa subclival disruption at the level the basion, type IIb subclival at the level of the odontoid, and type III thinning of the tectorial membrane.[14]

KINEMATICS

The atlas is a critical component in flexion and extension as it articulates with the occipital condyles. The CCJ accounts for approximately 60% of cervical rotation; the atlas provides about 50% of rotation as the atlas lateral masses rotate over the superior articulations of the axis.[1,7,8] The remaining flexion and extension occur primarily through the atlantooccipital joints and overall motion of the CCJ relative to the subaxial spine is about 40% to 45%.[8,9]

The susceptibility of CCJ to injury is related to the large lever arm and mass of the cranium, combined with the relative freedom of movement of the subaxial spine. Secondarily, the reliance on ligamentous structures rather than intrinsic bony stability for the maintenance of CCJ alignment also allows for a higher rate of injury.[8] Unlike the subaxial cervical spine, the atlantoaxial facets are oriented in the axial plane. They have no bony constraint to prevent them from dislocation and rely almost purely on ligamentous stability.[9,13] Injuries are three times more common in pediatrics than adults at the CCJ secondary to the horizontal plane of the articular surfaces and relative laxity of

the ligamentous structures combined with the presence of a relatively large head and higher affective fulcrum of the cervical spine relative to the neck and torso in pediatric patients.[5]

In children, fractures through the synchondrosis cartilage plates between the dens body are also possible as neural arches of the axis are potential weaknesses. These synchondroses do not ossify until the age of 7 to 10. A large head-to-body ratio with underdeveloped support musculature shifts the fulcrum of flexion-extension cephalad in comparison to adults.[15]

PHYSICAL EXAMINATION

Injuries to the CCJ should be suspected in all patients after high-energy trauma. In polytrauma patients, CCJ injuries can be hard to detect either due to distracting injuries or impaired consciousness, which precludes an adequate evaluation.[8] Low suspicion in patients presenting with multiple comorbidities, distracting injuries caused by concurrent life-threatening injuries, and lack of familiarity with the screening parameters of the CCJ all contribute to missed injuries or delays in diagnosis.[16]

A formal neurologic evaluation is important, if possible, including mental status and thorough neurologic extremity assessment using the American Spinal Injury Association (ASIA) score template. Neurologic injury at the level of the CCJ can range from complete paraplegia to incomplete neurologic injury. Assessment should include examination of spontaneous muscle tone, response to painful stimuli, reflexes, and anal sphincter tone.[1] Incomplete paraplegia, such as hemiplegia cruciata, characterized as ipsilateral arm and contralateral leg weakness and cruciate paralysis, presenting in a similar fashion to central cord syndrome, can manifest as unusual neurologic presentations.[6,7] Up to 20% of patients with AOD may have a normal neurologic exam on presentation.[5]

Other clinical presentations of CCJ can include sphincter disturbances, lower cranial nerve dysfunction, and respiratory distress. Untreated sequelae include myelopathy, respiratory failure, vertebral artery dissection, neurologic compromise, and rarely quadriplegia or death.[13] The examination therefore should include an assessment for any evidence of stroke or cranial nerve dysfunction in the vertebral artery distribution such as vertigo, dizziness, blurred vision, and nystagmus. The abducens and hypoglossal nerves are most commonly affected by CCJ injuries; other presentations such as Collet-Sicard syndrome, which refers to unilateral lesions of cranial nerves, may be present.[8] Posterior neck tenderness, ecchymosis, and interspinous crepitus or gapping are key findings to the physical examination. Other potential findings include epidural hematoma formation, hyperemic inflammatory tissues disrupted by trauma, and occult esophageal or aortic injuries.[6] In patients presenting with incomplete spinal cord injuries, mean arterial pressure support of 85 mm Hg is recommended to maintain adequate blood flow to the spinal cord. The duration of pressure support remains controversial.[7]

Additional examination findings in CCJ injury patients can include spasms, tenderness, abnormal head position with possible rotatory instability or atlantoaxial injury, and torticollis.[5] Patients may complain of base of the skull pain, limitation of movement, especially rotation, and the sense of instability with occipital condyle fractures, traumatic AAD, and other subtle injuries that may be missed.[1] In addition to pain, CCJ injury patients may complain of numbness or weakness of extremities, which can lead to paralysis or death if the respiratory center is affected at the medulla.[12]

The proximity of CCJ injuries to the brain stem may lead to diaphragmatic paralysis, which may then result in respiratory distress. An accompanied retropharyngeal hematoma can cause dysphagia with an associated increased risk of aspiration. This may be more commonly encountered in patients with advanced age.[3,4] Assessment of airway swelling prior to postoperative extubation and a low threshold for delaying extubation until airway swelling has diminished are important early postoperative management issues. Temporary loss of the patient's gag reflex should also be taken into consideration in the initial postoperative period and maintenance of intubation may be ideal in order to minimize risk of aspiration.[7]

DIAGNOSTIC IMAGING

Plain Radiographs

Plain radiographs have a limited role in the initial evaluation of a patient with CCJ due to their limited sensitivity in demonstrating injuries at the CCJ. The presence of prevertebral soft-tissue swelling in the lateral cervical radiograph may be the first clue for the presence of an unstable cervical lesion but is not routinely recommended as a first-line imaging study with rapid CT screening protocols.[4]

Computed Tomography

Computed tomography (CT) is the recommended imaging of choice as an initial radiographic method to identify CCJ injuries. In a patient with an identified injury at the CCJ, it is recommended to perform imaging of the entire spinal column due to the possibility of noncontinuous spinal column injuries, which may occur in up to 10% to 34% of patients.[3] Improved screening protocols for patients sustaining high-energy trauma include implementation of routine full spine helical CT scans for spinal clearance and head CT scans with inclusion of the suboccipital region.[4,8] Traditional CT axial images are oriented perpendicular in the midportion of the subaxial spine, which creates an oblique and distorted view in the upper cervical spine. Therefore, it should be requested that the axials be reconstructed to run in line with the C1 ring. Coronal CT images may also need to be reformatted to run parallel to the odontoid, and can be used to directly assess the congruency of the occipital cervical junction.[1,7,8]

CT angiogram (CTA) is indicated in the presence of injuries in the CCJ. Vascular injuries can occur in any distractive upper cervical injury, such as atlantoaxial dissociation or atlantoaxial rotatory subluxation. In addition, vertebral artery injuries should be suspected in any displaced fracture involving the transverse foramen of the atlas or axis.[1,16]

Clearance of cervical spine injuries is a process. CCJ injuries should be suspected in patients sustaining high-energy trauma. First-line evaluation with helical CT of the entire spine, with sagittal and coronal reformatted views must be obtained in order to clear the patient's CCJ. The second phase involves a secondary review of all spine imaging studies after an attempted clinical reevaluation. In the absence of any radiographic sign of injury, the third phase is initiated which includes upright lateral spine radiograph to assess for the presence of a new-onset deformity. If the patient is able to participate in a full exam after completing all three phases of clearance, their spine is then cleared and the collar and precautions are removed.[6]

In patients with severe ligamentous injuries at the CCJ, supine imaging obtained immediately postinjury can falsely indicate maintained alignment because of spontaneous reduction of the injury.[9] Typical fracture patterns suggestive of distraction include type I odontoid fractures or type III occipital condyle may be due to an alar ligament avulsion. Horizontal cleavage fracture of the anterior atlas has been implicated as being indicative of a high-energy pattern that is associated with CCJ injuries.[7,8]

The atlantooccipital joint space measures 0.6 mm with the upper 95% confidence interval of 1 mm at the most anterior or posterior aspect of the joint in the coronal plane. The atlantoaxial joint space measures 0.6 mm with the upper 95% confidence interval of 1.2 mm at the lateral aspect of the joint on the coronal image only. Consistently narrow joint spaces were found in the atlantooccipital and atlantoaxial joint space and any distance longer than 1.2 mm at the lateral, atlantoaxial joint on the coronal image or longer than 1 mm at the atlantooccipital joint would be outside of the 95% confidence interval for the uninjured population.[17] Adults presenting with more than 2 mm distraction between the atlantooccipital joint indicates craniocervical instability.[7,8]

Radiographic criteria for instability following CCJ injuries include: atlantodens interval (ADI) greater than 3 mm, posterior atlantodens interval (PADI) less than 13 mm, lateral mass displacement greater than 6.9 mm, craniocervical interval (CCI) greater than 1.5 mm, odontoid fractures with angulation greater than 8° or anterior translation greater than 3 mm, hangman combination fractures with C2, C3, and angulation greater than 11°, bony avulsion of the TAL insertion on CT or introligamentous TAL rupture on magnetic resonance imaging (MRI)[18] (Table 1).

The cord compression index is calculated as follows: diameter of the normal cord minus the diameter of the cord at the narrowest level divided by the diameter of the normal cord multiplied by 100%. The cord decompression rate is calculated as the diameter of the cord narrowest level after surgery minus the diameter of the corner level before surgery divided by the diameter of the normal cord minus the diameter of the normal cord at the nearest level before surgery multiplied by 100%. Severely compressed patients demonstrated ADIs of greater than 3 mm in space available for the cord less than 13 mm preoperatively.[19]

Magnetic Resonance Imaging

MRI is indicated if the fracture pattern does not match the neurologic examination of the patient, or in the setting of an obtunded patient. Routine MRI is recommended for any patient with cervical spinal cord injury and/or screening a patient with a possible occult spine injury. Common findings in CCJ injuries can include significant prevertebral soft-tissue swelling, increased joint edema at the atlantooccipital or atlantoaxial joints, tectorial membrane disruption, subarachnoid hemorrhage, and ligamentous injury to the alar ligaments. MRI may be overly sensitive and must be interpreted in relation to the mechanism, clinical presentation, and CT findings.[1,6]

Normal atlantooccipital metric parameters in the setting of unexplained perimesencephalic subarachnoid hemorrhage do not eliminate the

Table 1 Radiographic parameters of the CCJ		
Radiographic Parameters	**Description of Measurements**	**Normal Range**
Prevertebral swelling	AP distance of the soft tissue at the C3 level	<7 mm at C3
Wackenheim line	Projection from the caudal posterior projection of the clivus toward the upper cervical spine	2 mm of the odontoid tip
Atlanto-dens interval (ADI)	Distance between anterior odontoid cortex and posterior cortex of C1 arch	<3 mm
Basion-dens interval (BDI)	Distance from basion to odontoid tip	<12 mm
Harris lines	Measure the BAI and BDI	Both lines <12 mm in adults
Combined lateral mass overhang	Distance from the lateral border of C1 to the lateral border of C2 combined distance	<7 mm

Data from Bransford RJ, Alton TB, Patel AR, Bellabarba C. Upper cervical spine trauma. *J Am Acad Orthop Surg* 2014;22(11):718-29. https://doi.org/10.5435/JAAOS-22-11-718.

possibility of missed or delayed diagnosis of injury to the CCJ. Cervical MRI without contrast is considered in patients with vertebral artery dissection or perimesencephalic subarachnoid hemorrhage. A case report of a patient with perimesencephalic subarachnoid hemorrhage with normal CT findings but subsequent MRI imaging of the CCJ demonstrated partial disruption of the atlantoaxial membrane, tectorial membrane, ligamentum flavum, and apical ligament. Intraoperative traction testing demonstrated distraction through the AOC joint confirming diagnosis.[20]

Dynamic Fluoroscopy

A positive intraoperative traction testing in the setting of instability will demonstrate greater than 2 mm of distraction between the occiput and atlas or between atlas. Traction during testing requires no more than 5 to 10 lb. Manual traction under continuous or fluoroscopic guidance can provide radiographic findings. In addition, there is also the combined association with tactile sensation of a firm endpoint point or lack thereof. The primary role of traction testing has been to confirm whether there remains sufficient ligamentous integrity of the CCJ to proceed with nonoperative treatment in situations in which imaging studies have shown potential features for CCJ instability.[1,9] Traction testing has served to decrease the diagnosis of CCJ injury in situations when the diagnosis would otherwise have been made on strict interpretation of static imaging parameters, thus saving patients from the morbidity of unnecessary occipital cervical fusion[8] (**Fig. 2**).

CRANIOCERVICAL DISSOCIATIONS
Mechanism of Injury

AOD is one type of injury to the CCJ, yet there are other patterns of injury regarding craniocervical dissociations (CCD) that would not fall under the pure definition of AOD. The most common mechanism responsible for CCD is hyperextension resulting in rupture of the tectorial membrane from blunt injury mechanisms such as motor vehicle crashes, falls, and collisions.[1] CCD may account for 6% to 20% of fatal high-speed blunt trauma accidents.[21] For pediatric patients, child-restraint mechanisms leave the head exposed to major whiplash during deceleration drama. Such a scenario would likely entail hyperextension with disruption of the tectorial membrane and a lateral or hyperflexion with disruption of the alar ligaments and posterior atlantooccipital ligament. CCD can be a variable presentation that can range from a single ligament rupture, such as an isolated alar ligament injury that is unlikely to give atlantooccipital instability; to other cases of CCD such as extreme distraction with a high mortality rate.[4,22]

Classification

The Harborview classification system (**Table 2**) for AOD seeks to differentiate an injury based on the severity of ligamentous instability in a manner that is analogous to the injury used for extremities in a three-tiered system.[7] Type I are isolated structural injuries with most structures unaffected and can be treated nonoperatively. This includes unilateral type III occipital condyle injuries or isolated alar ligament tears. Type II injuries may be missed or difficult to characterize.

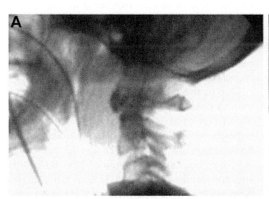 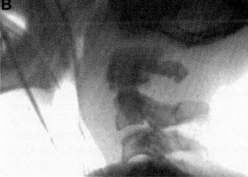

Fig. 2. Traction test fluoroscopic views. (*A*): prior to traction; (*B*): Same patient with 10lbs of traction demonstrating a positive traction test. (*From* Cheng CW, Bellabarba C, Bransford RJ. Craniocervical Injuries: Atlas Fractures, Atlanto-Occipital Injuries, and Atlantoaxial Injuries. SKELETAL TRAUMA: Basic science, management, and reconstruction, 2 vol. set. ELSEVIER; 2019; with permission.)

Table 2 Harborview classification of craniocervical dissociations (CCD)	
Stage	**Description of Injury**
I	MRI evidence of injury to CCD stabilizers; CCJ alignment within 2 mm of normal; distraction of 2 mm or less with dynamic fluoroscopy
II	MRI evidence of injury to CCD stabilizers; CCJ alignment within 2 mm of normal; distraction of more than 2 mm with dynamic fluoroscopy
IIIA	CCJ malalignment of more than 2 mm on static radiographic studies and survives
IIIB	CCJ malalignment of more than 2 mm on static radiographic studies and does not survive within 24 h of injury

Data from Cheng CW, Bellabarba C, Bransford RJ. Cranio-cerivcal Injuries: Atlas Fractures, Atlanto-Occipital Injuries, and Atlantoaxial Injuries. SKELETAL TRAUMA: Basic science, management, and reconstruction 2 vol set ELSEVIER; 2019; With Permission.

Type II injuries can have similar degrees of displacement as partially reduced or fully reduced, yet represent highly unstable injuries. The differentiation between the stable type I versus unstable type II is a challenge and can be differentiated by performing a dynamic traction test. Type II injuries are consistent with complete CCDs with initial lateral radiographs showing borderline screening measurement values. Type II injuries however have features of complete disruption of key ligaments of the CCJ and are unstable. Potential signs of instability are translation or distraction of more than 2 mm in any plane, neurologic injury, or concomitant cerebrovascular trauma. Type III complete disruption of all interconnecting ligaments with obviously unacceptable instability; patients are subclassified on the basis of whether they survive for at least 24 hours from the time of their injury. Type IIIA injuries demonstrate obvious major CCD displacement on plain radiographs, while type IIIB injuries identify death from CCD in the first 24 hours.[1,4] Change in protocols to include the CCJ in trauma CT scans increase the rate of detection of occipital condyle and type I odontoid fractures, which may be an indicator for CCD also.[4]

Imaging

Plain radiographs have limited use in the detection of CCD and have been superseded by CT scanning. Prevertebral soft-tissue swelling on the lateral cervical plain radiograph may be a key finding and a potential indicator of a more significant injury even in the setting of physiologic alignment.

Routine helical CT and suboccipital imaging obtained on routine head CT may improve the identification of injuries of CCD. The inclusion of the foramen magnum in routine craniocervical CT scans has increased the rate of detection of type III occipital condyle and type I odontoid fractures, which may be indicators of CCD as well.[7] The cost-effective impact on patient health through different radiation exposures remains to be assessed. In CCD patients, rapid completion of imaging with CT and possibly MRI is standard. Additional dynamic testing may be necessary in order to identify questionable cases.[4] Studies implementing standard imaging protocol for trauma patients found that 84% of patients were diagnosed on initial cervical spine imaging following the change, 74% were diagnosed within 24 hours, 22% were diagnosed between 24 and 48 hours, and one at 3% was diagnosed later than 48 hours. In comparison, preprotocol, 24% were diagnosed on initial cervical spine imaging, 24% were diagnosed within 24 hours of presentation, 52% were diagnosed between 24 and 48 hours, and 24% experienced a delay of greater than 48 hours.[11] Missed craniocervical injuries and improved education and awareness of these injuries among survivors of high-energy trauma have played a greater role in rapid diagnosis and thus appropriate treatment. Diagnosis of CCD is often missed on plain radiographs with the sensitivity ranging from .57 to .76.[7] The American Academy of the College for Radiology recommends that MRI imaging can be used to evaluate the cervical spine in patients who are unable to have assessment of their neurologic status within 48 hours of injury, including those with normal CT.[23]

Due to the difficulty in the initial evaluation of trauma patients, many radiographic parameters have been established in order to identify CCD patients with CT scan imaging. In uninjured patients, both the BAI and BDI are 12 mm or less in 95% of adults (aka the rule of 12s). Bellabarba and colleagues noted that 35% of patients may have normal BAIs and BDIs and yet still have a CCD. Thus, relying on Harris lines is not completely reliable and may have a higher specificity than sensitivity in detecting CCD.[1]

A gap greater than 2 mm between the occipital condyles and atlas lateral masses (CCI) indicates CCJ injury. Further sensitivity studies regarding CCI have tried to establish the sensitivity cut off. Recent investigations have recommended the sum of CCI with the normal defined as less than 4 mm, sensitivity at 100% for a cut off of 1.5 mm in comparison the CCI minimum greater than 2 mm resulting in 90% sensitivity rate, and using a BDI of less than 10 mm instead of 12 mm as more sensitive assessment of CCJ injuries.[1,11,24] Another study proposed to measure the actual distance between the articular surfaces of the occiput and superior facet of the atlas on the true lateral sagittal CT scan to ensure proper measurements.[4,23] CCI may have limitations in identification of CCD. A case report of concomitant AOD and AAD was unidentified using the method of CCI to diagnose the AOD. The diagnosis of AAD was made using the BDI and other methodologies including an MRI following the recognition. The current recommendations for using the CCI method solely may not diagnose an AOD in the presence of an AAD and another methodology should be applied. CCJ injury can occur with a minimum widening, as seen in a patient with a CCI of 1.6 mm. The CCI is the most sensitive and specific method to diagnose AOD.[25,26] The average CCI interval increases in the first several years of life, the largest in the 2- to 4-year range, and then decreases through late childhood and adolescence. As a single threshold for CCI doesn't detect AOD it may not be sensitive or specific enough for all age groups in pediatric patients. The main sagittal and coronal CCI increased in the first years of life to the largest involving 2.4 mm on average in the sagittal plane and 2.5 mm in the coronal plane. The prevalence of the medial occipital condyle notch may cause the variability in the measurement. This variability decreases in late childhood and adolescence.[27]

With using BDI and BAI in identifying CCD, there were no reported patients diagnosed with a CCD that were missed using the criteria of a BDI greater than 10 mm or CCI greater than 4 mm. The normal maximum values for institutions defined as BDI have less than 9.1 mm, CCI less than 3.5 mm, and AOI less than 2.1 mm. Seven patients had a BDI greater than 10 mm, two of which had a CCI greater than 4 mm. Five of them were qualified as an AOD and two as an AAD. Three diagnoses of AOD and two diagnoses of AAD were not reported. A BDI greater than 9.1 and/or a CCI greater than 3.5 may warrant an emergent MRI. This study concluded a

BDI greater than 10 mm and/or a CCI greater than 4 mm should be of greater concern for AOD versus AAD.[28,29] A case description of a 38-year-old female with AOD presenting with right-sided hemiparesis showed imaging of AOD with bilateral nondisplaced C1 lateral mass fractures and a BDI of 13 mm and CCI of 10 mm with a powers ratio of 1.1.[30] Parameters for diagnosis run on a CT scan with PDI greater than 10 mm, PAI greater than 12 mm, and CCI greater than 1.4.[31] Interobserver reliability of values measured on CT imaging to identify CCD include: BDI, Xline, sun ratio, BAI, and powers ratio had sensitivities of 72%, 54%, 32%, and 26%, respectively.[24]

If the CT is unable to identify an injury to the CCJ or there are questionable findings, an MRI may be warranted to identify ligamentous injuries, intramedullary changes, and hematoma in the epidural or prevertebral spaces.[7] A randomized controlled trial of patients identified with AOD was compared with control groups, in relation to the reliability of MRI to identify alar ligament injuries. Unsatisfactory interobserver reliability and intraobserver reliability in the valuation of alar ligament disruption on an MRI were found. No satisfactory or statistical significance was found in the difference in categorical analysis of the AOD versus non-AOD groups.[32]

Nonoperative Management

In true CCD, any nonoperative care assumes the role of temporary stabilization as a bridging measure until definitive surgical care is performed. Realignment with a halo vest has been suggested as preferable for acute temporary stabilization but may be inadequate in immobilization and may have an undesired distractive effect.[1] In 10% of cases of halo placement, neurologic worsening was noted.[4] In another temporary stabilization procedure, the patient's head may be sandbagged and taped down, as opposed to a neck collar which is usually highly undesirable due to the distractive effect of such a device. It should be clearly emphasized that any patient with CCD is at high risk for secondary neurologic deterioration until definitive fixation.[16]

Key restraints to CCJ instability identified by cadaveric studies are the alar ligaments, tectorial membrane, and atlantooccipital joint capsules. In stage 2 Harborview classification, any true substantial restraint to dissociation (ie, negative traction test <2 mm of displacement) allows a trial of nonoperative treatment and potential for healing, scarring of the junction, and a low risk of catastrophic treatment failure. The atlantooccipital joint capsules are a last line of defense in the CCD, a key component of the capsular ligament strength, and likely the reason for the all-or-none phenomena seen in this injury. The traction test requires no more than 10 lb to demonstrate injury to the restraints of dissociation.[7,11,33]

Operative Management

Patients with CCD should have the CCJ immobilized and definitively stabilized emergently to reduce the chance of progressive neurologic deficit. Many of the ligamentous stabilizers of the CCJ extend caudally to the atlas. For this reason, ending fixation constructs short of the axis would be ineffective, even if the primary distractive injury were identified between the occiput and atlas. Occiput to axis fusion for this injury is a reliable technique, with no patient, in a series of 48 patients with CCD, developing pseudoarthrosis or hardware failure. Posterior instrumentation to the axis is recommended for rare cases where concomitant distraction is present between the occipit and atlas, as well as distraction between the atlas and axis.[8,11,34]

The surgical procedure for stabilization should include maintaining full spine precautions during intubation with a glidescope or awake fiberoptic intubation. The patient is positioned supine on the Jackson flat top. Baseline SSEPs and MEPs are recorded. The patient is then turned into a prone position with the turning mechanism of the table to try to minimize cervical motion.[16] Modern segmental screw constructs enable rigid short-segment fixation and provide adequate stability to achieve successful fusion.[35] Posterior segmental instrumentation is then performed from the occiput to atlas.

Other approaches can be performed for surgical stabilization of CCD. A cadaver-based technique description study of anterior atlantooccipital transarticular screw fixation can be used as a bail out in these situations.[36] This technique may assist in situations where posterior atlantooccipital fixation may not be possible or may require supplemental fixation in cases such as congenital hyperplasia, absent posterior bony elements, and revision surgery. The screw entry point on sagittal plane was at the lower third of the midline of the lateral mass to achieve an ideal entry and the trajectory passes through the main point of the atlantooccipital joint, and points to the posterior inferior of the canal of the hypoglossal nerve.[36] Rare cases of AOD with superimposed congenital occipitalization of the atlas have also been reported. Occipitalization probably leads to the abnormal joint

mechanics at the CCJ ,which have altered the amount of force required to fracture and then therefore produced the CCD. The atlas lateral masses were not able to be instrumented, therefore the construct was extended to C3.[37]

Outcomes and Associated Injuries

CCD can be a devastating diagnosis in the trauma population; however, greater radiologic dissociation was not associated with increased mortality. Historically CCD has a low survivable incidence, but CCD survivors have been increasing secondary to resuscitative parameters and from advanced technology in car safety.[35] As a result of improvement in prehospital resuscitation and mobilization, over 30% of patients with CCD will make it to the hospital and 36% of those patients will survive. All of the nonsurvivors presented to the ED with a GCS of 3 and were undergoing CPR.[38]

Increased soft-tissue edema at the level of C1 greater than 10.86 mm is associated with hospital death. Edema was greater for nonsurvivors at 12.37 mm versus 7.86 mm for survivors. In order to determine an increased rate of mortality, a 75% specificity and sensitivity were found with edema at 10.86 mm. Various reports have cited CCD patients' presentations, with 33% mortality in the hospital, 67% surviving hospital discharge, with a statistically insignificant increased Glasgow Coma Scale (GCS) score for patients who survived.[39]

Identification of predictors of mortality in CCD patients has identified decreased GCS and increased ISS as predictors for increased mortality. A GCS odds ratio of 0.7 was the only independent predictor of death after AOD and time to AOD diagnosis was less than 6 hours in all patients.[40] Another cohort of CCD demonstrated 6 patients who died with complete high cervical spinal cord injuries, and mortality was associated with the presence of complete neurologic deficit, a high basion–dens interval (BDI) greater than 16 mm, and a high ISS. Of this cohort, 43% ultimately died and 57% survived after adequate stabilization. There was no significant association between PDI greater or less than 16 mm. However, if a patient presented with a BDI greater than 16 mm and complete quadriplegia, mortality was associated. The median ISS for patients who died was 75, compared to 34 for survivors.[38,41] The time to neurosurgical intervention was not predictive of survival. A total of 38% of patients were dead on arrival and excluded. Logistic regression analysis identifying predictors of mortality were older age, tachycardia on admission, lower GCS, higher AIS, and need for an exploratory laparotomy.[42] Lower GCS score, worse neurologic function as assessed by Asia score, and missed diagnosis is statistically associated with increased mortality. The average NDI was found to be 30, which is comparable to the mean 16-month NDI for an ACDF.[31]

A missed CCD diagnosis was the strongest predictor of mortality; while younger age, lower GCS, lower ISS, and worse initial ASIA scores were significantly associated with greater neurologic improvement. Early diagnosis and treatment resulted in better outcomes, while missed diagnosis is associated with poor outcomes. When the diagnosis of CCD was delayed by a mean of 2 days, almost 40% of these patients suffered profound neurologic deterioration before CCD was clinically recognized.[1] ASIA motor scores improved and the number of patients with useful motor function increased from 26% preoperatively to 55% postoperatively.[11]

Retrospective studies report up to 30% of patients with a delay in diagnosis of CCD and a potential for serious secondary neurologic deterioration with potentially life-threatening injuries.[4,6] The outcome of survivors is therefore highly dependent on the type and severity of the associated injuries, the severity of the neurologic injury, and the timeliness with which the diagnosis of craniocervical dissociation is recognized and thus operatively stabilize.[16] Outcomes of CCD depend on the type and severity of associated injuries, such as intracranial and cerebrovascular injuries, the severity of neurologic deficit and the timeliness of diagnosis.[8]

CCDs are caused mostly by high-energy mechanisms, and with distractive injuries appear to have a relatively high rate of vertebral artery and carotid artery injuries. It is therefore essential to obtain either a CTA or vascular study in these patients.[1] In a retrospective review of CCD managed operatively, 52% of patients had blunt cerebrovascular injuries, including 16 vertebral artery and 14 carotid injuries.[7] An additional cohort identified blunt cerebrovascular injury (BCVI) in more than 50% of patients, with major strokes occurring in 20%.[43] Additional signs and symptoms of concurrent vascular injuries in CCD can present as locked-in syndrome, with patients revealing a diffuse subarachnoid hemorrhage and intraparenchymal hemorrhage.[44]

In CCD cases with closed treatment in a halo vest, 27% demonstrated failure of closed management either due to neurologic worsening or failure to achieve stable healing.[4] In contrast with patients who were operatively treated with posterior fusion, there were no cases of CCD arthrosis or hardware failure. The caveat of posterior fusion is that there is a limit to motion, and successful treatment of CCD in a halo vest would potentially lead to retained motion after removal.[11]

Concomitant injuries in the cervical spine have been identified in CCD case reports. Compared with patients with AOD, patients with atlantoaxial rotatory dislocations have less severe degree of displacement of the AC joints and a better clinical outcome. Alternative presentations can include dynamic instability in occult injuries with AOD and associated AAD demonstrating reduction with flexion cervical spine radiographs.[45,46] Other concomitant cervical injuries below the atlas may require the extension of the fusion to the lowest disrupted level.[5] Additional concomitant injuries in CCD patients include C1 lateral mass fracture, TAL injuries, and type C1 anterior arch horizontal and sagittal split fractures.[47]

Despite the availability of diagnostic testing, patients with CCD continue to be subject to a critical delay in diagnosis. If patients survive CCD there's a trend toward improvement neurologically, with some patients even returning to normal but most having long-term neurologic deficit.[7]

OCCIPITAL CONDYLE FRACTURE

Mechanism of Injury

Occipital condyle fractures can be caused by direct trauma to the skull or rapid head deceleration during high-velocity motor vehicle collisions.[1] A variety of mechanisms involve impaction or axial loading, distraction with avulsion, or direct blows to the head and associated skull fractures that extends to the occipital condyle.[7]

Classification

Historically, the vast majority of occipital condyle fractures were treated with some form of bracing due to a lack of diagnosis caused by incomplete imaging.[16] Anderson and Montesano in 1988 described a fracture classification of occipital condyle fractures based on a limited cohort of patients:

Type I fractures are caused by impaction or axial load and may be comminuted. Type II injuries are associated with basilar skull fractures that extend into the occipital condyle. Type III injuries are avulsion injuries with the alar ligaments "pulling off" a bony piece of the occipital condyle typically because of distraction. These may be potentially unstable and associated with CCD.

The Mueller classification for occipital condyle fractures is described as: type I is unilateral, type II is bilateral, and type III is occipital fracture with associated CCD.[1,18]

Imaging
Plain x-ray imaging has a limited role in the characterization of occipital condyle fractures due to challenges with recognition of these injuries. Helical CT of the cranial skull base is standard to identify patients with occipital condyle fractures. Type III Montesano classification injuries may need an MRI to identify the presence of an associated CCD.[1]

Nonoperative Management
Management of occipital condyle fractures is dependent on whether there's an associated CCD. CCJ instability can be identified where there is a displacement of the occipital condyle and C1 lateral mass or by a positive traction test. Type I injuries can be treated conservatively and are stable with minimal risk of displacement or neurologic injury.[7]

Type II injuries can be treated in a collar. If a type III injury is identified or suspected, an MRI of the CCJ can help assess the degree of instability and help ascertain the presence or absence of an associated CCD. A collar or halo vest can be used if the injury is stable.[1]

Operative Management
Indications for surgical stabilization of occipital condyle fractures include: presence of CCD with atlantooccipital joint displacement greater than 2 mm on static imaging studies, provocative traction testing, or the presence of a neurologic injury. Occiput to C2 is preferred even if distraction is between occiput to atlas due to possible occult atlantoaxial instability or concurrent injury. An additional clue to the presence of unstable occipital cervical fractures can be provided by detecting avulsion fractures of the alar ligament which, along with the tectorial membrane, serve as one of the two primary stabilizers of the CCJ.[1,6]

Outcomes and Associated Injuries
Unilateral occipital condyle fractures are present in 77% of cases, with more than one-third of patients presenting with an additional cervical spine fracture. Only 18% with avulsion injuries had associated unstable CCD. A common complaint in patients with occipital condyle fractures treated nonoperatively is the development of high cervical pain and limited skull mobility

due to the development of posttraumatic arthritis.[1]

Associated traumatic brain injury, present in up to 50% of patients, can influence long-term results rather than the occipital condyle fracture alone. No patient with nonoperatively treated occipital condyle fractures developed late instability or required other treatment.[7,8]

Cranial nerve impairment of the abducens, the glossopharyngeus, hypoglossal, and the vagus nerve have been described in association with up to a third of patients with occipital condyle fractures. Torticollis may result from chronic atlantooccipital subluxation following an untreated fracture.[16]

ATLAS FRACTURES AND TRANSVERSE LIGAMENT INJURIES
Mechanism of Injury
Atlas fractures can occur in 3% to 25% of CCJ injuries, 2% to 13% of cervical injuries, and 1% to 3% of all spine fractures. Atlas fractures can be caused by traumatic falls, or flexion or extension mechanisms with direct head impaction injuries. Posterior arch fractures of the atlas are seen in the elderly with concomitant odontoid fractures due to an extension mechanism as the patient falls and strikes their head. Another extension injury is the "plow fracture," where the dens strikes through the anterior C1 arch secondary to the hyperextension force. This fracture can be associated with posterior atlantoaxial dislocation. Traumatic rupture of the TAL leading to atlantoaxial instability is caused by high-energy injuries typically resulting from hyperflexion of the neck. Comminuted atlas fractures are caused by combined axial compression and lateral flexion forces, with an avulsion fracture of the TAL with corresponding ipsilateral anterior and posterior arches.[1,48,49]

Classification
Jefferson was first to classify atlas fractures based on the axial compression mechanism. The Jefferson classification of atlas fractures is as follows: type I isolated fractures of either the anterior or posterior arch, type II involves both the anterior and posterior arches (previously characterized as Jefferson 3–4 part fractures), and type III involves fracture of the lateral mass. Fractures occur at the weakest points of the ring which are the anterior and posterior arches.[1]

Unstable type II atlas fractures are distinguished from stable fractures by a concomitant injury of the transverse ligament, characterized by the outward spread of the lateral masses under axial compression. Type II atlas fractures are an important minority of atlas fractures, which are usually caused by the axial loading of the head to the occiput. The projecting occipital condyles support is simultaneously lost, resulting in a concomitant failure of the vertical ligamentous tension. Because of the loss of CCJ height, there is a loss of ligamentous restraint of the tectorial membrane, the cruciate ligament, the alar ligaments, the capsular ligaments, the apical ligament, and the atlantoaxial anterior and posterior membranes.[50] The TAL is the major ligamentous structure providing stabilization for the atlantoaxial articulation. If the TAL is disrupted by the separation of the lateral masses in an atlas fracture, then the stability of the AA relationship is lost.[1]

The Gehweiler classification and the Revised European Atlas Fracture Classification are as follows: type 1 isolated anterior arch fracture, type 2 isolated bilateral fracture of the posterior arch, type 3 anterior and posterior arch fracture, type 3a stable injuries with intact TAL, type 3b disrupted TAL, type 4 lateral mass fractures, and type 5 isolated C1 transverse process fractures.[1,49]

TAL injuries can be further characterized by the Dickman classification into: type 1 intrasubstance TAL injuries, type 1A midsubstance ruptures, and type 1B periosteal insertion injuries. Type 2 is avulsion injuries of the TAL, type 2A is associated with comminuted lateral mass fractures, and type 2B is an intact lateral mass.[1]

Other unique atlas fractures have been further identified. Bransford and colleagues identified patients with atlas unilateral sagittal split fractures of the lateral mass with an intact TAL who were initially treated with external immobilization alone. These patients developed significant loss of neck rotation, a "cock-robin deformity," and severe neck pain that ultimately required traction and occipitocervical fusion.[1] Another case report of patients demonstrating a similar unilateral lateral mass sagittal split fracture, which resulted in a late cock-robin deformity. A sagittal split fracture has a propensity to result in the late cock-robin deformity and thus require surgical correction of the deformity with occipital cervical instrument at fusion (**Fig. 3**). All patients demonstrated an intact transverse atlantal ligament. Additional secondary CCJ unilateral subsidence and settling leads to loss of motion and unacceptable coronal alignment.[51]

Unilateral or bilateral transverse process fractures are a result of avulsion injuries with lateral bending. These are benign injuries but may be associated with vertebral artery injury. Another avulsion fracture of the atlas may involve a transverse fracture of the inferior pole, which usually results from avulsion injuries of the longus colli muscle and is caused by a distraction mechanism with neck hyperextension.[51]

Imaging

Plain films, including an open-mouth odontoid view, can assist in the characterization of the amount of displacement of the lateral masses of the atlas in relation to the axis. This imaging has been replaced more readily by helical CT scans and use of MRI to better characterize TAL disruption.[51] Disruption of the TAL occurs with total C1 lateral mass displacement (>7 mm). Furthermore, retropharyngeal soft-tissue swelling greater than 5 mm at C3 with posterior arch fracture is highly suggestive of an atlas burst fracture.[1,51]

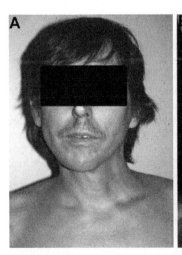
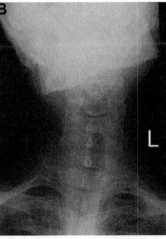

Fig. 3. (*A*): Fifty-year-old male with a C1 lateral mass sagittal split fracture with clinical portrait of cock-robin deformity. (*B*): AP radiograph of the same patient demonstrating radiographic representation of cock-robin deformity. (*From* Bransford R, Falicov A, Nguyen Q, Chapman J. Unilateral C-1 lateral mass sagittal split fracture: an unstable Jefferson fracture variant. *J Neurosurg Spine* 2009;10(5):466-73. https://doi.org/10.3171/2009.1. SPINE08708; with permission.)

Based on the biomechanical cadaver study, the "rule of Spence" characterizes lateral mass displacement that is greater than 6.9 mm, suggesting injury to the TAL.[48] An amendment to this rule was proposed by Heller that the displacement should be adjusted to 8.1 mm for the radiographic magnification factor.[49] Lateral mass displacement (LMD) less than 6.9 mm was not sensitive enough to exclude a TAL injury, but greater than 6.9 mm was able to identify all TAL injured. This, however, was limited to the identification of concurrent atlantoaxial injuries. The Dickman classification is more sensitive in identifying TAL injuries in which there is concurrent atlantoaxial instability. In Dickman type I TAL injuries, 100% failed to restore the atlantoaxial stability and 85% succeeded in Dickman type II TAL injuries. Dickman's classification of TAL is superior to the rule of Spence in terms of accuracy and predicting atlantoaxial stability and nonoperative treatment of atlas fractures.[52]

MRI imaging in atlas fractures can be used as an opportunity to provide for identifying intrasubstance tears of the TAL. T2 gradient MRI imaging will indicate whether there is disruption of the TAL, and can include areas of signal heterogeneity within the injured ligament.[34]

A novel measurement technique to identify TAL disruption in atlas fractures is the C1:C2 ratio. The C1:C2 ratio was measured using open-mouth odontoid and first taken trauma radiographs. The combined overhang of lateral mass and C1:C2 ratio was calculated. No patients with a reported ratio of 1.15 had an intact TAL; whereas a ratio greater than 1.1 captured 80% of ligament injuries.[53]

Nonoperative Management

TAL integrity may contribute to the stability of atlas fractures, which can be determined by measuring total LMD and ADI on either radiographs or a CT. Nondisplaced and displaced bilateral or unilateral lateral mass fractures with intact TAL are also managed in a rigid cervical collar for 6 to 12 weeks. Sagittal split fracture of the lateral mass should be observed closely to look for further displacement or development of cock-robin deformity, persistent severe neck pain, and difficulty with range of motion.[1] Gehweiler types 1, 2, 3A, and 5 are stable and require cervical spine mobilization with a hard collar.[18,49]

Operative Management

The ideal treatment of unstable type II atlas fractures is to preserve the function of the atlantoaxial joint and maintain alignment of the spine to allow healing of the atlas. If nonoperative management fails, surgery is warranted to prevent the risk of further displacement of lateral mass and unacceptable atlantooccipital alignment with the development of a pseudoarthrosis.[1,54] Operative Gehweiler type 3B with an intraligamentous TAL rupture, also known as Dickman type 1A, is treated with a fusion of C1–C2 versus type 3B fracture with bony avulsion of the TAL, known as Dickman type 2, which can be treated with direct osteosynthesis.[18,49]

Direct osteosynthesis can be performed in unstable atlas burst fractures. The purpose of this procedure is to restore the height between the occiput and axis by restoring vertical ligamentous tension via reduction of atlas lateral mass fractures. Direct osteosynthesis is used to maintain stability despite TAL incompetence, while preserving motion in the upper cervical spine and avoiding fusion (Fig. 4). Anterior transoral approaches for direct reduction of the fracture have been described, but come at the risk of increased postoperative infections and retropharyngeal complications.[1,50,55]

In a subsequent study, direct osteosynthesis use has been expanded to include both types of TAL injuries. In one cohort, the TAL was found to be disrupted with type I or type II injuries with an average displacement of 7.1 mm with postoperative reduction averaging 2.4 mm. No patients developed atlantoaxial instability on final flexion extension cervical x-rays. Also, no patients had complications that resulted in neurologic deficit or vascular injury within the procedure, and no patients demonstrated malunion or loss reduction. Although direct osteosynthesis was a contraindication for intrasubstance TAL injuries, this cohort determined successful treatment. An important note is that maintaining the integrity of the secondary stabilizers of the atlantoaxial joint, while restoring the axial ligamentous tension and height of the CCJ, is the main goal of this technique and success in treatment.[56]

In a comparison of occipital cervical versus atlantoaxial fusion in the treatment of unstable Jefferson fractures, no patient developed postoperative upper cervical spine instability or loss of reduction following surgery based on radiographic review. There was only one nonunion in the occipital cervical fusion group. No differences between outcome studies or patient reported parameters for any of the groups.[57]

Outcomes and Associated Injuries

Failed nonoperative management of atlas fractures is common. Seventeen percent of nonunion of atlas fractures were initially treated by immobilization alone. Nonoperative

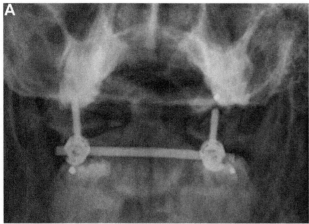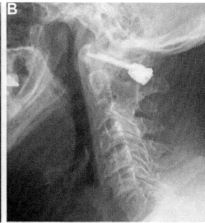

Fig. 4. (*A*): Open-mouth radiograph; (*B*): lateral cervical radiograph demonstrating C1 osteosynthesis. (*From* Cheng CW, Bellabarba C, Bransford RJ. Craniocervical Injuries: Atlas Fractures, Atlanto-Occipital Injuries, and Atlantoaxial Injuries. SKELETAL TRAUMA: Basic science, management, and reconstruction, 2 vol. set. ELSEVIER; 2019; with permission.)

outcomes are associated with stiffness in 8% to 20%, mild pain in 14% to 80%, and the rate of limitations is 34% in failed management.[1] The overall success rate for conservative treatment of Dickman type 2 injuries was 66%.[52] Patients with greater than 7 mm of LMD had poorer long-term outcomes compared to those who did not.[8]

Direct osteosynthesis patients' outcomes reported low neck pain and good physiologic cervical range of motion.[8] Successful treatment of 1-year follow-up of patients with CT scans and plain radiographs with flexion and extension views demonstrated maintained alignment, bony healing, and no atlantoaxial instability.[50] VAS and NDI scores postoperatively and at final follow-up showed significant improvement.[58]

Atlas fractures are associated with head injuries, and 50% are associated with other cervical spine fractures. These fractures include dens fractures, hangman's fractures, teardrop fractures of the axis, and cervical burst and lateral mass fractures of the cervical lower spine. Collet-Sicard syndrome refers to unilateral lesions of cranial nerves.[1,49,54] Vertebral artery injury was independently and positively associated with an injury of the transverse ligament with an 8.5 odds ratio. TAL injury was independently associated with an increased ADI, increased LMD, and male sex.[48]

ATLANTOAXIAL INJURIES
Mechanism of Injury
Atlantoaxial injuries can be associated with multiple causes including traumatic injuries, inflammatory disease, or congenital abnormalities. Nontraumatic causes of atlantoaxial injuries are excluded from the context of this article. Traumatic atlantoaxial subluxation or dislocation (AAD) is due to forced rotation, distraction or flexion–extension injury resulting in disruption of the TAL. AAD can also involve simultaneous disruption of the alar and apical ligaments, resulting in complete disarticulation between the atlas and the dens. Posterior dislocation injuries are hypothesized to be the result of the hyperextension and are often accompanied by type II odontoid fracture.[1,59,60]

AAD can be described as directional and are either anterior, posterior, or rotational. Concurrent ligament tears are common, often resulting from rupture of the TAL or deformity of the dens. Posterior AAD is relatively uncommon and often associated with an odontoid fracture.[12] A rare form of ADD involves an intact odontoid process ventral to the ring and associated soft-tissue swelling to the upper cervical spine, often requiring emergency intubation. Most cases of posterior AAD have successfully been managed by closed reduction, which is technically challenging to relocate the odontoid process back to the osseous ring.[60]

Another extension injury is the plow fracture, where the dens impact through the interior C1 arch secondary to a hyperextension force. This fracture pattern is usually associated with posterior AAD. Patients routinely complain of base of the skull discomfort and a sense of instability on presentation. With intact TAL, atlantoaxial articulation can rotate approximately 65° before the narrowing of the neural canal, and cause potential damage to the spinal cord. Alternatively, with a deficient TAL, unilateral condylar dislocation in AAD will result in approximately 45°

rotation with injury into the spinal cord resulting in myelopathy or paralysis. In patients with AAD, 50% of patients will present with neck pain or a limited range of motion, and 70% with weakness or paresthesia in their extremities.[8]

Segmentation abnormalities such as assimilated C1 and C2–3 are noted to be significantly higher in cases with irreducible AAD. Bony anomalies were seen in 96% of patients with irreducible AAD compared to 63% of patients with reducible AAD. The most common bony anomaly in irreducible AAD was atlas assimilation in 79% of cases, followed by 74% of C2–3 fusion cases. Vertebral artery anomalies were found in 26% of patients with irreducible AAD compared to 7% with reducible AAD. Bifid atlas with assimilation was seen in irreducible lateral angular AAD.[61]

Classification

The AAD Fielding classification is determined by the direction of the dislocation and accounts for the integrity of the TAL and position of the facet joints. Type I is pure rotational injury and is the most common, typically caused by low-energy trauma such as a same-level fall in the elderly. Type II involves both rotatory malalignment with less than 3 mm to 5 mm anterior displacement of the atlas relative to the axis. Mild TAL deficiency occurs with unilateral anterior displacement of atlas lateral mass, with the opposite intact joint acting as a pivot. Type III injuries are rotatory subluxation, with greater than 5 mm anterior displacement of the atlas of the axis; the greater anterior displacement suggests complete TAL deficiency. Type IV injuries are uncommon rotational and posterior displacements, possibly due to a deficient odontoid. Type V injuries are very rare and involve both AA and AO rotatory fixation, and were added to the classification by Levine and Edwards.[1,8,12]

White and Punjabi described AAD classification as type A bilateral anterior displacement, type B bilateral posterior dislocation, type C rotatory dislocation of the atlas around the ipsilateral facet joints, and type D as rotatory displacement around the contralateral. Type E is bilateral displacement on the center of the odontoid.[62]

Another unique description of AAD is called a Haralson dislocation. It is caused by hyperextension of the neck following a blow to either the face or the posterior torso, which causes the trunk to accelerate forward as the head extends back. Haralson dislocation is categorized by a traumatic posterior AAD without fracture of the odontoid process and a grade 4 retrolisthesis of the atlas on the axis or complete posterior AAD.[27] There is classification of two types of Haralson dislocations depending on the integrity of the transverse ligament after MRI: type I with intact TAL and type II with torn TAL.[63]

The Wayne classification system of AAD provides a practical means to diagnose and treat. The Wayne classification categorizes AAD into four types: instability type 1, reducible dislocation type 2, irreducible dislocation type 3, and bony dislocation type 4.[13]

Imaging

Plain radiographs can show evidence of asymmetry of the lateral masses with an open-mouth odontoid view. The lateral masses of the atlas override on axis joints on one side with normal joint alignment on the contralateral side, also known as the "wink" sign. Plain film on the lateral view will show an increased ADI with a decreased space available for the cord and anterior dislocation of the atlas.[1,8] If the space available for the spinal cord is less than 14 mm it predicts the development of paralysis.[13] The space available for the cord at the level of the outlet was about one-third of the spinal canal. In posterior dislocation the reduced canal area, being less than 36%, is sufficient to avoid cord compression.[64]

ADI can be a variable determinant on age. An ADI less than 3 mm in adults and 4 mm in adolescence is considered normal. An ADI between 3 mm and 5 mm indicates a transverse ligament rupture. An ADI between 5 mm and 10 mm indicates a rupture of the transverse and other assisting ligaments such as the alar ligament. An ADI from 10 mm to 12 mm indicates a rupture of all ligaments and joint capsules.[19] An LMI greater than 2.6 mm should alert to the possibility of distraction injury.[1,8,65] Open-mouth odontoid views with the patient's head rotated 15° to each side will determine whether or not there is a fixed rotational deformity.[12]

Standard trauma protocol is with helical CT and inclusion of the CCJ on imaging to determine if an AAD is present. CT can potentially produce a false-negative injury in AAD if the patient's head is rotated during the scan; it is necessary to ensure the patient is looking straight forward, which can be assessed on scout imaging. Advanced imaging with an MRI can determine if there are disruptions of the alar, apical ligaments, and TAL. Distraction of the atlantoaxial joint was found in patients who sustained high-energy trauma and can also present with additional fracture of the odontoid process.[62]

To determine the extent of AAD reducibility identification of motion on dynamic x-rays, along with a malunion ruled out on CT, make a direct posterior reduction for locked facets feasible. The degree of difficulty increases in remote fractures due to increased fibrosis at the joints. Vertebral artery injury detected on preoperative CT angiogram reduces the chances of iatrogenic injury during intraoperative reduction. If unilateral vertebral artery injury is identified, only a unilateral approach opposite to the injured vertebral arteries is planned.[62,66]

Nonoperative Management

AAD nonoperative management can include attempted closed reduction under general anesthesia with spinal cord monitoring. The reduction mechanism consists of the first operator applying moderate traction and hyperextension with a Mayfield/Gardner clamp, while the second operator manually pushes the odontoid transorally. Manipulation of the head is first done with hyperextension and then flexion of the neck under fluoroscopic guidance. There is potential for use of bivector traction with the patient in a supine position with a horizontal force applied to the traction of the head and a perpendicular force applied to the neck. It is important to avoid the serious pitfall of closed reduction techniques and overdistraction in elderly patients; a maximum traction of 12 kg should be applied. Major complications include iatrogenic vertebral artery injury, iatrogenic cervical spine instability, and life-threatening distraction lesions due to skull traction by halo frame.[12,59,63,65]

Operative Management

There is not one definitive classification that assists in guiding surgical management in AAD. In cases in which atlantoaxial angulation is found to be greater than 30°, significant displacement of 10% to 100%, or associated neurologic symptoms, early surgery may be indicated as it is possible that these are all indicators of ligamentous instability.[15] Surgical CCJ stabilization is indicated for all patients with CCJ displacement of greater than 2 mm on static imaging studies or with provocative traction testing in the presence of neurologic injury.[20] This is analogous to CCD and should be treated using similar guidelines.[34] Surgical intervention is generally recommended for unstable symptomatic AAD in order to avoid progressive neurologic symptoms, respiratory failure, and death.[1] Other studies have isolated treatment algorithms based on case presentations such as Haralson dislocation case series in

which they advocate for successful close reduction and conservative treatment with type I Haralson dislocations, while type II Haralson dislocations require atlantoaxial internal fixation or fusion.[63] Some resources state that surgical treatment is recommended, even for an asymptomatic AAD, to avoid development of myelopathy due to concerns of increased morbidity and mortality.[13]

The first step in correcting AAD is an attempted reduction of dislocation. In the final setting of traction, the release phase consists of switching to an extension posture and slowly releasing traction with gradual weight reduction and finally compressing with a Mayfield during definitive fixation. Assessment of the reducibility of the AAD is critical prior to proceeding with a posterior fusion alone to optimize adequate decompression and restoration of physiologic alignment.[13,65] If irreducible, a two-step procedure with a transoral release is performed first, with reduction via traction then a secondary posterior spinal fusion being performed in the single anesthesia. Avoiding fixing the patient with persistent dislocation is the key to limiting postoperative failure.[12,64] In the setting of single approaches to irreducible AAD, DeAndre and McNabb described a bilateral lateral retropharyngeal approach. This is a rarely used lateral approach and has an advantage because the atlantoaxial joint exposure is excellent and the option exists to perform anterior transarticular fusion.[67] Factors implicated in the irreducibility of AAD are entrapment of the transverse ligament at the base of the odontoid, jagged margins of the fracture line, bony spicule, or locked facet joints.[66,68]

In type I rotatory dislocation, the alar ligaments are usually disrupted as well as the facet capsule of the dislocated joint, and treated with closed reduction with posterior instrumentation. In terms of posterior fixation types, the Harms technique is advantageous in comparison to transarticular fixation for AAD. Primarily, the risk of relapse and dislocation may increase intraoperatively if the transarticular screws inserted into the atlas are possibly pushing the atlas away. Secondly, especially in young patients, the violation of atlantoaxial joints has led to be an avoidance in order to remove implants after consolidation instead of fusion.[62]

Outcomes and Associated Injuries

AAD prevalence rates must nonetheless be interpreted in the light of the likelihood that some patients die before radiological examination. Previous reports state a 7.3% prevalence of AAD among cervical spine injuries, 2.7% pure dislocations, versus those combined with odontoid fractures at 4.7%. The diagnosis of AAD is rare and probably underestimated secondary to immediate death, with mortality with AAD reportedly 60% to 80%.[12,65]

Type II odontoid fractures are the most common fracture associated with AAD at 72%, followed by atlas fractures, then hangman fractures.[19] Even more rare combinations have been reported in cases with concurrent AOD with AAD, which increases the delay in diagnosis.[69] Dickman and colleagues reported an overall complication rate of 9.4% during transoral surgery, including cerebral spinal fluid leakage, wound infection, pneumonia, and death. The postoperative incidence of degenerative disc disease after fixation of an AAD has also been reported in the setting of nonphysiologic lordosis. In such cases, the apex was found near the subaxial sagittal curvature at C6–7 rather than at the adjacent level fusion. Patients undergoing a retropharyngeal approach in a postoperative study were found to have an uneventful recovery with significant improvement in neurologic function.[13]

The AAD prognosis is largely contingent on the neurologic status at the time of injury. Severe neurologic injury at this level is incompatible with life due to cardiorespiratory compromise; patients who survive the injury generally have a favorable neurologic prognosis.[34] Sequelae of AAD may include myelopathy, sphincter disturbances, lower cranial nerve dysfunction, respiratory failure, vertebral artery dissection, neurologic compromise, and rarely quadriplegia or death if left untreated.[8] Certain presentations, such as Foville syndrome, produce ipsilateral horizontal gaze, facial nerve palsy, and contralateral hemiparesis.[65]

Patients presenting with AAD can develop incomplete quadriplegia and show significant improvement in neurologic exam after closed reduction with head holter traction at 10% of body weight.[64] There is a high risk of delayed myelopathy for patients with AAD who do not undergo timely surgical treatment. An operative intervention was performed and resulted in no neurologic or vascular complications; as well as no screw failure or pseudoarthrosis. Irreducible AAD with late presentation can result in scar tissue and prevent reduction via traction. Irreducible AAD requires a decompression anteriorly via the transoral approach with a posterior decompression and occipital cervical fusion.[19]

Segmentation defects, such as an assimilated arch of the atlas and C2–3 fusion, can present with anomalous vertebral arteries and are found to be the causes of irreducible rather than reducible AAD.[61] Accompanying vascular injuries affect the vertebral artery but may also involve the carotid arteries. Patients with a high-riding variant of the vertebral artery are at risk for vessel dissection or rupture because the artery is limited by the restriction of the bony structures.[62] A CT angiogram demonstrating the relationship of the vertebral artery is necessary for perioperative planning.[66] Unfortunately there is no current preoperative prediction modeled for patients with irreducible AAD; a poor preoperative JOA score was seen in one-fifth of patients with irreducible AAD, although mean JOA scores were similar between reducible and irreducible AAD.[61]

ODONTOID FRACTURES
Mechanism of Injury
Odontoid fractures account for between 10% and 20% of all cervical spine fractures. There is a well-described bimodal age distribution of patients, with a smaller peak occurring in younger, physically active, and healthy usually male patients. A second larger peak occurs in the elderly, with approximately 85% over the age of 65, with a larger number of female patients. A less common injury cohort is seen in children under the age of 7; with disruption of the unossified synchondrosis of the dens and often associated with a hyperflexion mechanism. Fractures of the odontoid have been associated with mortality rates as high as 14% in a 30-day period and 44% by 2 years, which are comparable with literature on the mortality of hip fractures in the aging population.[3,70,71] Rates of neurologic injury with odontoid fractures present with 82% neurologically intact, 8% had minimal sensory disturbances over the scalp or limbs, and 10% had significant neurologic deficits. Odontoid fractures have an associated 16% rate of noncontiguous spine fractures in the trauma population.[72]

The increased prevalence of arthrosis between the tip of the dens and the clivus, as well as its articulation with the C1 ring, in combination with a relative increase in stiffness of the subaxial spine, increases biomechanical stresses on the upper motion segments at the CCJ. Cervical spondylosis with preserved atlantoaxial joints places an increased rotational moment arm on the base of the odontoid during deceleration trauma, which leads to fracture. The microarchitecture of the axis has a decreased volume of cancellous bone, with poorer trabecular interconnections and decreased cortical thickness in the lower regions of the dens at its connections with the base with advancing age. This creates an area of weakness that leads to odontoid fractures with relatively low-energy trauma.[3]

Classification
Odontoid fractures classified by D'Alonzo are classified into three types. Type I fractures occur near the tip of the odontoid process above the transverse ligament. This is the least common type of odontoid fracture and likely a result of an alar ligament avulsion. Type I odontoid fractures can be associated with an unstable CCD that can result from bilateral avulsion of the alar ligaments. Type I acute fractures may also be mistaken for an os odontoideum or vice versa.[3]

Type II odontoid fractures are the most common injuries of the axis, occurring in 38% to 46% of cases in the general population, with this number rising to 82% to 95% in elderly patients. Type IIa subtype of classification by Hadley describes the comminution frequency at the base of the odontoid direction of fracture type anterior oblique 16%, posterior oblique 34%, or horizontal at 50%.[3] A revised classification by Grauer refines the D'Alonzo classification with a type IIa fracture defined as a transverse fracture with less than 1 mm of displacement. Type IIb fractures pass from anterior superior to posterior inferior. Transverse fractures that are displaced greater than 1 mm are generally amenable to anterior screw fixation. Type IIc fractures are oriented from anterior inferior to posterior superior and have the highest degree of comminution.[71] One distinction of the type IIa Grauer classification that is different from the Hadley description of type IIa is that Hadley fractures are comminuted. Instability of type II injuries can be anticipated with anteroposterior displacement >5 mm, angulation greater than 11°, and fracture gap >2 mm.[3]

Type III odontoid fractures, in contrast to type II, extend below the level of the bony recess along the medial edge of the superior articular plafond. Most type III fractures are considered inherently stable and are associated with a relatively high union rate due to the preeminent fracture location involving cancellous bone.[3]

Imaging
Plain films and CT scans can identify odontoid fractures following both high-energy and low-energy trauma. A high-riding transverse foramen can by present in at least 18% of patients and may prohibit the placement of transarticular screws. It is recommended to obtain a CT angiogram prior to surgical invention, if surgery is anticipated, to identify these potential variants.[72] An MRI should be used in the setting of odontoid fractures with concurrent neurologic deficit or suspicion of noncontiguous cervical spine injuries.[3]

Nonoperative Management
Surgical versus nonsurgical intervention demonstrated radiographic union was achieved in only 50% of patients treated in a cervical collar versus 90% of patients that achieved radiographic stability in type II odontoid fractures. Traditionally, the goals of treatment have been pain relief and structural stability for a nonunion. Twenty-three percent of patients with nonunions underwent surgical intervention within 1 year of injury. In general, male sex, older age, the presence of a neurologic injury, and initial nonsurgical management have all been associated with high treatment failures. The complication rate of halo fixation, including pins and infection, is most common at up to 35%. Patients greater than 65 years of age with halos have increased mortality, secondary to pulmonary complications, with mortality rates as high as 21% to 40%. Halo treatment failure has been associated with a fracture gap greater than 1 mm, posterior displacement greater than 5 mm, delayed start to treatment of .4 days, and posterior displacement greater than 2 mm. Nonoperative management mean time to union is approximately 13 weeks.[71] Conversely, nonsurgical treatment in a series of patients with type II odontoid fractures treated in the halo vest for 6 weeks followed by hard collar for 4 weeks reported a union rate of 82%. A systematic review of 12 papers including 714 fractures indicated a nonunion rate equivalent between halo and cervical collar. Complications were higher in patients treated with a halo at 34% compared to 15% with a collar. The rates of healing with nonoperative treatment with type III fractures is 85% to 100%. Type III fractures should be treated surgically if there is greater than 5 mm displacement.[72]

Operative Management
Identified parameters for operative treatment are: patient age greater than 50, comminuted fractures, and posterior or significant displacement >5 mm.[73] Current surgical indications for odontoid fracture fixation that most surgeons would agree upon include: neurologic deficits resulting from the dens fracture and associated unstable subaxial spine injuries that require surgical fixation.[3,70]

It has been proposed that anterior odontoid screw fixation is a relative indication in multiply injured patients, associated closed head injury, initial displacement of 4 mm or more, angulation of 10° or more, delayed presentation greater than 2 weeks, multiple risk fractures for non-unions, associated cranial or thoracoabdominal injury or other medical factors, and the presence of associated upper cervical fractures. Grauer type IIB, which is a displaced fracture extending from anterior superior to posteroinferior, is ideal for an anterior screw. The desirable screw starting spot for anterior odontoid screw fixation is properly recessed into the center of the C2–3 anterior disc space, with a properly performed lag screw technique following the longitudinal axis of the odontoid. If there is significant comminution at the odontoid waist present and/or a reverse oblique fracture is identified, then posterior C1–2 arthrodesis is preferred over attempts at anterior odontoid fixation. A lack of anatomic reduction or inability to achieve interfragmentary compression across the fracture can greatly impair the efficacy of the odontoid screw fixation. Anterior procedures in the elderly for placement of odontoid screws should not be done due to the risk of significant swallowing complications and the risk of failure from screw out or loss of fixation secondary to osteoporosis.[3] Use of anterior screw fixation was found to have 87% bony unions, 9.6% stable nonunions, and 3.2% unstable nonunions, suggesting that high stability and low mechanical failure rates can be achieved. Sasso and colleagues determined that the load failure was equivalent in biomechanical studies using either one or two screws.[71,72]

Outcomes and Associated Injuries

Odontoid fractures in functionally active patients can result in nonhealing fractures, secondary displacement, pain, dysfunction, and even serious neurologic injury or death. Spinal cord injury—either of a primary or secondary nature—is relatively rare, perhaps a benefit of the capacious spinal canal found between the foramen magnum and the C2–3 disc space. Because of the growing geriatric demographic population, improved odontoid fracture care algorithms for the elderly can cause significant improvements from societal and economic perspectives.[3]

The surgical intervention union rate of type II odontoid fractures is upwards of 93% to almost 100%. Paired anterior and posterior ascending arteries arise from the vertebral arteries and form anastomosis at the tip of the odontoid, supplying much of the region's blood supply, creating a plexus at the base of the odontoid

and are disrupted in type II fractures. The disruption of the arcade weakens the biologic environment for osseous union potentially contributing to a relatively high nonunion rate.[71]

A case report identified an occult CCD where initial imaging of the cervical spine failed to illustrate displacement of atlantooccipital or atlantoaxial articulation. Cervical spine CT from the outside facility demonstrated a moderately distracted but relatively well aligned type 2 dens fracture. Soft-tissue swelling measured 16.7 mm at the level of the axis, accompanied with a type III occipital condyle and the distractive type II dens fracture, led to a higher concern for a more substantive injury.[11]

Geier deformity, with a stooped-forward position, is named after the pathology resembling the distinct features of a vulture's neck. This deformity develops after odontoid fractures with clinical findings that include: anterior displacement of the upper cervical spine with the occiput in reference to C7 and a decreased lordosis, increased kyphosis of C2–7 resulting in a loss of physiologic alignment, and a stooped-forward posture. The deformity is associated with an oblique posterior fracture pattern of odontoid fractures and nonunion. The underlying pathomechanism may be disequilibrium of the anterior load and posterior muscle forces in the upper cervical spine. Fracture morphology was found to have a significant impact on the radiological outcome; the union rate for surgical cases with a posterior oblique fracture was 86% and significantly higher than that of surgical cases with a transverse fracture pattern at 40%. The neural canal balance was determined by angulation by McCrae's line, a line drawn from the basion to the opisthion, representing the level of the foramen magnum and tangent to the lower endplate of C7. Displacement was determined by the distance between the opisthion and the mid-vertebral level of the C7 spinolaminar line. Neural canal angulation at follow-up varied according to the fracture pattern; 64° in transverse versus oblique posterior at 67° and differed from fracture union at 62° versus nonunion 71°.[73]

The associated nonunion rate with nonoperative management is believed to be caused by the higher instability of the odontoid fracture pattern. A watershed region of blood supply is present at the odontoid base, thus producing decreased healing potential. There is also associated arthrosis at the C1–2 interface as well as in the subaxial cervical spine which places excessive stress on the fracture. Patients with a symptomatic nonunion fracture can present with persistent neck pain, myelopathy, or both. Nonunion rates of type II odontoid fractures treated in a halo vest and with a fracture displacement of <6 mm or >6 mm, ranged from 26% to 67% respectively.[73] Furthermore, halo vest use in the elderly has been associated with complications in the range of 26%, including poor reduction maintenance, swallowing difficulties, aspiration pneumonia, pin tract infection, and even death.[3]

In a comparison between surgical versus nonsurgical treatment of type II odontoid fractures, the bony proportion of fusion is significantly higher in the surgical fixation group. There were no significant differences in the primary surgical fixation group and conservative treatment between long-term failure with pseudoarthrosis or neck pain. Survival rates of all patients at 30 days, 6 months, and 12 months were 84%, 78%, and 73%, respectively, with 67% of patients having severe comorbidities.[70]

In another study, type II odontoid fractures were associated with higher nonunion rates, and surgical intervention for type II fractures in the elderly population is associated with a higher union rate and less mortality. Overall immediate postoperative dysphagia with anterior odontoid screw fixation is upwards of 35%. Patients found with greater than a 1-week delay in treatment had a 37.5% increased risk of fixational failure in a fracture gap greater than 2 mm. If surgical treatment of odontoid fractures is performed, this allows cervical collar removal in the elderly population while eating to reduce the risk of aspiration.[71] Type II fractures over the age of 60 treated surgically were found to have a decreased risk of short-term and long-term mortality without an increased risk of complication versus those treated conservatively. Another study found equivalent mortality rates, but a 50% increase in the complication rate, such as pneumonia or UTI in the surgical group.[72] Concomitant fractures with type II odontoid are the most common including the atlas, and it is recommended to surgically treat if the odontoid has greater angulation or an ADI greater than 5 mm.[18]

HANGMAN FRACTURES
Mechanism of Injury
Hangman fracture, also known as traumatic spondylolisthesis of the axis, with bilateral pars interarticularis fractures, is caused by hyperextension and distraction or hyperextension and compression. Hangman fractures account for 15% to 20% of all cervical spine fractures with a component of combined atlantoaxial injuries, and is 2:1 more common in males versus females.[74,75]

Classification
The Levine classification (updated to the Levine, Eismont, Starr, and Effendi) of hangman fractures includes type 1 injuries defined as nonangulated fractures with displacement less than 3 mm. These injuries likely result from an extension axial loading mechanism that fractures the axis, but does not disrupt the C2–C3 disc or the anterior-posterior ligamentous complex. Atypical type 1A, later added to the hangman fractures classification by Eismont and Starr, is described as a unilateral pars fracture and the contralateral body and/or vertebral foramen fracture, and has more spinal cord injuries. Atypical hangman fractures are associated with significant spinal canal narrowing and an increase in neurologic injury with a coronal fracture line through the posterior vertebral body that allows for canal narrowing to occur with injury anterolisthesis through the C2–C3 space.[18,74,75]

Type 2 injuries demonstrate angulation of greater than 11° and an average displacement of 5 mm. There is a combined mechanism of axial loading and extension followed by a flexion compression. Type 2A injuries are proposed to be predominantly flexion distraction injuries. This subtype 2A fracture is caused predominantly by a flexion force that is imparted on the C2 vertebra and leads to a more unstable injury pattern.[18,74,75]

Type 3 injuries are flexion compression injuries often associated with severe neurologic injury with distraction of the C2–C3 disc resulting in complete dislocation with facet dislocation. The neural arch is completely free of the damage of the posterior capsules.[18,74,75]

Imaging
Standard plain films, including upright cervical spine films, can demonstrate hangman fracture patterns. Patients sustaining high-energy trauma should undergo further evaluation with CT and potentially CT angiogram, as vertebral artery injury must be ruled out.[34] Atypical hangman fractures are better identified with a CT scan. Serial upright imaging to determine progressive anterolisthesis of the C2-3 level may guide surgical treatment. MRI has potential for identifying disc and ligamentous disruption of types 2 or 3 hangman fractures and in patients presenting with a spinal cord injury.[76]

Nonoperative Management

Evaluation of hangman fractures is done with upright x-rays in order to determine stable extension types 1 and 2 fractures which can be treated with external immobilization, such as a hard collar or halo vest. Atypical hangman variance (type 1A), great vigilance, and close clinical observation are paramount as nonoperative treatment is given due to the potential neurologic compressions fracture pattern. In one cohort, 3% of the atypical hangman fractures in the series required surgical fixation.[75,77]

Operative Management

Surgical treatment of hangman types 2A and 3 fractures is generally reserved, constituting a greater treatment challenge due to their atypical fracture orientation and the amount of displacement and associated ligamentous injury. Unstable type 1A also may require operative intervention if it fails trial nonoperative management. It is important to avoid distraction in type 2a injuries which will accentuate the kyphotic deformity.[34]

Type 2 significant kyphotic angulation and translation greater than 3 mm can be treated with an anterior cervical discectomy and fusion (ACDF) at C2–3. Type 2A severe angulation without translation requires surgical intervention, while type 3 with severe angulation displacement with the facet dislocation requires posterior fixation and/or fusion. Care should be taken to avoid traction of type 2A, especially in halo vest treatment, as it accentuates the deformity. The type of fixation may depend on the extent of facet dislocation; either posterior C1–3 instrumentation and fusion versus ACDF C2–3, and the necessary incorporation of the atlas segment from posterior is limited unless a direct pars fracture with internal fixation screws is feasible. Anterior C2–3 fixation with an ACDF offers preservation of the atlantoaxial motion.[6,18,75]

Outcomes and Associated Injuries

A cohort of hangman fractures in all subtypes were analyzed, with 30% managed operatively. The minimum displacement of operative fractures was 3.7 mm and greater than 11° of angulation based on surgeon discretion. In this cohort, there was a reported 82% union rate with operative and nonoperative, with no significant difference in nonunion rate.[74] However, in subsequent studies a reduced chance of nonunion was reported in patients treated surgically, with a union rate of 99.3%. There was no significant difference in mortality between patients treated surgically or nonsurgically. Both authors advocate surgery of unstable types 2, 2A, and 3 fractures.[78]

In a comparison of ACDF versus posterior fixation at C2–3 for treatment of unstable hangman fractures, the results showed statistically significant differences in surgical time, operative blood loss, pain-free status postsurgery, and hospital stay between the 2 groups. There were no statistically significant differences in clinical or radiologic outcomes between the surgical types at final follow-up, and no differences in the rates of fusion.[77] When performed, there was no difference in fusion rates, complications, mortality, and/or treatment failure with patients undergoing a ACDF versus posterior fixation or combined.[78]

SURGICAL FIXATION OF CRANIOCERVICAL INJURIES

Anesthetic Principles

Positioning

The basic recommendation in positioning is to seek a neutral craniocervical alignment and avoid the temptation to fix the CCJ in a forward-flexed position that would induce compensatory hyperlordosis of the cervical spine.[4] The nonphysiologic relationship of the head to the CCJ after fusion, with a change greater than 10° compared with preoperative neutral position, can result in a myriad of complications including: dysphagia, dyspnea, loss of horizontal gaze, and acceleration of adjacent segment degeneration caudal to the stabilization construct.[2] When positioning the head, in order to determine accurate fusion of the CCJ, the angle formed between the McGregor line and the inferior endplate of C2, normal angles range from 10° to 20°. This is very difficult to visualize with intraoperative fluoroscopic guidance and was found to be variable among individuals of different ages, and a consistent value to target was not suggested. Therefore, others have advocated for easily reproducible evaluation. In one study, a simpler way to ensure the proper alignment of the head and CCJ during fusion was using the angle between the posterior of the mandible with the anterior cortex of C2 (**Fig. 5**).[1,2] Intraoperative reverse Trendelenburg position should be avoided as it causes a distraction force between the cranium and cervical spine.[7]

Neuromonitoring

Approach and technique. The goals of surgical fixation in CCJ trauma include: internal fixation should only be involved in the unstable

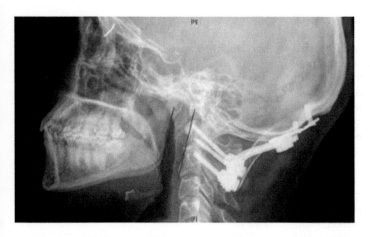

Fig. 5. Demonstration of the parallel lines of the posterior mandible and the anterior body of C2 angle. (*From* Cheng CW, Bellabarba C, Bransford RJ. Craniocervical Injuries: Atlas Fractures, Atlanto-Occipital Injuries, and Atlantoaxial Injuries. SKELETAL TRAUMA: Basic science, management, and reconstruction, 2 vol. set. ELSEVIER; 2019; with permission.)

segments; internal fixation does not require access to the vertebral canal or intracranial space; decompression can be performed simultaneously while performing fixation; and providing sufficient mechanical stability with no additional need for external fixation.[36] It is important to remember that a specific injury entity must be seen in the context of its possible association with upper cervical injuries. Combination injuries are not uncommon and a detailed assessment of the entire spine as a functional unit is required with subsequent comprehensive treatment to optimize the result.[6]

A comparison bone graft study reported no cases of pseudoarthrosis found in operatively managed patients with allograft extenders versus local autograft. Modern rigid craniocervical fusion techniques using screw and rod constructs with structural grafts have almost resolved the issue of pseudoarthrosis and loss of fixation associated with wire constructs.[1]

For the approach for instrumentation at the CCJ, place the head in a neutral position, with the Mayfield head holder with the chin tucked to open up the CCJ to aid with access. Gentle cervical traction is used to aid with the reduction of the lateral mass if atlas fractures are present, but care should be taken to not overdistract in the setting of CCD. It is important to avoid venous plexus between the poster ring of C1 in the laminate of C2. Electrocautery can be used to begin the subperiosteal exposure of the posterior ring of C1. As a more lateral exposure is performed, one must be careful to avoid injury to the venous plexus below and the vertebral artery above as the course is cranial to the atlas. The lamina of C2 should also be exposed until the lateral masses are reached.[55]

Occipital plating

The latest generation of fixation devices have eliminated the shortcomings of the previous generations of occipitocervical plates with modular connections between the occipital plate and cervical screws. Current constructs bridge the cervical spine fixation to an independently placed plate with locking screws into the occiput. Bridge plating the CCJ via contoured rods that connect to an independently placed occipital plate secured with locking screws is a newer technology that assists in fusion. The occipital plate can be applied to the midline of the occipital bone where the thick midline keel provides the greatest resistance to pull out with blunt tip locking screws placed. The thickest occipital portion located in the midline at the superior nuchal line was reported to measure up to 17.5 mm. Drilling above the level of the inion should be avoided to steer clear of the hardware prominence and possible injury to the transverse sinus or the confluences of the sagittal sinus with potentially fatal consequences to the patient. The technique for screw placement involves sequential drilling starting with an 8 mm stop and progressing by 2 mm increments to ensure bicortical fixation to the occiput but avoidance of the dural penetration and cerebrospinal fluid leak.[1,8,79]

Posterior occipital atlantoaxial fixation techniques have generally concluded that the presence of a transarticular screw or pedicle screw improves the stability of the construct provided by other constructs, such as posterior wiring.[4]

A structural tricortical bone graft can be placed between plates over the posterior occiput and straddled over the decorticated spinous process of the axis and atlas. Grafts are secured against the occiput in the C2 segment with a cable fixation to enhance the graft healing compressive effect.[16] Allograft extenders or a morselized autograft can be used also to fill the void surrounding the structural graft. In a recent review of 48 patients with operatively managed CCDs, there were no cases of pseudoarthrosis using structural graphs in concert with allograft extenders or local autograph.[7]

C1 screw options
Seeman introduced C1–2 transarticular screw stabilization in the late 1980s. This procedure provided immediate and superior fixation, especially in axial rotation and lateral bending, which were mechanically inferior with stand-alone posterior wiring. Transarticular screw placement, however, is technically demanding and anatomically cannot always safely be placed due to the necessary approach angle and the large medial vertebral artery channels at C2, hypoplastic C2 pars, and malalignment of the C1–2 intrinsic anatomy.[3,79] Careful evaluation of preoperative CT scans is important to evaluate the medial trajectory of the C1 lateral mass relative to the transverse foramen in the vertebral artery. It is critical to identify whether or not the patient has an arcuate foramen, or bony bridge, also known as "ponticulus posticus," covering the vertebral artery as it passes along the superior aspect of the posterior ridge of C1.[55]

Goel, Melcher, and Harms first described the placement of a C1 lateral mass screw. After C1 and C2 are adequately exposed, the sharp edge of a penfield can be used to continue the periosteal elevation along the inferior ridge of the C1 posterior ring and careful retraction of the C2 nerve root distally. The starting point for the screw is on the posterior aspect of the C1 lateral mass caudal to the prominence where the posterior arch meets the lateral mass. Exposure of the pars interarticularis of the C2 also helps serve as a general guide to the appropriate starting point. The drill is slowly advanced, utilizing the lateral fluoroscopic view to estimate the depth in the correct trajectory as needed. Radiographic studies have shown that the anterior cortex of the lateral mass becomes engaged when the screw tip lies an average of 6–7 mm posterior to the anterior tip of the arch of C1 lateral radiographs.[50,55] Depending on the manufacture of the polyaxial screw, approximately 10 mm is added to the screw length and addition of a smooth portion of the screw shaft in order to avoid C2 nerve root irritation; the most common length is

30 mm. It is imperative not to place a screw that is too long as the internal carotid artery and the hypoglossal nerve are located just anterior to the C1 cortex of the lateral mass. A recommended target on the lateral fluoroscopic is to aim just below the midpoint of the anterior C1 rings.[55] In these patients, it is key to protect the vertebral artery on the superior side. The complications associated with C1 lateral mass screw placement include, as with transarticular screws, injury to the vertebral artery, injury to the ICA, injury to the hypoglossal nerve, irritation of the C2 dorsal root ganglion, or medial penetration causing a dural tear or cord injury.[15,55,79]

Descriptive techniques prefer C1 screw starting points that are somewhat more cranial, only located at the junction of the posterior ring to the lateral mass. The starting point usually requires burring down the overhang edge of the posterior arch at the level of the lateral mass. This method allows for the screw to be placed further away from the C2 nerve root. The screw is directed in the sagittal plane toward the middle of the anterior margin of the C1 anterior ring on the lateral fluoroscopic view. A medial angulation of 0° to 10° is desirable to achieve optimal C1 lateral mass purchase, while avoiding a lateral course which may result in a vertebral artery or hypoglossal nerve injury.[8]

Despite C1 lateral mass screws being a documented safe technique, there are some instances where the patient's anatomy may not allow the placement of the screw. In that case, there are various other techniques that allow C1 instrumentation. A C1 hook or sublaminar wiring may be used instead. In comparison, studies between C1 hook versus sublaminar wire placement showed that there were no significant differences between the two groups in any outcome for patient-reported scores including the VASSNP, neck stiffness, patient satisfaction, or NDI. The C1 laminar hook was safer than subliminal wiring to reduce the risk of spinal cord and venous plexus injury, although no complications of either were demonstrated. No vertebral artery malformation, such as high riding of the vertebral artery, is possible with either of these techniques. Blood loss was less when the C1 hook was used in comparison to the sublaminar wire. The transarticular screw fixation technique was more effective in preventing lateral bending and axial rotation than the cable fixational technique, but less effective in preventing flexion and extension. The conclusion was found that the number of fixation points is associated with a significant increase in axial rotation in translation—confirming a biomechanical advantage to including as many C1–C2 fixation points as possible.[80] A comparison study was performed between C1–C2 transarticular screws with laminar hook comparison to C1 lateral mass screw with C2 pedicle screw. There were no complications related to the surgical approach or instrumentation in either group. Fusion rates were 100% for both groups. The neurologic status greatly improved in both groups with no difference in functional outcome scores between the two groups.[81] Clinical outcome studies comparing C1 laminar hook use instead of C1 lateral mass screws due to vertebral artery anatomy that will not allow C1 lateral mass type of fixation. C1 laminar hook can theoretically avoid vertebral artery injury and is less technically demanding. C1 laminar hooks reportedly achieved biomechanical stability similar to those achieved by C1 lateral mass screws with a C2 pedicle screw, although this is inferior to 3-point fixation systems, such as transarticular screw fixation with a C1 laminar hook. The only differences between the gold standard and comparison group were reduced operative times and blood loss. This technique has strict indications, which means that a C1 lateral mass screw accompanied with a C2 pedicle screw should be the primary technique and should only be used when the vertebral artery does not allow instrumentation.[82]

C2 screw options

Techniques used for posterior C2 fixation include pedicle screw fixation, transarticular screw fixation, pars interarticularis fixation, and translaminar screw fixation. A safety study determining C2 screw safe placement, defined as safe or completely within bone, showed that less than half the diameter of the screw violates the surrounding cortex with a clear violation of the transverse foramen or spinal canal. Within the first cohort of placed screws, 98% to 100% were accurately placed between transarticular, laminar, and pars screws. Of the screws that were unacceptably placed, 2 were placed medially and 6 were encroaching on the vertebral foramen. One patient had a VA occlusion and another had a dissection.[83] Particular attention needs to be paid to the course of the vertebral arteries, the dimensions of the C2 lateral masses, and their corresponding trajectories. The sizes of the C2 pedicles are visualized on preoperative CT scans and/or MRI scans.[79]

Anatomic characteristics that may limit the placement of the C2 screws include large,

immediately located vertebral arteries, hypoplastic axis pars, inability to obtain an anatomic reduction of the atlantoaxial joint, and substantial thoracic kyphosis that precludes the necessary angle approach. The C2 translaminar technique is a described method in which screws are placed in the lamina of C2 in a crossed trajectory. The translaminar C2 screw technique is a viable option for fixation, particularly in patients with unsuitable anatomy for pars or pedicle screws. This technique may also be used in patients with unilateral vertebral artery injury secondary to trauma or iatrogenic injury.[9] More descriptive case techniques to avoid iatrogenic vertebral artery injury involve the use of a penfield dissector to properly mobilize the vertebral artery inferior to the pathway and pave the way for the C2 pedicle screw placement.[84]

There is a slightly more medial trajectory to follow the angle of the C2 pedicle and enter the body, thus staying well away from the vertebral artery foramen. In conclusion, C2 pars screws follow the identical trajectory of C2 pedicle screws, but are much shorter and used as an alternative in patients with anatomy deemed too dangerous to attempt pedicle screws or transarticular screws. Usually, pars screws will have about a 20° to 25° medial trajectory compared to the 10° medial trajectory utilized with the transarticular screws.[79]

In the event that there is a vertebral artery injury intraoperatively, completion of the intended surgery then subsequent interventional angiography with an attempt at stenting the injury site or embolization is recommended to minimize local bleeding and to diminish the risk of embolic stroke or emergence of an AV fistula.[3] The treatment of asymptomatic vascular injuries in this region remains controversial, with proponents for observation versus aspirin or anticoagulation therapy.[34]

SUMMARY

Injuries to the CCJ are complex, involving both intricate bony and ligamentous connections. They display a wide spectrum of occult versus high-energy fractures. Careful evaluation including helical CT and MRI of the CCJ allows for classification of these injuries. Approaching the CCJ with carefully placed screws surrounding difficult anatomy is the main challenge to achieving stability. The goals of surgical fixation include internal fixation only of the involved unstable segments that do not require access to the vertebral canal or intracranial space with simultaneous decompression, while performing fixation and providing sufficient mechanical stability with no additional need for external fixation.

CLINICS CARE POINTS

- A delay in the diagnosis of craniocervical dissociation and the potential for serious secondary neurologic deterioration with potentially life-threatening injuries. The outcome of survivors is therefore highly dependent on the type and severity of the associated injuries, the severity of the neurologic injury, and the timeliness with which the diagnosis of craniocervical dissociation is recognized and thus operatively stabilized.

- Clearance of cervical spine injuries is a process. CCJ injuries should be suspected in patients sustaining high-energy trauma. First-line evaluation with helical CT of the entire spine, with sagittal and coronal reformatted views must be obtained in order to clear the patient's CCJ. The second phase involves a secondary review of all spine imaging studies after an attempted clinical reevaluation.

- The susceptibility of CCJ to injury is related to the large lever arm and mass of the cranium, combined with the relative freedom of movement of the subaxial spine. Secondarily, the reliance on ligamentous structures rather than intrinsic bony stability for the maintenance of CCJ alignment also allows for a higher rate of injury

- Within CCJ injuries is a spectrum of instability, ranging from isolated nondisplaced occipital condyle fractures treated nonoperatively to highly unstable injuries with severely distracted craniocervical dissociation.

- Approaching the craniocervical junction with carefully placed screws surrounding difficult anatomy is the main challenge in achieving stability.

DISCLOSURE

The authors have nothing to disclose.

REFERENCES

1. Bransford R, Manoso M, Bellabarba C. Occipital-cervical spine injuries. In: Browner B, Jupiter J, editors. Skeletal trauma. 5th edition. Philadelphia: Elsevier; 2014. p. 813–28.

2. Bellabarba C, Karim F, Tavolaro C, et al. The mandible-C2 angle: a new radiographic assessment of occipitocervical alignment. Spine J 2021; 21(1):105–13.

3. Chapman J, Patt J, Bransford R. Odontoid fractures. In: Benzel EC, editor. The cervical spine. 5th edition. Philadelphia, PA: Lippincott Williams & Wilkins; 2012.

4. Madrazo I, Zamorano C, Bransford R, et al. Craniocervical disruption: injuries of the occiput-C1-C2 region. In: Vaccarro A, Fehlings M, Dvorak M, editors. Spine and spinal cord trauma: evidence-based management. New York, NY: Thieme; 2010. p. 211–28.

5. Hall GC, Kinsman MJ, Nazar RG, et al. Atlanto-occipital dislocation. World J Orthop 2015;6(2): 236–43.

6. Chapman J, Richard R. Cervical spine trauma. Orthopaedic knowledge update 10. Rosemont, IL: AAOS Publications; 2011.

7. Bellabarba C, Bransford R, Chapman J. Occipitocervical and upper cervical spine fractures. In: Shen F, Samartzis D, Fessler RG, editors. The cervical spine. Philadelphia: Elsevier; 2014. p. 167–83.

8. Cheng CW, Bellabarba C, Bransford RJ. Craniocervcal injuries: atlas fractures, atlanto-occipital injuries, and atlantoaxial injuries. SKELETAL TRAUMA: basic science, management, and reconstruction, vol. 2. Philadelphia, PA: ELSEVIER; 2019.

9. Bransford RJ, Alton TB, Patel AR, et al. Upper cervical spine trauma. J Am Acad Orthop Surg 2014; 22(11):718–29.

10. Tavolaro C, Pulido H, Bransford R, et al. Traumatic Craniocervical Dissociation in Patients with Congenital Assimilation of the Atlas to the Occiput. Case Rep Orthop 2019;2019:2617379.

11. Shatsky JB, Alton TB, Bellabarba C, et al. Occult Cranial Cervical Dislocation: A Case Report and Brief Literature Review. Case Rep Orthop 2016; 2016:4930285.

12. Yin QS, Wang JH. Current Trends in Management of Atlantoaxial Dislocation. Orthop Surg 2015;7(3): 189–99.

13. Yang SY, Boniello AJ, Poorman CE, et al. A review of the diagnosis and treatment of atlantoaxial dislocations. Glob Spine J 2014;4(3):197–210.

14. Fiester P, Soule E, Natter P, et al. Tectorial membrane injury in adult and pediatric trauma patients: a retrospective review and proposed classification scheme. Emerg Radiol 2019;26(6):615–22.

15. Karamian BA, Campbell ST, Rinsky LA. Complete Atlantoaxial Dislocation After Odontoid Synchondrosis Fracture: A 2-Year Follow-up Study: A Case Report. JBJS Case Connect 2019;9(2):e0327.

16. Bransford RJ, Bellabarba C, Chapman JR. Cervicocranial Injuries. In: Albert T, Lee J, Lim M, editors. Cervical Spine Surgery Challenges. Diagnosis and

Management. New York, NY: Thieme; 2008. p. 172–82.

17. Radcliff KE, Ben-Galim P, Dreiangel N, et al. Comprehensive computed tomography assessment of the upper cervical anatomy: what is normal? Spine J 2010;10(3):219–29.

18. Alves OL, Pereira L, Kim SH, et al. Upper Cervical Spine Trauma: WFNS Spine Committee Recommendations. Neurospine 2020;17(4):723–36.

19. Wang L, Gu Y, Chen L, et al. Surgery for Chronic Traumatic Atlantoaxial Dislocation Associated With Myelopathy. Clin Spine Surg 2017;30(5): E640–7.

20. Souslian FG, Patel PD, Elsherif MA. Atlanto-occipital Dissociation in the Setting of Relatively Normal Radiologic Findings. World Neurosurg 2020;143: 405–11.

21. Kalani MA, Ratliff JK. Considering the diagnosis of occipitocervical dissociation. Spine J 2013;13(5): 520–2.

22. Ibrahim GM, Perrin RG. Traumatic craniocervical dissociation. Br J Neurosurg 2012;26(4):572–3.

23. Martinez-Del-Campo E, Kalb S, Soriano-Baron H, et al. Computed tomography parameters for atlantooccipital dislocation in adult patients: the occipital condyle-C1 interval. J Neurosurg Spine 2016; 24(4):535–45.

24. Gire JD, Roberto RF, Bobinski M, et al. The utility and accuracy of computed tomography in the diagnosis of occipitocervical dissociation. Spine J 2013; 13(5):510–9.

25. Abouelleil M, Siddique D, Dahdaleh NS. Failure of the Condyle-C1 Interval Method to Diagnose Atlanto-occipital Dislocation in the Presence of an Associated Atlanto-axial Dislocation: A Case Report. Cureus 2018;10(4):e2486.

26. Dahdaleh NS, Khanna R, Menezes AH, et al. The Application of the Revised Condyle-C1 Interval Method to Diagnose Traumatic Atlanto-occipital Dissociation in Adults. Glob Spine J 2016;6(6):529–34.

27. Smith P, Linscott LL, Vadivelu S, et al. Normal Development and Measurements of the Occipital Condyle-C1 Interval in Children and Young Adults. AJNR Am J Neuroradiol 2016;37(5):952–7.

28. Chaput C, Walgama J, Song J, et al. P85. Radiologic Criteria for Defining Atlantoaxial Dissociation (AAD) and Atlanto-Occipital Dissociation (AOD): The Reliability of CT Measurements and an Evaluation of the Effect of Age and Gende. Spine J 2009; 9(10). https://doi.org/10.1016/j.spinee.2009.08.344.

29. Chaput CD, Walgama J, Torres E, et al. Defining and detecting missed ligamentous injuries of the occipitocervical complex. Spine (Phila Pa 1976) 2011;36(9):709–14.

30. Goodwin CR, Iyer R, Abu-Bonsrah N, et al. Traumatic atlantooccipital dissociation. Spine J 2016; 16(3):e165–6.

31. Mendenhall SK, Sivaganesan A, Mistry A, et al. Traumatic atlantooccipital dislocation: comprehensive assessment of mortality, neurologic improvement, and patient-reported outcomes at a Level 1 trauma center over 15 years. Spine J 2015;15(11): 2385–95.

32. Dyas AR, Niemeier TE, McGwin G, et al. Ability of magnetic resonance imaging to accurately determine alar ligament integrity in patients with atlanto-occipital injuries. J Craniovertebr Junction Spine 2018;9(4):241–5.

33. Child Z, Rau D, Lee MJ, et al. The provocative radiographic traction test for diagnosing craniocervical dissociation: a cadaveric biomechanical study and reappraisal of the pathogenesis of instability. Spine J 2016;16(9):1116–23.

34. Chapman J, Bransford R. Upper cervical spine trauma. In: Devlin V, editor. Spine secrets plus. St. Louis, Missouri: Hanley and Belfus Publications; 2011.

35. Kasliwal MK, Fontes RB, Traynelis VC. Occipitocervical dissociation-incidence, evaluation, and treatment. Curr Rev Musculoskelet Med 2016;9(3):247–54.

36. Ji W, Xu X, Liu Q, et al. Anterior Atlantooccipital Transarticular Screw Fixation: A Cadaveric Study and Description of a Novel Technique. Spine (Phila Pa 1976) 2019;44(17):E1010–7.

37. Chaudhary N, Wang BH, Gurr KR, et al. A rare case of atlantooccipital dissociation in the context of occipitalization of the atlas, with a 2-year follow-up: case report. J Neurosurg Spine 2013;18(2): 189–93.

38. Cooper Z, Gross JA, Lacey JM, et al. Identifying survivors with traumatic craniocervical dissociation: a retrospective study. J Surg Res 2010;160(1):3–8.

39. Schellenberg M, Anderson GA, Owattanapanich N, et al. Radiologic predictors of in-hospital mortality after traumatic craniocervical dissociation. J Trauma Acute Care Surg 2020;89(3):565–9.

40. Filiberto DM, Sharpe JP, Croce MA, et al. Traumatic atlanto-occipital dissociation: No longer a death sentence. Surgery 2018;164(3):500–3.

41. Chaput CD, Torres E, Davis M, et al. Survival of atlanto-occipital dissociation correlates with atlanto-occipital distraction, injury severity score, and neurologic status. J Trauma 2011;71(2):393–5.

42. Schellenberg M, Inaba K, Cheng V, et al. Independent predictors of survival after traumatic atlantooccipital dissociation. J Trauma Acute Care Surg 2018;85(2):375–9.

43. Vilela MD, Kim LJ, Bellabarba C, et al. Blunt cerebrovascular injuries in association with craniocervical distraction injuries: a retrospective review of consecutive cases. Spine J 2015;15(3):499–505.

44. Desai R, Kinon MD, Loriaux DB, et al. Traumatic atlanto-occipital dissociation presenting as locked-in syndrome. J Clin Neurosci 2015;22(12):1985–7.

45. Robles LA, Mundis GM, Cuevas-Solorzano A. Atlanto-Occipital Rotatory Dislocation: A Case Report and Systematic Review. World Neurosurg 2018;110:106–14.

46. Wu TL, Jia JY, Chen WC, et al. Nontraumatic posterior atlantooccipital dislocation associated with atlantoaxial instability. Eur Spine J 2015;24(Suppl 4):S619–22.

47. Chang DG, Park JB, Song KJ, et al. Traumatic Atlanto-occipital dislocation: analysis of 15 survival cases with emphasis on associated upper cervical spine injuries. Spine (Phila Pa 1976) 2020;45(13):884–94.

48. Cloney M, Kim H, Riestenberg R, et al. Risk Factors for Transverse Ligament Disruption and Vertebral Artery Injury Following an Atlas Fracture. World Neurosurg 2021;146:e1345–50.

49. Kandziora F, Chapman JR, Vaccaro AR, et al. Atlas Fractures and Atlas Osteosynthesis: A Comprehensive Narrative Review. J Orthop Trauma 2017; 31(Suppl 4):S81–9.

50. Li L, Teng H, Pan J, et al. Direct posterior c1 lateral mass screws compression reduction and osteosynthesis in the treatment of unstable jefferson fractures. Spine (Phila Pa 1976) 2011;36(15):E1046–51.

51. Bransford R, Falicov A, Nguyen Q, et al. Unilateral C-1 lateral mass sagittal split fracture: an unstable Jefferson fracture variant. J Neurosurg Spine 2009;10(5):466–73.

52. Liu P, Zhu J, Wang Z, et al. Rule of Spence" and Dickman's Classification of Transverse Atlantal Ligament Injury Revisited: Discrepancy of Prediction on Atlantoaxial Stability Based on Clinical Outcome of Nonoperative Treatment for Atlas Fractures. Spine (Phila Pa 1976) 2019;44(5):E306–14.

53. Lin P, Chuang TC, Baker JF. C1:C2 ratio is a potential tool assessing atlas fracture displacement and transverse ligament injury. J Craniovertebr Junction Spine 2019;10(3):139–44.

54. Fiedler N, Spiegl UJA, Jarvers JS, et al. Epidemiology and management of atlas fractures. Eur Spine J 2020;29(10):2477–83.

55. Pittman J, Bransford R. C1-Ring osteosynthesis for unstable jefferson, burst fractures. In: Koller H, Robinson Y, editors. Cervical spine surgery: standard and advanced techniques. Europe: CSRS; 2019. p. 201–6.

56. Shatsky J, Bellabarba C, Nguyen Q, et al. A retrospective review of fixation of C1 ring fractures–does the transverse atlantal ligament (TAL) really matter? Spine J 2016;16(3):372–9.

57. Hu Y, Yuan ZS, Kepler CK, et al. Comparison of occipitocervical and atlantoaxial fusion in treatment of unstable Jefferson fractures. Indian J Orthop 2017;51(1):28–35.

58. Guo W, Lin Y, Huang J, et al. Treatment strategy of unstable atlas fracture: A retrospective study of 21 patients. Medicine (Baltimore) 2020;99(18):e20153.

59. Ghailane S, Alsofyani MA, Pointillart V, et al. Traumatic posterior Atlanto-axial dislocation: case report of an atypical C1-C2 dislocation with an anterior arch fracture of C1. BMC Musculoskelet Disord 2019;20(1):612.

60. Nowell M, Nelson R. Traumatic posterior atlantoaxial dislocation with associated C1 Jefferson fracture and bilateral vertebral artery occlusion without odontoid process fracture or neurological deficit. Eur Spine J 2019;28(Suppl 2):9–12.

61. Deepak AN, Salunke P, Sahoo SK, et al. Revisiting the differences between irreducible and reducible atlantoaxial dislocation in the era of direct posterior approach and C1-2 joint manipulation. J Neurosurg Spine 2017;26(3):331–40.

62. Meyer C, Eysel P, Stein G. Traumatic Atlantoaxial and Fracture-Related Dislocation. Biomed Res Int 2019;2019:5297950.

63. Hu D, Yang X, Wang J. Traumatic Posterior Atlantoaxial Dislocation Without Fracture of Odontoid Process: A Case Report and Systematic Analysis of 19 Cases. J Orthop Trauma 2015;29(9):e342–5.

64. Song R, Fan D, Wu H, et al. Management of Unusual Atlantoaxial Dislocation. Spine (Phila Pa 1976) 2017;42(8):573–7.

65. Pissonnier ML, Lazennec JY, Renoux J, et al. Trauma of the upper cervical spine: focus on vertical atlantoaxial dislocation. Eur Spine J 2013; 22(10):2167–75.

66. Salunke P, Sahoo SK, Savardekar A, et al. Factors influencing feasibility of direct posterior reduction in irreducible traumatic atlantoaxial dislocation secondary to isolated odontoid fracture. Br J Neurosurg 2015;29(4):513–9.

67. Moreau PE, Nguyen V, Atallah A, et al. Traumatic atlantoaxial dislocation with odontoid fracture: A case report. Orthop Traumatol Surg Res 2012;98(5):613–7.

68. Tian NF, Xu HZ, Wu YS, et al. Traumatic atlantoaxial dislocation with type II odontoid fracture. Spine J 2014;14(6):1067–9.

69. Chaudhary SB, Martinez M, Shah NP, et al. Traumatic atlantoaxial dislocation with Hangman fracture. Spine J 2015;15(4):e15–8.

70. Rizvi SAM, Helseth E, Harr ME, et al. Management and long-term outcome of type II acute odontoid fractures: a population-based consecutive series of 282 patients. Spine J 2021;21(4):627–37.

71. Goz V, Spiker WR, Lawrence B, et al. Odontoid Fractures: A Critical Analysis Review. JBJS Rev 2019;7(8):e1.

72. Carvalho AD, Figueiredo J, Schroeder GD, et al. Odontoid Fractures: A Critical Review of Current Management and Future Directions. Clin Spine Surg 2019;32(8):313–23.

73. Reinhold M, Bellabarba C, Bransford R, et al. Radiographic analysis of type II odontoid fractures in a geriatric patient population: description and

pathomechanism of the "Geier"-deformity. Eur Spine J 2011;20(11):1928–39.

74. Prost S, Barrey C, Blondel B, et al. Hangman's fracture: Management strategy and healing rate in a prospective multi-centre observational study of 34 patients. Orthop Traumatol Surg Res 2019;105(4): 703–7.

75. Turtle J, Kantor A, Spina NT, et al. Hangman's Fracture. Clin Spine Surg 2020;33(9):345–54.

76. Al-Mahfoudh R, Beagrie C, Woolley E, et al. Management of Typical and Atypical Hangman's Fractures. Glob Spine J 2016;6(3):248–56.

77. Patel JYK, Kundnani VG, Kuriya S, et al. Unstable Hangman's fracture: Anterior or posterior surgery? J Craniovertebr Junction Spine 2019; 10(4):210–5.

78. Murphy H, Schroeder GD, Shi WJ, et al. Management of Hangman's Fractures: A Systematic Review. J Orthop Trauma 2017;31(Suppl 4):S90–5.

79. Bransford R, Michael J. Contemporary Fixation Techniques in Posterior Cervical Spine Surgery. Contemp Spine Surg 2009;10(7):1–6.

80. Zhao W, Wu Y, Hu W, et al. Comparison of Two Posterior Three-Point Fixation Techniques for Treating Reducible Atlantoaxial Dislocation. Spine (Phila Pa 1976) 2019;44(1):E60–6.

81. Ni B, Zhao W, Guo Q, et al. Comparison of outcomes BETWEEN c1-c2 Screw-Hook fixation AND C1-C2 screw-rod fixation for Treating Reducible Atlantoaxial Dislocation. Spine 2017;42(20):1587–93.

82. Han Z, Yang J, Chen Q, et al. C2 Pedicle Screws Combined With C1 Laminar Hooks for Reducible Atlantoaxial Dislocation: An Ideal Salvage Technique for C1-C2 Pedicle Screws. Oper Neurosurg (Hagerstown) 2020;19(2):150–6.

83. Bransford RJ, Russo AJ, Freeborn M, et al. Posterior C2 instrumentation: accuracy and complications associated with four techniques. Spine (Phila Pa 1976) 2011;36(14):E936–43.

84. Guo Q, Zhou X, Guo X, et al. C2 partial transpedicular screw technique for atlantoaxial dislocation with high-riding vertebral artery: A technique note with case series. Clin Neurol Neurosurg 2021;200: 106403.

Thoracolumbar Spine Trauma

William Hunter Waddell, MD, Rishabh Gupta, BA, Byron Fitzgerald Stephens II, MD*

KEYWORDS
• Thoracolumbar spine trauma • Posterior ligamentous complex • Computed tomography

KEY POINTS
• The thoracolumbar region has a unique anatomy which influences both the extent and management of trauma.
• Thoracolumbar trauma is evaluated using the McAffee classification, Dennis classification, Allen/Ferguson scale, Thoracolumbar Injury Classification and Severity Scale (TLICS), and AO thoracolumbar fracture classification.
• Patients should acquire imaging, undergo the ATLS primary survey as well as a motor/sensory/reflex exam to determine extent of neurologic damage.
• Nonoperative management includes bracing and physical therapy. Operative management is most commonly done via a posterior approach.
• Medications and bracing are commonly used to manage osteoporotic vertebral fractures. Vertebroplasty is not recommended by AAOS guidelines while kyphoplasty is a potential option.

INTRODUCTION/HISTORY/DEFINITIONS/BACKGROUND

An estimated 75% to 90% of spine fractures involve the thoracolumbar region, 26% of which result in neurologic injury.[1,2] The prevalence and clinical implications of thoracolumbar spine trauma makes it particularly important for clinicians to understand optimal treatment strategies for each injury pattern.

Anatomy of the Thoracolumbar Spine
The thoracolumbar spine consists of the thoracic (T2-10), thoracolumbar junction (T11-L2), and lumbosacral (L3-S1) regions. The thoracic region is kyphotic, typically between 20 to 50°.[3] Kyphosis predisposes the posterior tension band to disruption and the anterior vertebral bodies to compression forces. The thoracic spine's relatively narrow spinal canal also increases the spinal cord's injury risk.[4] In spite of these risks, less than a quarter of all thoracolumbar injuries are in the thoracic region due to the stabilization provided by the rib cage and coronal orientation of the facets.[5,6] In contrast, the thoracolumbar junction (T11-L1) is the most commonly injured region of the thoracolumbar spine.[5] This is primarily due to the increased biomechanical stress in the region as a result of it being a transitional zone between the kyphotic, rigid thoracic spine and the lordotic lumbar spine.[6] This can make non-operative management somewhat difficult.

The facet joints' sagittal orientation makes the lumbosacral region particularly mobile. The 40 to 60° of lordosis shifts the center of gravity posteriorly and increases the tensile forces across the vertebral bodies and compressive forces across the facet joints.[7] This minimizes kyphotic forces and kyphotic misalignment during traumatic injury and makes the region more inherently stable and amenable to non-operative treatment. Additionally, the lumbosacral region contains the cauda equina, a portion of the central nervous system better able to recover compared to the spinal cord or conus medullaris.[8]

Department of Orthopedics, Vanderbilt University Medical Center, Suite 4200, 1215 21st Avenue South, Nashville, TN 37212, USA
* Corresponding author.
E-mail address: byron.stephens@vumc.org

Orthop Clin N Am 52 (2021) 481–489
https://doi.org/10.1016/j.ocl.2021.05.014
0030-5898/21/© 2021 Elsevier Inc. All rights reserved.

There are additional anatomic considerations to consider when evaluating the thoracolumbar spine. Pedicle diameter is narrowest at T4 and increases cranially and caudally from here.[9,10] In regard to soft tissue, the posterior ligamentous complex (PLC) is critical. The PLC extends throughout the thoracolumbar spine and includes the facet joint capsules, interspinous ligaments, supraspinous ligaments, and ligamentum flavum. The posterior tension band includes the PLC as well as posterior osseous elements. Injury to the posterior tension band can result in an unstable injury.[11]

Mechanism of Traumatic Thoracolumbar Injuries

Many forces contribute to thoracolumbar trauma, including distraction, flexion, extension, shear, and translational/rotation. 65% of all traumatic thoracolumbar spine injuries are due to motor vehicle accidents and falls.[6] It is important to note that traumatic thoracolumbar injuries are also associated with abdominal injuries. Chapman and colleagues[12] found approximately 30% of patients with flexion-distraction injuries have concomitant intraabdominal injuries.

Classification of Traumatic Thoracolumbar Injuries

An unstable spine cannot withstand a normal load without causing deformity, pain, or neurologic injuries. Assessing spine stability is important when deciding between operative and non-operative treatment. Many classification systems and treatment algorithms are available to help determine the appropriate treatment plan.

The McAffee classification uses CT imaging to divide injuries into six categories: wedge-compression, stable burst, unstable burst, Chance, flexion-distraction, and translational injuries.[13] The Denis classification system divides injuries into compression fractures, burst fractures, flexion-distraction injuries (including Chance fractures), and fracture-dislocations. Denis also classified injuries based on three columns: the anterior column (anterior longitudinal ligament, anterior portion of the vertebral body/disk), the middle column (posterior half of vertebral body/disk, posterior longitudinal ligament), and the posterior column (neural arch, facets, posterior ligament complex). At least two columns must be affected for an injury to considered unstable.[14,15] Allen and Ferguson used forces of injury to categorize fracture types. Their categories include compressive-flexion, distractive flexion, lateral-

flexion, translational, torsional-flexion, vertical compression, and distractive-extension features.[16,17] Vacarro and colleagues developed the Thoracolumbar Injury Classification and Severity Scale (TLICS). TLICS sums three values representing injury morphology (1 = compression, 2 = burst, 3 = translational/rotations, 4 = distraction), neurologic status (0 = intact, 2 = nerve root injury, 2 = complete cord injury, 3 = incomplete cord injury, 3 = cauda equina injury), and the integrity of the PLC (0 = intact, 2 = suspected/indeterminate, 3 = injured). TLICS scores below four are considered stable and need nonoperative management, four is left to surgeon's discretion, and above four is an unstable injury requiring operative management.[18,19]

More recent is the AO thoracolumbar fracture classification. Here, traumatic injuries are assigned to one of three categories. Type A injuries are compression injuries and are subdivided as follows:

- A0 - Clinically insignificant injuries (ie, spinous or transverse process injuries).
- A1 - Wedge compression or impaction fractures involving one endplate but where the posterior vertebral body wall remains unaffected
- A2 – Involvement of both endplates but not the posterior vertebral wall
- A3 - Single endplate injury involving posterior vertebral body injury (incomplete burst fractures)
- A4 - Fractures of both endplates and the posterior vertebral body (burst fractures)

Type B injuries are distraction injuries where the anterior or posterior tension band fails but does not cause translational displacement. Type B injuries have a few subclassifications:

- B1 - Chance fractures (complete failure along a transverse plane from the posterior tension band through the vertebra)
- B2 - Flexion-distraction injuries involving failure of anterior elements in flexion and posterior elements fail in tension
- B3 – Hyperextension injuries typically resulting in failure of the anterior tension band (often due to ankylosing spondylitis or diffuse idiopathic skeletal hyperostosis)

Type C injuries involve translocation/dislocation resulting from failure of all three spinal columns. Surrounding tissue and stabilizers are often significantly damaged and these fractures are universally unstable.[20,21]

DISCUSSION

Imaging

Anteroposterior and lateral radiographs are routinely used to analyze thoracolumbar injuries. First, anteroposterior imaging should be examined to identify discontinuities in the pedicles, vertebral bodies, and spinous processes. Second, increased interpedicular and interspinous distance should be noted as they indicate a burst fracture and posterior tension band injury respectively. Third, the vertebral body edges and spinal canal (anterior vertebral body line, posterior vertebral body line, and spinolaminar line) should appear as continuous lines. Fourth, vertebral discs lacking continuous edges or are unexpectedly asymmetric hint at possible anterior longitudinal ligament (ALL) and/or posterior longitudinal ligament (PLL) failure. Finally, radiographs can determine the height and angular deformation of the vertebral bodies. A 50% or greater loss in the vertebral body height, more than 20° kyphotic angle, or larger than 3.5 mm of translation often indicate of an unstable injury.[22]

Most centers use computed tomography (CT) scans for initial screening of traumatic thoracolumbar injuries due to their high resolution.[23–25] CT scans allow for detection of subtle fractures, the degree of fragmentation, and the presence of osseous matter in the spinal canal. CT scans are particularly useful in differentiating compression and burst fractures and other features such as facet widening. Additionally, many trauma patients already receive a CT scans to assess damage in other anatomic structures making it more efficient for spine surgeons to examine.

Magnetic Resonance Imaging (MRI) allows clinicians to view soft tissue (PLC, ALL, PLL, discs), the neural elements, and fluid (epidural hematoma, cerebrospinal fluid, prevertebral edema).[26] It is recommended that MRIs be used alongside CT scans when evaluating the spinal canal, spinal cord, posterior tension band, and in cases where the neurologic examination does not correlate with CT findings.[19,27] Drawbacks of MRI imaging include the relatively long time to acquire images, high cost, and lack of high-resolution pictures of osseous structures.[28,29]

Evaluating Traumatic Thoracolumbar Injuries

Trauma patients should first be subject to the ATLS primary survey to assesses their airway, breathing, circulation, and neurologic status. Throughout standard evaluation of traumatic patients, spinal precautions are necessary. This includes keeping patients on a flat spine board and having them wear a cervical collar.[30,31]

A more thorough spine examination can be done during the ATLS secondary survey. Patients should be log rolled to gain visual access to the back and neck. One person should stabilize the head and one more should stabilize the torso to ensure minimal spine movement. The spine should then be thoroughly inspected. This includes looking for soft tissue injuries, palpating for tenderness, step offs, and/or ligament injury, and the presence of internal degloving injuries.[30]

A thorough neurologic examination is also necessary. Motor and sensory function can be tested by assigning each muscle group a score from five to zero:

- 5 – patient can resist through their entire range of motion
- 4 – patient can partially resist through their entire range of motion
- 3 – patient can complete a full range of motion against gravity but not added resistance
- 2 - patient cannot complete a full range of motion independently but can when effects of gravity are removed
- 1 - contraction of muscle group but no movement
- 0 - complete absence of function

Assessing anal sphincter tone is important. The sensory examination should be done in a dermatomal pattern and should test both point pressure and a gentle touch. Sensory testing around the perianal area is also important as it can be the sole indication of an incomplete SCI. We recommend using a standardized form when evaluating patients with traumatic thoracolumbar injury, such as the International Standards for Neurologic Classification of Spinal Cord Injury (ISNCSCI) form.[32]

Following a motor and sensory examination, a patient's reflexes can be tested. Hyporeflexia and hyperreflexia can indicate different pathology. Hyperreflexia may not be present in the period immediately following trauma even if there is injury of the upper motor neurons. The absence of the bulbocavernosus reflex arc can indicate spinal shock.[30,33] This involves stimulating the penis/clitoris (usually by tugging gently on the foley catheter) and examining the presence of simultaneous, involuntary anal contraction. Injures to the conus medullaris and cauda equina commonly cause prolonged loss of the bulbocavernosus reflex.

The ASIA motor score evaluates 20 muscle groups using the mentioned 0 to 5 motor scale. For this scale, the lowest functional spine level is defined as the most caudal level with intact sensation and at least 3/5 (antigravity) strength. The five AIS grades are:

1. A – complete spinal cord injury; no motor or sensory function below lowest functional spine level
2. B –incomplete spinal cord injury; preserved sensation but no motor function below lowest functional spine level
3. C –incomplete spinal cord injury; preserved sensation along with 50% of key muscle groups caudal to lowest functional spine level receiving a motor grade of 3/5 or less
4. D –incomplete spinal cord injury; preserved sensation along with 50% of key muscle groups caudal to lowest functional spine level receiving a motor grade of 3/5 or greater
5. E – normal neurologic function

The presence of incomplete or complete SCI can be determined by examining for sacral sparing or perianal sensations. The presence of either indicates an incomplete injury and has enormous implications on prognosis.[33]

Non-operative Treatment for Thoracolumbar Fractures

Thoracolumbar trauma with spinal stability, preserved neurologic function, and no significant deformity typically receive non-operative treatment.[34–37] Bracing is commonly utilized to limit motion across injured segments. That said, its efficacy is questionable.[38,39] In some studies, bracing reduces pain immediately following traumatic injury, which is a reasonable indication for its utilization. A thoracolumbar orthosis (TLSO) or Jewett brace can be used for injuries between T7 and L3, cervicothoracic orthosis (CTO) is used for injuries T6 and cephalad, and hip-thoracolumbosacral orthosis (HTLSO, also referred to as an LSO or TLSO with a thigh cuff) is used for injuries below L3. Upright radiographs of braced patients should be taken to ensure no spinal instability is present during normal physiologic loads. The prescribed time to wear a brace ranges from 6 to 12 weeks. The brace is removed when there is both radiographic evidence and clinical evidence of improvement. When the brace is removed, flexion and extension x-rays should be done to ensure spine stability. Physical therapy should follow brace removal.

Operative Treatment for Thoracolumbar Fractures

Neurologic deficits and/or mechanically unstable fractures require operative treatment to minimize secondary damage from ischemia and the inflammatory cascade.

The efficacy and timing for mean arterial pressure (MAP) goals in the setting of neurologic injury is controversial. Some preclinical data supports MAP goals.[40] Our institution has compromised on 48 hours postoperatively as the time allowed for MAP goals (typically >85 mm Hg) for SCI. The use of steroids is also highly debated. The National Acute Spinal Cord Injury Study (NASCIS) determined that a 30 mg/kg dose of IV methylprednisone followed by a 5.4 mg/kg/h steady infusion for an additional 23 hour, if given within 3 hours of the injury, resulted in improved long term neurologic outcomes.[41–43] The AO Spine North America guidelines noted a paucity of evidence for or against steroid administration within 8 hours of a spinal cord injury.[44] When considered with associated risks, steroids should be used sparingly.

Timing of surgery is important when evaluating patients with operative thoracolumbar injuries; however, current clinical understanding is limited. The Surgical Timing in Acute Spinal Cord Injury Study (STASCIS) demonstrated that decompression of cervical injuries within 24 hours of an SCI lead to an average two grade improvement in AIS scores at 6-month[45] It's unknown whether this translates to thoracolumbar trauma. Bellabarba and colleagues[46] found that early stabilization of thoracic fractures decreased ventilator dependence, ICU/hospital days, and respiratory morbidity, but only resulted in a decreased number of hospital days in early stabilization of lumbar fractures. The lack of convincing evidence makes it difficult to provide firm recommendations on this topic.

Thoracolumbar spine injuries are most commonly addressed through a posterior approach as it allows for neurologic decompression, correction of associated deformity, and adequate fixation. An advantage of the posterior approach is that it does not require an access surgeon while, in contrast, an anterior approach often does. Additionally, patients with thoracolumbar spine trauma often have severe abdominal/chest trauma and doing posterior spine surgery avoids these regions. The posterior approach is extensile in nature and allows for longer and more stable fixation than the anterior approach. This allows the surgeon to manipulate the spine in reduction scenarios to restore normal alignment. Pedicle screw and rod fixation is the typical construct used for the posterior approach. It is important to mention that pedicle screws are more biomechanically stable compared to hooks or standalone anterior instrumentation. The improved strength and stability of pedicle screws and rods allow for shorter constructs, sometimes limiting instrumentation to one level above and below the injury (short segment fixation). This is controversial with studies showing it places increased amount of stress on the posterior instrumentation from cantilever forces and increases hardware failure. It is because of this new data that it is recommended to limit short segment fixation use to the young patients with good bone quality. This same principal applies in highly comminuted fractures of the thoracolumbar spine. In injuries requiring reduction this can be done through cantilever rod bending, distraction/compression maneuvers, and rod bending techniques. Specifically, restoration of the vertebral body height is indirectly achieved by contouring the rods to correct the kyphosis due to the fracture. Surgeons can also indirectly decompress the spinal canal as a result of the ligamentotaxis effect caused by the attachment of retropulsed bony fragments to the annulus and PLL through intersegmental distraction.

Retropulsed bony fragments can be decompressed from a posterior approach although it is more technically demanding. It involves performing a laminectomy as well as at the minimum a unilateral facetectomy (in the lumbar spine where nerve roots can be retracted) or transpedicular/costrotransversectomy approach (at the spinal cord level). The surgeon will then use angled curettes and the Woodson elevator to push the retropulsed fragment anteriorly, away from the spinal cord/thecal sac.

Osteoporotic Vertebral Fractures

Osteoporotic vertebral fractures (OVF) are common and significantly diminish quality of life. An estimated 550,000 osteoporotic vertebral fractures occur annually in the United States.[47] The lifetime risk of developing a symptomatic osteoporotic vertebral fracture is 18% for women and 11% for men. Patients can experience progressive thoracic kyphosis as a result of collapse of the vertebral body which leads to significant morbidity. Hyperkyphotic posture results in more vertebral body fractures and pain, fatigue, decreased back extensor strength, respiratory complications, and depression. Additionally, the mortality of patients following an osteoporotic vertebral fracture is significantly higher,

even after controlling for confounding variables.[48]

Various medications can help patients manage pain and promote osseous healing after an OVF. These include bisphosphonates, PTH analogues such as teriparatide (Forteo), and calcitonin. The American Academy of Orthopedic Surgeons (AAOS) offers a limited strength recommendation for ibandronate and moderate strength recommendation for 4 weeks of calcitonin usage in treating patients with osteoporotic vertebral fractures.[49] There is no mention of teriparatide as a therapeutic agent in the AAOS recommendations; however, the literature indicates teriparatide is effective in healing OVFs and decreasing pain.[50–52] Teriparatide is not recommended for patients with hypercalcemia, current or prior skeletal malignancies, an additional bone disease, and a heightened risk of osteosarcoma.[51] Another possible nonoperative treatment option is the use of various types of bracing. High-quality studies evaluating the use of different types braces in improving outcomes for patients with OVF are sparse. As such, the AAOS has stated that they cannot provide a conclusive guideline on this matter.[49]

While success with non-operative treatment is ideal, a small proportion of patients require surgery. Cement augmentation procedures like vertebroplasty and kyphoplasty are commonly discussed. AAOS guidelines strongly recommends against vertebroplasty for OVF.[49] Two Level I studies noted no statistically significant decrease in pain.[53,54] Three additional Level II studies found similar results.[55–57] The AAOS offers a limited strength recommendation for using kyphoplasty in OVF patients.[49] In terms of pain, kyphoplasty has been shown to be effective in patients with subacute fractures up until at least 1 month but not at the 1-year timepoint. Patients with subacute fractures who receive kyphoplasty also have at least 3 to 6 months of better physical functioning post-operatively. These results translated to improved quality of life at 1 month and possibly extend to a year or more. It is fair to conclude that kyphoplasty provides short-term improvement in patients with subacute fractures and longer benefits with chronic fractures.[58–62]

One of the main indications for open surgical intervention for OVF patients is presence of neural element compression with a deficit. Three techniques can serve as an adjunct to posterior stabilization: (1) Cement augmentation of pedicle screws, (2) restoration of anterior column support for load-sharing purposes, (3) vertebroplasty at the level adjacent to the stabilization construct. Posterior fixation of the osteoporotic spine comes with risks including pedicle screw loosening, pseudoarthrosis, rod fracture, and junctional fractures. Cement can be injected into the vertebral body prior to screw placement or through cannulated screws which have already been placed. There is a risk of cement extravasation and embolization similar to that of when doing a vertebroplasty. Reconstruction of the anterior vertebral body fracture can provide anterior column support to decrease posterior instrumentation load and prevent hardware failure and kyphotic deformity. Anterior column reconstruction can be done via vertebroplasty or kyphoplasty. Interbody devices also achieve anterior column support. Adjacent segment vertebroplasty is something that has been used to try to diminish the rigidity of an instrumented spine relative to the adjacent non instrumented spine. The long-term effectiveness of this procedure is not clear. Raman and colleagues[63] performed a prospective cohort study that concluded that although a two adjacent level vertebroplasty decreases the incidence of proximal junctional kyphosis 2 years post operatively, it had no effect on PJK at 5 years. It remains unclear if using adjacent level cement augmentation techniques improves functional outcomes after a posterior instrumented fusion for osteoporotic compression fractures.

Penetrating Spinal Injuries

Missile penetrating spinal injuries (PSIs) are increasing in incidence and are now a leading cause of civilian spinal injury just behind falls and motor vehicle accidents.[64–67] The size, composition, and design of the bullet contribute to the damage it inflicts; however, the most important variable is the missile's velocity. Damage is caused by three mechanisms: direct damage to the tissue, the shock wave created by bullet impact, and temporary cavitation.[68] As such, bullets which do not directly pass through the spinal cord can indirectly cause trauma, an entity known as spinal cord concussion. Approximately 45% of the military GSI patients and 60% of civilian GSI patients have complete spinal cord injury.[69]

Sagittal, axial, and coronal reconstructions of CT scans are typical imaging techniques used as they allow for visualization of bullet fragments and the extent of damage to osseous elements. MRIs allows for a more in-depth examination of soft tissue elements and the spinal cord. The most obvious risk of using an MRI in GSI patients is introducing metal bullet fragments into the scanner. Prior studies concluded that steel bullets, not metal alloy or lead, are at risk for movement.[70] Caution must be taken when conducting an MRI on GSI patients, especially if bullet fragments are close to vital structures.

Three treatments are provided to patients with gunshot injuries: tetanus prophylaxis, antibiotics prophylaxis, and potentially skin debridement. Patients with unknown tetanus status require both tetanus toxoid and immunoglobulin.[71] The literature does not firmly conclude how long antibiotic prophylaxis should be provided for penetrating spinal injuries. In patients with concomitant gastrointestinal injury, 7 to 14 days of broad-spectrum antibiotics may be advisable; however, a course less than 48 hours could be sufficient for patients without hollow viscus injury.[72] Surgical intervention is also an option and is done to aid spine stability, decompress neurologic structures, repair CSF leaks, and remove bullet fragments. Very few civilian gunshot injuries require spine stabilization.[73]

Surgical intervention to improve neurologic status can be done in specific situations. The first is if the neurologic deficits are progressive due to a migrating intracanal bullet fragment. A potential second situation is when an intracanal bullet fragment is in the lumbar spine. Some evidence indicates that motor symptoms improve in patients who have bullet fragment removal and decompression at the T12 to L4/5 levels; however, the same procedures did not result in statistically significant improvement in motor function when done in the cervical and thoracic levels.[74,75] In general, we do not recommend surgical decompression in this scenario as the damage done by the bullet's passage through/near the spinal cord far outweighs the damage done by fragments in the canal. Finally, surgery to remove a bullet fragment is occasionally an option to treat lead toxicity. Patients with embedded bullets should be closely followed with annual venous lead levels to ensure they are below the limit of 5 μg/mL. New symptoms should warrant immediate blood testing.[76] In cases where lead levels are increasing, bullet fragment removal is recommended along with medicine consultation for chelation therapy.

CLINICS CARE POINTS

- Bracing is a non-operative treatment option in patients with spinal stability and preserved neurologic function, although efficacy is questionable.

- Given the lack of evidence for steroid use after spinal cord injury and their associated risks, we advise caution in their administration.
- Posterior approach to the spine is the most common due to there not being a need for an access surgeon, allows for stable fixation constructs, and can avoid the abdomen which could be a significant zone of injury in a poly-trauma patient.

DISCLOSURE

Dr B.F. Stephens is a consultant for Dupuy Synthes Spine and Stryker Spine. All other authors have no disclosures.

REFERENCES

1. Patel AA, Vaccaro AR. Thoracolumbar Spine trauma classification. J Am Acad Orthop Surg 2010;18(2):63–71.
2. Katsuura Y, Osborn JM, Cason GW. The epidemiology of thoracolumbar trauma: a meta-analysis. J Orthop 2016;13(4):383–8.
3. Boseker EH, Moe JH, Winter RB, et al. Determination of "normal" thoracic kyphosis: a roentgenographic study of 121 "normal" children. J Pediatr Orthop 2000;20(6):796–8.
4. Panjabi MM, Takata KO, Goel V, et al. Thoracic human vertebrae. Quantitative three-dimensional anatomy. Spine 1991;16(8):888–901.
5. Magerl F, Aebi M, Gertzbein SD, et al. A comprehensive classification of thoracic and lumbar injuries. Eur Spine J 1994;3(4):184–201.
6. Rajasekaran S, Kanna RM, Shetty AP. Management of thoracolumbar spine trauma: an overview. Indian J Orthop 2015;49(1):72–82.
7. Lee ES, Ko CW, Suh SW, et al. The effect of age on sagittal plane profile of the lumbar spine according to standing, supine, and various sitting positions. J Orthop Surg 2014;9(1):11.
8. Brouwers E, van de Meent H, Curt A, et al. Definitions of traumatic conus medullaris and cauda equina syndrome: a systematic literature review. Spinal Cord 2017;55(10):886–90.
9. Kretzer RM, Chaput C, Sciubba DM, et al. A computed tomography-based morphometric study of thoracic pedicle anatomy in a random United States trauma population. J Neurosurg Spine 2011;14(2):235–43.
10. Chadha M, Balain B, Maini L, et al. Pedicle morphology of the lower thoracic, lumbar, and S1 vertebrae: an Indian perspective. Spine 2003;28(8):744–9.
11. Oxland TR, Panjabi MM, Southern EP, et al. An anatomic basis for spinal instability: a porcine trauma model. J Orthop Res 1991;9(3):452–62.
12. Chapman JR, Agel J, Jurkovich GJ, et al. Thoracolumbar flexion-distraction injuries: associated morbidity and neurological outcomes. Spine 2008;33(6):648–57.
13. McAfee PC, Yuan HA, Fredrickson BE, et al. The value of computed tomography in thoracolumbar fractures. An analysis of one hundred consecutive cases and a new classification. J Bone Joint Surg Am 1983;65(4):461–73.
14. Denis F. The three column spine and its significance in the classification of acute thoracolumbar spinal injuries. Spine 1983;8(8):817–31.
15. Denis F. Spinal instability as defined by the three-column spine concept in acute spinal trauma. Clin Orthop Relat Res 1984;(189):65–76.
16. Ferguson RL, Allen BL. A mechanistic classification of thoracolumbar spine fractures. Clin Orthop Relat Res 1984;(189):77–88.
17. Ferguson RL, Allen BL. An algorithm for the treatment of unstable thoracolumbar fractures. Orthop Clin North Am 1986;17(1):105–12.
18. Vaccaro AR, Lehman RA, Hurlbert RJ, et al. A new classification of thoracolumbar injuries: the importance of injury morphology, the integrity of the posterior ligamentous complex, and neurologic status. Spine 2005;30(20):2325–33.
19. Vaccaro AR, Baron EM, Sanfilippo J, et al. Reliability of a novel classification system for thoracolumbar injuries: the Thoracolumbar Injury Severity Score. Spine 2006;31(11 Suppl):S62–9 [discussion S104].
20. Reinhold M, Audigé L, Schnake KJ, et al. AO spine injury classification system: a revision proposal for the thoracic and lumbar spine. Eur Spine J 2013;22(10):2184–201.
21. Vaccaro AR, Oner C, Kepler CK, et al. AOSpine thoracolumbar spine injury classification system: fracture description, neurological status, and key modifiers. Spine 2013;38(23):2028–37.
22. Radcliff K, Su BW, Kepler CK, et al. Correlation of posterior ligamentous complex injury and neurological injury to loss of vertebral body height, kyphosis, and canal compromise. Spine 2012;37(13):1142–50.
23. Hauser CJ, Visvikis G, Hinrichs C, et al. Prospective validation of computed tomographic screening of the thoracolumbar spine in trauma. J Trauma 2003;55(2):228–34 [discussion 234-5].
24. Inaba K, Munera F, McKenney M, et al. Visceral torso computed tomography for clearance of the thoracolumbar spine in trauma: a review of the literature. J Trauma Acute Care Surg 2006;60(4):915–20.
25. Sheridan R, Peralta R, Rhea J, et al. Reformatted visceral protocol helical computed tomographic

scanning allows conventional radiographs of the thoracic and lumbar spine to be eliminated in the evaluation of blunt trauma patients. J Trauma 2003;55(4):665–9.

26. Adam F, Schwartz E, Croul S. MRI of Spinal trauma. In: Magnetic resonance imaging of the brain and spine. Philadelphia, PA: Wolters Kluwer; 2017. p. 1686–763.

27. Lee JY, Vaccaro AR, Schweitzer KM, et al. Assessment of injury to the thoracolumbar posterior ligamentous complex in the setting of normal-appearing plain radiography. Spine J 2007;7(4):422–7.

28. Rihn JA, Fisher C, Harrop J, et al. Assessment of the posterior ligamentous complex following acute cervical spine trauma. J Bone Joint Surg Am 2010;92(3):583–9.

29. Vaccaro AR, Rihn JA, Saravanja D, et al. Injury of the posterior ligamentous complex of the thoracolumbar spine: a prospective evaluation of the diagnostic accuracy of magnetic resonance imaging. Spine 2009;34(23):E841–7.

30. ATLS Subcommittee, American College of Surgeons' Committee on Trauma, International ATLS working group. Advanced trauma life support (ATLS®): the ninth edition. J Trauma Acute Care Surg 2013;74(5):1363–6.

31. Schmidt OI, Gahr RH, Gosse A, et al. ATLS® and damage control in spine trauma. World J Emerg Surg 2009;4(1):9.

32. Kalsi-Ryan S. International Standards for Neurological Classification of Spinal Cord Injury (ISNCSCI). In: Vaccaro AR, Fisher CG, Wilson JR, editors. 50 Landmark papers. 1st edition. Boca Raton, Florida: CRC Press; 2018. p. 83–6.

33. Maynard FM, Bracken MB, Creasey G, et al. International Standards for neurological and functional classification of spinal cord injury. American Spinal Injury Association. Spinal Cord 1997;35(5):266–74.

34. Cantor JB, Lebwohl NH, Garvey T, et al. Nonoperative management of stable thoracolumbar burst fractures with early ambulation and bracing. Spine 1993;18(8):971–6.

35. Moller A, Hasserius R, Redlund-Johnell I, et al. Nonoperatively treated burst fractures of the thoracic and lumbar spine in adults: a 23- to 41-year follow-up. Spine J 2007;7(6):701–7.

36. Mumford J, Weinstein JN, Spratt KF, et al. Thoracolumbar burst fractures. The clinical efficacy and outcome of nonoperative management. Spine 1993;18(8):955–70.

37. Weinstein JN, Collalto P, Lehmann TR. Thoracolumbar "burst" fractures treated conservatively: a long-term follow-up. Spine 1988;13(1):33–8.

38. Mulcahy MJ, Dower A, Tait M. Orthosis versus no orthosis for the treatment of thoracolumbar burst fractures: a systematic review. J Clin Neurosci 2021;85:49–56.

39. Linhares D, Pinto BS, Ribeiro da Silva M, et al. Orthosis in thoracolumbar fractures: a systematic review and meta-analysis of randomized controlled trials. Spine 2020;45(22):E1523.

40. Martin ND, Kepler C, Zubair M, et al. Increased mean arterial pressure goals after spinal cord injury and functional outcome. J Emerg Trauma Shock 2015;8(2):94–8.

41. Bracken MB, Shepard MJ, Collins WF, et al. A randomized, controlled trial of methylprednisolone or naloxone in the treatment of acute spinal-cord injury. Results of the Second National Acute Spinal Cord Injury Study. N Engl J Med 1990; 322(20):1405–11.

42. Bracken MB. Steroids for acute spinal cord injury. Cochrane Database Syst Rev 2012;2012(1): CD001046.

43. Bracken MB, Shepard MJ, Holford TR, et al. Administration of methylprednisolone for 24 or 48 hours or tirilazad mesylate for 48 hours in the treatment of acute spinal cord injury. Results of the Third National Acute Spinal Cord Injury Randomized Controlled Trial. National Acute Spinal Cord Injury Study. JAMA 1997;277(20):1597–604.

44. Fehlings MG, Wilson JR, Tetreault LA, et al. A clinical practice guideline for the management of patients with acute spinal cord injury: recommendations on the use of methylprednisolone sodium succinate. Glob Spine J 2017;7(3 Suppl): 203S–11S.

45. Fehlings MG, Vaccaro A, Wilson JR, et al. Early versus delayed decompression for traumatic cervical spinal cord injury: results of the Surgical Timing in Acute Spinal Cord Injury Study (STASCIS). PLoS One 2012;7(2):e32037.

46. Bellabarba C, Fisher C, Chapman JR, et al. Does early fracture fixation of thoracolumbar spine fractures decrease morbidity or mortality? Spine 2010; 35(9 Suppl):S138–45.

47. Burge R, Dawson-Hughes B, Solomon DH, et al. Incidence and economic burden of osteoporosis-related fractures in the United States, 2005–2025. J Bone Miner Res 2007;22(3):465–75.

48. Nguyen ND, Ahlborg HG, Center JR, et al. Residual lifetime risk of fractures in women and men. J Bone Miner Res 2007;22(6):781–8.

49. Esses SI, McGuire R, Jenkins J, et al. The treatment of symptomatic osteoporotic spinal compression fractures. J Am Acad Orthop Surg 2011;19(3): 176–82.

50. Tsuchie H, Miyakoshi N, Kasukawa Y, et al. The effect of teriparatide to alleviate pain and to prevent vertebral collapse after fresh osteoporotic vertebral fracture. J Bone Miner Metab 2016;34(1):86–91.

51. Iwata A, Kanayama M, Oha F, et al. Effect of teriparatide (rh-PTH 1–34) versus bisphosphonate on the healing of osteoporotic vertebral compression

fracture: a retrospective comparative study. BMC Musculoskelet Disord 2017;18(1):148.

52. Hadji P, Zanchetta JR, Russo L, et al. The effect of teriparatide compared with risedronate on reduction of back pain in postmenopausal women with osteoporotic vertebral fractures. Osteoporos Int 2012;23(8):2141–50.

53. Buchbinder R, Osborne RH, Ebeling PR, et al. A randomized trial of vertebroplasty for painful osteoporotic vertebral fractures. N Engl J Med 2009;361(6):557–68.

54. Kallmes DF, Comstock BA, Heagerty PJ, et al. A randomized trial of vertebroplasty for osteoporotic spinal fractures. N Engl J Med 2009;361(6): 569–79.

55. Neer RM, Arnaud CD, Zanchetta JR, et al. Effect of parathyroid hormone (1-34) on fractures and bone mineral density in postmenopausal women with osteoporosis. N Engl J Med 2001;344(19):1434–41.

56. Voormolen MHJ, Mali WPTM, Lohle PNM, et al. Percutaneous vertebroplasty compared with optimal pain medication treatment: short-term clinical outcome of patients with subacute or chronic painful osteoporotic vertebral compression fractures. The VERTOS study. AJNR Am J Neuroradiol 2007;28(3):555–60.

57. Diamond TH, Bryant C, Browne L, et al. Clinical outcomes after acute osteoporotic vertebral fractures: a 2-year non-randomised trial comparing percutaneous vertebroplasty with conservative therapy. Med J Aust 2006;184(3):113–7.

58. Wardlaw D, Cummings SR, Van Meirhaeghe J, et al. Efficacy and safety of balloon kyphoplasty compared with non-surgical care for vertebral compression fracture (FREE): a randomised controlled trial. Lancet 2009;373(9668):1016–24.

59. Grafe IA, Da Fonseca K, Hillmeier J, et al. Reduction of pain and fracture incidence after kyphoplasty: 1-year outcomes of a prospective controlled trial of patients with primary osteoporosis. Osteoporos Int 2005;16(12):2005–12.

60. Grohs JG, Matzner M, Trieb K, et al. Minimal invasive stabilization of osteoporotic vertebral fractures: a prospective nonrandomized comparison of vertebroplasty and balloon kyphoplasty. J Spinal Disord Tech 2005;18(3):238–42.

61. Liu JT, Liao WJ, Tan WC, et al. Balloon kyphoplasty versus vertebroplasty for treatment of osteoporotic vertebral compression fracture: a prospective, comparative, and randomized clinical study. Osteoporos Int 2010;21(2):359–64.

62. De Negri P, Tirri T, Paternoster G, et al. Treatment of painful osteoporotic or traumatic vertebral compression fractures by percutaneous vertebral augmentation procedures: a nonrandomized comparison between vertebroplasty and kyphoplasty. Clin J Pain 2007;23(5):425–30.

63. Raman T, Miller E, Martin CT, et al. The effect of prophylactic vertebroplasty on the incidence of proximal junctional kyphosis and proximal junctional failure following posterior spinal fusion in adult spinal deformity: a 5-year follow-up study. Spine J 2017;17(10):1489–98.

64. Heary RF, Vaccaro AR, Mesa JJ, et al. Thoracolumbar infections in penetrating injuries to the spine. Orthop Clin North Am 1996;27(1):69–81.

65. Chittiboina P, Banerjee AD, Zhang S, et al. How bullet trajectory affects outcomes of civilian gunshot injury to the spine. J Clin Neurosci 2011;18(12):1630–3.

66. Farmer JC, Vaccaro AR, Balderston RA, et al. The changing nature of admissions to a spinal cord injury center: violence on the rise. J Spinal Disord 1998;11(5):400–3.

67. Jaiswal M, Mittal RS. Concept of gunshot wound spine. Asian Spine J 2013;7(4):359–64.

68. Patil R, Jaiswal G, Gupta TK. Gunshot wound causing complete spinal cord injury without mechanical violation of spinal axis: case report with review of literature. J Craniovertebr Junction Spine 2015;6(4):149–57.

69. Güzelküçük Ü, Demir Y, Kesikburun S, et al. Spinal cord injury resulting from gunshot wounds: a comparative study with non-gunshot causes. Spinal Cord 2016;54(9):737–41.

70. Dedini RD, Karacozoff AM, Shellock FG, et al. MRI issues for ballistic objects: information obtained at 1.5-, 3- and 7-Tesla. Spine J 2013;13(7):815–22.

71. Jakoi A, Iorio J, Howell R, et al. Gunshot injuries of the spine. Spine J 2015;15(9):2077–85.

72. Mahmood B, Weisberg M, Baribeau Y, et al. Duration of antibiotics for penetrating spine trauma: a systematic review. J Spine Surg 2020;6(3):606–12.

73. Staggers JR, Niemeier TE, Neway WE, et al. Stability of the subaxial spine after penetrating trauma: do classification systems apply? Adv Orthop 2018; 2018:6085962.

74. Bono CM, Heary RF. Gunshot wounds to the spine. Spine J 2004;4(2):230–40.

75. Waters RL, Adkins RH. The effects of removal of bullet fragments retained in the spinal canal. A collaborative study by the National Spinal Cord Injury Model Systems. Spine 1991;16(8):934–9.

76. Towner JE, Pieters TA, Maurer PK. Lead toxicity from intradiscal retained bullet fragment: management considerations and recommendations. World Neurosurg 2020;141:377–82.

Statement of Ownership, Management, and Circulation
(All Periodicals Publications Except Requester Publications)

UNITED STATES POSTAL SERVICE®

1. Publication Title
ORTHOPEDIC CLINICS OF NORTH AMERICA

2. Publication Number
950 – 920

3. Filing Date
9/18/2021

4. Issue Frequency
JAN, APR, JUL, OCT

5. Number of Issues Published Annually
4

6. Annual Subscription Price
$347.00

7. Complete Mailing Address of Known Office of Publication (Not printer) (Street, city, county, state, and ZIP+4®)
ELSEVIER INC.
230 Park Avenue, Suite 800
New York, NY 10169

Contact Person
Malathi Samayan

Telephone (Include area code)
91-44-4299-4507

8. Complete Mailing Address of Headquarters or General Business Office of Publisher (Not printer)
ELSEVIER INC.
230 Park Avenue, Suite 800
New York, NY 10169

9. Full Names and Complete Mailing Addresses of Publisher, Editor, and Managing Editor (Do not leave blank)
Publisher (Name and complete mailing address)
DOLORES MELONI, ELSEVIER INC.
1600 JOHN F KENNEDY BLVD. SUITE 1800
PHILADELPHIA, PA 19103-2899

Editor (Name and complete mailing address)
LAUREN BOYLE, ELSEVIER INC.
1600 JOHN F KENNEDY BLVD. SUITE 1800
PHILADELPHIA, PA 19103-2899

Managing Editor (Name and complete mailing address)
PATRICK MANLEY, ELSEVIER INC.
1600 JOHN F KENNEDY BLVD. SUITE 1800
PHILADELPHIA, PA 19103-2899

10. Owner (Do not leave blank. If the publication is owned by a corporation, give the name and address of the corporation immediately followed by the names and addresses of all stockholders owning or holding 1 percent or more of the total amount of stock. If not owned by a corporation, give the names and addresses of the individual owners. If owned by a partnership or other unincorporated firm, give its name and address as well as those of each individual owner. If the publication is published by a nonprofit organization, give its name and address.)

Full Name	Complete Mailing Address
WHOLLY OWNED SUBSIDIARY OF REED/ELSEVIER, US HOLDINGS	1600 JOHN F KENNEDY BLVD. SUITE 1800 PHILADELPHIA, PA 19103-2899

11. Known Bondholders, Mortgagees, and Other Security Holders Owning or Holding 1 Percent or More of Total Amount of Bonds, Mortgages, or Other Securities. If none, check box ▶ ☐ None

Full Name	Complete Mailing Address
N/A	

12. Tax Status (For completion by nonprofit organizations authorized to mail at nonprofit rates) (Check one)
The purpose, function, and nonprofit status of this organization and the exempt status for federal income tax purposes:
☒ Has Not Changed During Preceding 12 Months
☐ Has Changed During Preceding 12 Months (Publisher must submit explanation of change with this statement)

PS Form **3526**, July 2014 [Page 1 of 4 (see instructions page 4)] PSN: 7530-01-000-9931 PRIVACY NOTICE: See our privacy policy on www.usps.com

---

13. Publication Title
ORTHOPEDIC CLINICS OF NORTH AMERICA

14. Issue Date for Circulation Data Below
JULY 2021

15. Extent and Nature of Circulation

		Average No. Copies Each Issue During Preceding 12 Months	No. Copies of Single Issue Published Nearest to Filing Date
a. Total Number of Copies (Net press run)		201	175
b. Paid Circulation (By Mail and Outside the Mail)	(1) Mailed Outside-County Paid Subscriptions Stated on PS Form 3541 (Include paid distribution above nominal rate, advertiser's proof copies, and exchange copies)	64	53
	(2) Mailed In-County Paid Subscriptions Stated on PS Form 3541 (Include paid distribution above nominal rate, advertiser's proof copies, and exchange copies)	0	0
	(3) Paid Distribution Outside the Mails Including Sales Through Dealers and Carriers, Street Vendors, Counter Sales, and Other Paid Distribution Outside USPS®	98	93
	(4) Paid Distribution by Other Classes of Mail Through the USPS (e.g., First-Class Mail®)	0	0
c. Total Paid Distribution [Sum of 15b (1), (2), (3), and (4)] ▶		162	146
d. Free or Nominal Rate Distribution (By Mail and Outside the Mail)	(1) Free or Nominal Rate Outside-County Copies included on PS Form 3541	22	16
	(2) Free or Nominal Rate In-County Copies Included on PS Form 3541	0	0
	(3) Free or Nominal Rate Copies Mailed at Other Classes Through the USPS (e.g. First-Class Mail)	0	0
	(4) Free or Nominal Rate Distribution Outside the Mail (Carriers or other means)	0	0
e. Total Free or Nominal Rate Distribution (Sum of 15d (1), (2), (3) and (4)) ▶		22	16
f. Total Distribution (Sum of 15c and 15e) ▶		184	162
g. Copies not Distributed (See Instructions to Publishers #4 (page #3)) ▶		17	13
h. Total (Sum of 15f and g) ▶		201	175
i. Percent Paid (15c divided by 15f times 100) ▶		88.04%	90.12%

* If you are claiming electronic copies, go to line 16 on page 3. If you are not claiming electronic copies, skip to line 17 on page 3.

16. Electronic Copy Circulation

	Average No. Copies Each Issue During Preceding 12 Months	No. Copies of Single Issue Published Nearest to Filing Date
a. Paid Electronic Copies ▶		
b. Total Paid Print Copies (Line 15c) + Paid Electronic Copies (Line 16a) ▶		
c. Total Print Distribution (Line 15f) + Paid Electronic Copies (Line 16a) ▶		
d. Percent Paid (Both Print & Electronic Copies) (16b divided by 16c × 100) ▶		

☒ I certify that 50% of all my distributed copies (electronic and print) are paid above a nominal price.

17. Publication of Statement of Ownership
☒ If the publication is a general publication, publication of this statement is required. Will be printed in the OCTOBER 2021 issue of this publication.   ☐ Publication not required.

18. Signature and Title of Editor, Publisher, Business Manager, or Owner

Malathi Samayan - Distribution Controller   *Malathi Samayan*

Date 9/18/2021

I certify that all information furnished on this form is true and complete. I understand that anyone who furnishes false or misleading information on this form or who omits material or information requested on the form may be subject to criminal sanctions (including fines and imprisonment) and/or civil sanctions (including civil penalties).

PS Form **3526**, July 2014 (Page 3 of 4)   PRIVACY NOTICE: See our privacy policy on www.usps.com

Moving?

Make sure your subscription moves with you!

To notify us of your new address, find your **Clinics Account Number** (located on your mailing label above your name), and contact customer service at:

Email: journalscustomerservice-usa@elsevier.com

800-654-2452 (subscribers in the U.S. & Canada)
314-447-8871 (subscribers outside of the U.S. & Canada)

Fax number: 314-447-8029

Elsevier Health Sciences Division
Subscription Customer Service
3251 Riverport Lane
Maryland Heights, MO 63043

*To ensure uninterrupted delivery of your subscription, please notify us at least 4 weeks in advance of move.

Printed and bound by CPI Group (UK) Ltd, Croydon, CR0 4YY

08/05/2025

01864723-0012